Contents

PART THREE

Treating the Complications of Diabetes

NATURAL SUPPLEMENTS FOR DIABETES

Practical and Proven Health Suggestions
for Types 1 and 2 Diabetes

REVISED & UPDATED

FRANK MURRAY

Foreword by Len Saputo, M.D.

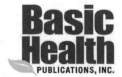

Basic
Health
PUBLICATIONS, INC.

The information contained in this book is based upon the research and personal and professional experiences of the author. It is not intended as a substitute for consulting with your physician or other healthcare provider. Any attempt to diagnose and treat an illness should be done under the direction of a healthcare professional.

The publisher does not advocate the use of any particular healthcare protocol but believes the information in this book should be available to the public. The publisher and author are not responsible for any adverse effects or consequences resulting from the use of the suggestions, preparations, or procedures discussed in this book. Should the reader have any questions concerning the appropriateness of any procedures or preparation mentioned, the author and the publisher strongly suggest consulting a professional healthcare advisor.

Basic Health Publications, Inc.
28812 Top of the World Drive
Laguna Beach, CA 92651
949-715-7327 • www.basichealthpub.com

Library of Congress Cataloging-in-Publication Data
Murray, Frank.
    Natural supplements for diabetes : practical and proven health suggestions for types 1 and 2 diabetes / Frank Murray. — Rev. ed.
        p. cm.
    Includes bibliographical references and index.
    ISBN 978-1-59120-206-6
    1. Diabetes—Alternative treatment. 2. Dietary supplements. I. Title.

    RC661.A47M87   2007
    616.4'62—dc22

                                                            2007019851

Editor: John Anderson
Typesetting/Book design: Gary A. Rosenberg
Cover design: Mike Stromberg

Printed in the United States of America

10   9   8   7   6   5   4   3   2   1

Foreword

There is an alarming increase in the incidence of diabetes. Neither the billions of dollars spent on medical research nor the arsenal of pharmaceutical drugs and medical devices that have subsequently emerged have been able to curb this epidemic. Too many people are suffering, and we cannot sustain the skyrocketing costs that support these therapies. Fortunately, there is a better way.

Americans are becoming proactive about their health. We are also entering an exciting integrative era that is blending the best of conventional and alternative medicine with the ancient wisdom of indigenous healing systems. Never before in our history have we had the opportunities that are possible today. We are in the process of changing from a "disease care" into a "health care" medical model, shifting our focus to optimizing health by preventing disease and promoting wellness. Lifestyle enhancement and the use of natural therapies are emerging as powerful tools that can achieve these goals.

While we all recognize and highly value the achievements of modern technology, we are becoming less dependent on the "miracles" of high-tech medicine. Despite its technological brilliance, modern medicine has not solved the epidemic of chronic diseases; its lack of safety has become a frightening reality, and it has become unaffordable for too many of us. There are just too many health problems and too few solutions.

Natural Supplements for Diabetes is a rich compendium of extensively referenced information that is practical, effective, safe, and affordable. Put simply, you can use it. Frank Murray's commonsense wisdom inspires confidence so that you can take responsibility and realistically expect to optimally manage, or even prevent, diabetes for yourself and for your loved ones.

The book begins by providing an easy to understand view of what diabetes is and highlights the importance of identifying risk factors that predispose one to its development or progression. For example, more than fifty million Americans suffer from the so-called Syndrome X, or "metabolic syndrome," which many experts feel is the prelude to the development of overt diabetes. There are also sections on obesity, hypertension, cholesterol, smoking, diet, and exercise and diabetes. Valuable information will help you protect the target organs that are particularly vulnerable to the complications of diabetes—heart, brain, eyes, feet, kidneys, and thyroid gland.

The book goes far beyond mainstream medical approaches to help reverse the underlying problems leading to the development of diabetes. Natural therapies that promote healing and allow the body to help restore normal physiology are offered. As they reverse the severity of the diabetic state, these insights also enhance overall health. Although these simple and effective tools are fully compatible with pharmacological drugs, typically, dosages can be dramatically reduced or, in some instances, entirely eliminated.

The value of specific vitamins, minerals, and supplements is also addressed in this book. The science behind their use is thoroughly documented, and a strong rational basis for using them is established. There is an enormous database of modern, cutting-edge biochemical research supporting the concept that many complications of diabetes are related to increased oxidative stress—the chemical damage of vital structures within the cell that result in premature aging. Reducing oxidative stress is certainly one of the major keys that can not only slow the development of aging, but also improve health and vitality. Simple and powerful natural substances can be used to prevent and repair oxidative stress.

While it is wise to include your health-care practitioner in the decision-making process when considering changes in therapy, *Natural Supplements for Diabetes* makes it possible for you to begin the process of creating your own program to minimize the manifestations of diabetes and maximize health. Today's health care is transforming into a collaborative process in which dialogue between patients and physicians is the norm. We are learning that the best way to ensure good health comes from taking responsibility for making decisions about our individual health-care needs while considering the advice of our health-care practitioners. Now that information is so readily available from the news, books, magazines, and the Internet, it is realistic to partner with your practitioner and contribute the potentially important information that emerges from your research.

Len Saputo, M.D.
Co-founder and Medical Director
Health Medicine Institute
Lafayette, California

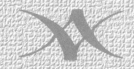

PART ONE

Diabetes—
An Epidemic
in the Making

CHAPTER 1

What Is Diabetes?

Diabetes develops when there is too much glucose (sugar) in the blood. The body's cells require glucose for fuel, but when glucose builds up in the blood instead of going into the cells, the cells are starved for energy. High blood sugar levels can eventually harm your eyes, nerves, kidneys, and heart.

The nature of diabetes is still being investigated today, but we know that the disease is a disorder of metabolism—that is, the way our bodies use digested food for energy. Most of the food we ingest is broken down into glucose, the form of sugar in the blood and the main source of fuel for the body. After food is digested, glucose passes into the bloodstream, where it is needed by cells for growth and energy. However, in order for glucose to enter the cells, it must have insulin, which is a hormone produced by the pancreas.

The pancreas is located behind the lower part of the stomach and is about the size of a human hand. It makes insulin so that the body can use glucose for energy and it also makes enzymes that help the body digest food. Spread over the pancreas are areas called the islets of Langerhans. The cells in these areas have a special purpose: alpha cells make glucagon, which raises the level of glucose in the blood, beta cells make insulin, and delta cells make somatostatin, a hormone that is thought to control the release of insulin and glucagons.

After we eat, the pancreas should automatically produce the correct amount of insulin to move glucose from the blood into the body's cells. In people with diabetes, the pancreas either manufactures little or no insulin or the cells of the body do not respond to the insulin produced. When this occurs, glucose accumulates in the blood, overflows into the urine, and passes out of the body. The body loses its main source of fuel, even though the blood still has large amounts of glucose.[1]

Symptoms of diabetes include increased thirst and urination, blurred vision, weight loss, fatigue, and other conditions. Out-of-control diabetes can lead to blindness, heart and blood vessel diseases, strokes, kidney failure, amputations, and nerve damage. Regular monitoring is essential.

Types of Diabetes

The three main types of diabetes are type 1 diabetes (formerly called insulin-dependent or juvenile diabetes), type 2 diabetes (formerly called non-insulin-dependent or adult-onset diabetes), and gestational diabetes, which affects pregnant women.

Type 1 Diabetes: Type 1 diabetes is an autoimmune disease that results when the body's system for fighting infection—the immune system—turns against a part of the body. For diabetics, the immune system

---

ALL ABOUT GLUCOSE

Glucose is the main sugar that the body makes from proteins, fats, and carbohydrates (mostly from carbohydrates). It is the major source of energy for the body's cells and is carried to the cells via the bloodstream. Cells cannot use glucose without the help of insulin. The body also uses **glycogen,** a substance made up of sugars and the chief source of stored fuel in the body. It is stored in the liver and muscles and is released into the blood when needed by the cells.

Glucagon is a hormone that raises the level of glucose (sugar) in the blood. The alpha cells of the pancreas (in the islets of Langerhans) make glucagon when the body needs to put more sugar into the blood.

Hyperglycemia is when there is too high a level of glucose in the blood, a sign that diabetes is out of control. It occurs when the body does not have enough insulin or cannot use the insulin it does have to turn glucose into sugar. Signs of hyperglycemia are great thirst, dry mouth, and a need to urinate often. **Hypoglycemia** is when there is too low a level of sugar in the blood. This occurs when a person with diabetes has injected too much insulin, eaten too little food, or has exercised without extra food. The person may feel nervous, shaky, weak, or sweaty and have a headache, blurred vision, and hunger. Taking small amounts of sugar, sweet juice, or food with sugar, will usually help the person feel better within 10 to 15 minutes.

attacks the insulin-producing beta cells in the pancreas and destroys them. The pancreas then produces little or no insulin, which requires the diabetic to take insulin daily. Scientists aren't sure exactly what causes the immune system to attack the pancreas, but both genetic factors and environmental factors (such as viruses) are probably involved. Type 1 diabetes accounts for about 5 to 10 percent of diagnosed diabetes in the United States.[2]

Type 1 diabetes develops generally in children and young adults, but this disorder can appear at any age. Symptoms of the disease usually develop over a short period, although beta cell destruction can begin years earlier. Symptoms of type 1 diabetes include increased thirst and urination, constant hunger, weight loss, blurred vision, and extreme fatigue. If the disease is not diagnosed and treated with insulin, the patient can lapse into a life-threatening diabetic coma (diabetic ketoacidosis).

Type 2 Diabetes: This is the most common form of diabetes mellitus, affecting 90 to 95 percent of the people diagnosed with the disease. It usually develops in adults at age forty and older and is commonly found in adults over the age of fifty-five. Roughly 80 percent of those with type 2 diabetes are overweight. This disorder is usually part of a metabolic syndrome that includes obesity, elevated blood pressure, and high levels of blood fats. Unfortunately, as more children become overweight, type 2 diabetes is becoming more common in young people.

With type 2 diabetes, the pancreas is usually producing enough insulin, but the body cannot use the insulin effectively—this is called insulin resistance. After several years, insulin production decreases and the result is the same as for type 1 diabetes—glucose builds up in the blood and the body cannot make efficient use of it.[3] Symptoms of type 2 diabetes develop gradually, and some people have no symptoms. Typical symptoms may include fatigue, nausea, frequent urination, unusual thirst, weight loss, blurred vision, frequent infections, and the slow healing of wounds and sores. While these diabetics may often be treated with diet and exercise, they may require insulin or other oral medications.

Gestational Diabetes: This type of diabetes develops in up to 5 percent of non-diabetic women during the later stages of their pregnancy. Those most often affected are African-Americans, American Indians, Hispanic Americans, and those with a family history of diabetes. Although gestational diabetes usually disappears after delivery, the mother is at increased risk of getting type 2 diabetes later in life.

Diabetes in History

Writings from the earliest civilizations in Asia Minor, China, Egypt, and India have documented the problems with diabetes mellitus, referring to patients with boils, infections, excessive thirst, loss of weight, and passing copious amounts of honeysweet urine, which often drew ants and flies. The term *diabetes* is derived from the Greek work meaning "siphon," or the passing through of water, and *mellitus* comes from the Latin word for "honeysweet." The Papyrus Ebers, an Egyptian paper dated about 1550 B.C., recommended that those afflicted with the disease go on a diet of beer, fruits, grains, and honey, which was said to stifle the excessive urination. Indian writings from the period attributed diabetes to overindulgence in food and drink.[4]

In northern European countries during the 15th, 16th, and 17th centuries, meals consisted primarily of roasted meats dripping in fat, sugary pastries, and plenty of butter and cream, but only small amounts of whole-grain breads or green, leafy vegetables. "It is, therefore, not surprising that many cases of diabetes were reported during these times of abundance. It is noteworthy, too, that during this period doctors had to taste the urine of patients for sweetness in order to detect the disease."[5]

Eventually, doctors centered on two schools of thought concerning diet. One school suggested dietary replacement of the sugar lost in the urine, while the other camp believed in restriction of carbohydrates in order to reduce the effects attributed to an excess of sugar. The first school was exemplified by Thomas Willis, a British physician who, in 1675, recommended a diet limited to milk, barley water, and bread. The diet was high in carbohydrates but low in calories. The other school was promoted by Dr. Rollo, a British military surgeon who, in 1797, began the trend toward high-fat, high-protein, and low-carbohydrate diets by prescribing mainly meat and fat. Some of the patients apparently were helped by the diets, as evidenced by reductions in the amounts of sugar spilled in the urine. Caloric restriction appears to have been the most effective therapy, since a French physician named Bouchardat found that the limited availability of food in Paris during the Franco-Prussian War of 1870–1871 brought marked reductions in the sugar spilled by his diabetic patients.

A major breakthrough in understanding the pathology of diabetes came in the latter part of the 19th century when Paul Langerhans, a German pathologist, while examining a pancreas under a microscope, discovered tiny cells that were different from the rest of the pancreatic tissue; these were later named the islets of Langerhans. Many physicians attempted to cure diabetes with extracts of the pancreatic islets, but these attempts were unsuccessful. This was because the extracts were contaminated with digestive juices from the pancreas that destroyed the activity of insulin, which is a protein.

In 1921, Frederick G. Banting and Charles H. Best, working at the University of Toronto, in Canada, discovered that they could obtain biologically active insulin from dogs and that the insulin cured the diabetes in dogs who had had their pancreases removed. The insulin was later given to a male diabetic human, who experienced a remarkable recovery. The use of insulin brought a dramatic drop in deaths due to diabetic coma and greatly increased the years of survival following detection of the disease. However, the insulin initially used brought sharp drops in blood sugar levels (hypoglycemia), which resulted in distressing symptoms.

New forms of the hormone were developed by chemically modifying the substance so as to slow its action. One modification was developed in 1936 by a Danish researcher named Hagedorn, who added protamine, a protein-like substance. This and other modifications of insulin made it possible to use only one daily injection, instead of the three or four originally required.

The Diabetes Epidemic

In 2002, the American Diabetes Association calculated that 18.2 million Americans—6.3 percent of the population—had diabetes. That number has continued to climb, making diabetes the fifth deadliest disease in the United States. The study further revealed these grim statistics:

- About 210,000 people under the age of twenty have diabetes.

- An estimated 8.7 million men and 9.3 million women aged twenty and older are diabetic.

- An estimated 8.6 million people sixty years of age or older are diabetic.

- Diabetes affects all ethnic groups: 12.5 million non-Hispanic whites

(8.4 percent of this population age twenty or older) have the disease; 2.7 million African-Americans (11.4 percent of this population age twenty or older) are diabetic; and 2 million Hispanic/Latino-Americans have the disease (8.2 percent of this population age twenty or older). Of the American Indians and Alaska Natives who receive care from the Indian Health Service, 107,775 are diabetic (14.5 percent of this population age twenty or older).[6]

Diabetes costs an estimated $132 billion in health-care expenditures. The annual per capita costs of health care for those with diabetes rose from $10,071 in 1997 to $13,243 in 2002, an increase of over 30 percent.[7]

The prevalence of diabetes in the United States continues to rise by epidemic proportions, according to Samuel Klein and colleagues at Washington University School of Medicine, in St. Louis, Missouri, and other facilities. The increase parallels the rising rates of obesity and over-weight observed over the past decade. They've found that as the body mass index (BMI) increases (a measure of obesity), the risk of develop-ing type 2 diabetes increases in a dose-dependent manner.[8] The preva-lence of type 2 diabetes in obese adults is three to seven times that in normal-weight people, and those with a BMI over 35 are twenty times as likely to develop diabetes as are those with a BMI between 18.5 and 24.9. In addition, weight gain during adulthood is directly correlated with an increased risk of type 2 diabetes.

Type 2 diabetes is a common and serious condition associated with reduced life expectancy and increased illness, reported Charlotte Glumer, M.D., Ph.D., and colleagues at the Steno Diabetes Center, in Centofte, Denmark, and the Prince of Wales Hospital, in Sydney, Australia. Recent estimates have suggested that 195 million people around the world have diabetes and that this number will increase to over 330 million by 2025. About 50 percent of the people with diabetes are under-diagnosed. Since type 2 diabetes can remain undetected for years, many people already have one or more complications by the time the disease is discovered.[9]

Complications of Diabetes

In addition to the health difficulties posed by diabetes itself, it can also lead to a number of serious illnesses and complications.

- Cardiovascular Disease—Diabetes increases the risks of microvascular complications, such as retinopathy (disease of the small blood vessels in the retina of the eye), nephropathy (disease of the kidneys), and neuropathy (diseases of the nervous system). Diabetics also have a marked increased risk of myocardial infarction (heart attack) and stroke, when compared to those without diabetes, and cardiovascular disease is the chief cause of death among type 1 and type 2 diabetics.[10] High blood pressure is reported with greater frequency in type 1 and type 2 diabetics than in the general population. Uncontrolled diabetes contributes to the buildup of fatty deposits in the arteries (atherosclerosis), which plays a prominent role in the development of high blood pressure.[11]

• High Cholesterol and Triglycerides—Blood levels of cholesterol and triglycerides are elevated in diabetes during periods of weight gain or low thyroid activity and with other conditions of depressed metabolism.

• Eye Problems—The most serious eye problems for diabetics are glaucoma, cataracts, retinopathy, and macular degeneration.

DIABETES AND AFRICAN AMERICANS

The disparity in the prevalence of cardiovascular disease and type 2 diabetes between African Americans and whites has been well-established. Ethnic differences in several risk factors for the diseases are evident in childhood, according to Christine H. Lindquist and colleagues at the University of Alabama, at Birmingham. They concluded that African-American children showed a greater disease risk than did white children, even after body composition, social class background, and dietary patterns were adjusted for.[12] The study involved ninety-five African-American and white children with a mean age of 10. Cardiovascular disease and type 2 diabetes risk were determined on the basis of total cholesterol, triglycerides, and insulin sensitivity in which cells remain responsive to insulin's action. Insulin sensitivity has been reported to be nearly 50 percent lower, and insulin secretion higher, in African-American children than in whites, especially in girls.

A study by the U.S. Department of Agriculture (USDA), in Washington, D.C., found that on the Healthy Eating Index (HEI), computed on a regular basis by the USDA, the mean HEI score for African-Americans was 59 compared to 64 for whites and 65 for other racial groups, including Asian/Pacific Islander Americans, American Indians, and Alaskan Natives. Only 5 percent of African Americans, compared with 11 percent of whites, had a good diet. Overall, 28 percent of African Americans had a poor diet compared with 16 percent of whites and 14 percent of other racial groups.[13]

- Foot Problems—Foot problems usually happen when there is nerve damage in the feet and when blood flow is poor, according to the American Diabetes Association. About one in five diabetics who enter the hospital have foot problems.[14]

- Kidney Disease—Kidney failure is a serious potential complication for long-standing diabetes. Damage to the small blood vessels in the nephrons can lead to progressive kidney failure, which is characterized by the excretion of protein and other nutrients in the urine.[15]

- Hypothyroidism—Hypothyroidism is more frequent in diabetics than in non-diabetics.

- Impotence—Impotence or erectile dysfunction is three times more common in men with diabetes in all age groups.[16]

- Depression—Numerous reports have indicated that diabetics are 1.5 to 2 times more likely to be depressed when compared to those without the disease. Patients with diabetes and depression have been known to have poorer self-management in following a diet and exercise program, and in checking blood glucose. In addition, they have significantly more relapses in refilling oral hypoglycemic, lipid-lowering and antihypertensive medications. Depressed patients with diabetes are also more likely to have three or more cardiac risk factors, such as smoking, obesity, and sedentary lifestyles.[17]

- Dementia—Elderly people with type 2 diabetes have an 8.8 percent increased risk of developing dementia, including Alzheimer's disease.[18]

- Restless Leg Syndrome—Restless leg syndrome is a common complaint of type 2 diabetics, and it can be a major cause of sleep disruption. In a Brazilian study, restless leg syndrome was reported in 27 percent of the patients, and poor sleep quality was found in 45 percent of the volunteers. Restless leg syndrome is a disabling and uncomfortable process that may interfere with falling asleep and lead to sleep deficit.[19]

In Part Three of this book, we will examine these complications in more detail and provide information on how to treat them with natural supplements and other strategies.

CHAPTER 2

What Causes Diabetes?

While the cause of type 1 diabetes—the autoimmune form of the disease—is still under investigation, it is thought to be influenced by both genetics and the environment. Type 2 diabetes, on the other hand, has a number of causes and risk factors, including obesity and the metabolic syndrome, hyperglycemia, dietary factors, and smoking.

Obesity

Obesity is the epidemic of the 21st century. The World Health Organization (WHO) estimates that there are over 1 billion overweight adults in the world, 300 million of whom are obese. In the United States in 2001, 20.9 percent of adults were said to be obese.[1] Obesity and overweight increase the risk of type 2 diabetes, cardiovascular disease, hypertension, strokes, and high levels of cholesterol and triglycerides.

Some clinical studies suggest that obesity and weight gain are associated with an increased risk of diabetes, according to Ali M. Mokdad, Ph.D., at the National Center for Chronic Disease Prevention and Health Promotion, in Atlanta, Georgia. In 2000, the prevalence of obesity in the U.S. was 19.8 percent; of diabetes, 7.3 percent; and the prevalence of both combined was 2.9 percent. Mississippi had the highest rate of obesity at 24.3 percent and of diabetes at 8.8 percent.[2]

The prevalence of obesity is rapidly increasing and is projected to soon become the leading cause of death in the United States. Body mass index (BMI) may be an effective way to predict diseases such as type 2 diabetes. According to researchers, the more overweight or obese a person is, the greater the degree of insulin resistance. In this condition, type 2 diabetics may produce enough insulin, but their bodies do not respond normally to the action of insulin. This is one of the main causes of type 2 diabetes.[3]

"Obesity and physical inactivity are well-established risk factors for the development of type 2 diabetes, and it is estimated that for every one-kilogram (2.2 pounds) increase in weight, the prevalence of diabetes increases by 9 percent," reports Patrick W. Sullivan, Ph.D., and colleagues at the University of Colorado Health Sciences Center, in Denver. "Physical inactivity is associated with increased insulin resistance and poorer glycemic control independent of body weight."[4]

The epidemic of obesity is no longer confined to well-fed, high income countries, but is spreading rapidly among developing nations. From the streets of China to the Siberian tundra, people are eating diets higher in fat while becoming more sedentary—a sure-fire recipe for increasing the risk of heart disease, type 2 diabetes, and other diseases related to obesity. Countries that are ill-equipped to deal with these illnesses are faced with the burden of understanding and controlling this life-threatening trend.[5]

"Urbanization, rapid shifts in technology, and increasing availability of processed foods are altering the way people in many developing countries are living, and these changes are fueling the obesity epidemic," adds Barry Popkin, Ph.D., of the University of North Carolina, at Chapel Hill. Each culture has its own response to these pressures, and it is not unusual to have obese individuals coexisting with undernourished ones, sometimes in the same household.

In a 2003 sample from low-income, rural regions of Mexico, the combined prevalence of overweight and obesity was nearly 60 percent for women, and more than 50 percent for men, according to Lia C. Fernald, Ph.D., of the University of California at Berkeley. This was slightly lower than the prevalence found in the nationally representative sample from 2000—67 percent in women and 61 percent in men—but this difference was not statistically significant.[6]

If, as many experts believe, under-nutrition in childhood can set the stage for obesity later in life, addressing the nutritional requirements of children in developing countries becomes an even more pressing concern.[7] It is hoped that taking into account the underlying cultural and biological factors that influence the rise of obesity in a country will help each nation's policymakers design approaches that successfully address these problems.

Fat Levels and Insulin

Fat cells (adipocytes) are critical for health and well-being as repositories of free fatty acids, but they also release hormones that, in lean people, modulate body fat mass. As a person gets heavier and the adipocytes enlarge, these control mechanisms become dysregulated and inflammation ensues. The regulators of free fatty acid storage and oxidation in fat cells are also critical regulators of metabolic balance in general. Fat cells are apparently active endocrine organs that play multiple roles. The body's metabolic rate changes as fat cells enlarge with increasing obesity. Also, researchers are just beginning to understand the interplay of inflammation and obesity.

While the dramatic worldwide increase in the incidence of obesity and, consequently, in the incidence of type 2 diabetes has been recognized, the exact causal link between these remains unclear, reports Marieke B. Snijder and colleagues at the VU University Medical Center,

SWEETENED DRINKS AND OBESITY

The high consumption of sugar-sweetened drinks has been associated with weight gain in the United States, according to Maira Bes-Rastrollo at the University of Navarra, in Pamplona, Spain. The trend may also be affecting populations with different eating patterns who increasingly are adopting typical U.S. dietary patterns.[8] In the U.S., the consumption of fast food and sugar-sweetened soft drinks has increased—a 68 percent increase in carbonated soft drink consumption from 1977 to 1997—parallel to the obesity epidemic. The researchers noted that soft drinks contain easily absorbable carbohydrates, and because of the lower satiety associated with liquid foods. a larger quantity may be consumed. In addition, cola-based drinks contain caramel that is rich in glycated end products, which may increase insulin resistance.

Sweetened fruit juices might also promote weight gain if they are consumed in large amounts, although the evidence is scarce. Soft drink and fast-food consumption are at least markers of an unhealthy dietary pattern that promotes overweight and obesity. This dietary pattern has the potential of being used as a quick screening test for an increased risk of overweight and obesity.

in Amsterdam, Netherlands, and other facilities. In the Hoorn Study—a population-based study of glucose tolerance among 2,484 men and women, fifty to seventy-five years of age, which was started in 1989—the waist-to-hip ratio (WHR) and not body mass index (BMI) was an important predictor of diabetes.[9] This suggests that fat distribution may be a better predictor for progression in type 2 diabetes. The accumulation of visceral fat is assumed to play a role in the etiology by overexposing the liver to free fatty acids, which results in insulin resistance and high levels of insulin in the blood.[10]

Studies show that a special risk for the development of type 2 diabetes is what's known as visceral or truncal obesity, in which excess fat is carried mainly in the area of the abdomen and around the hips and thighs, reports Porter Shimer, author of *New Hope for People with Diabetes*. Since more fat is near the liver, the fat has a tendency to find its way into the liver's blood supply, thereby interfering with sensitive hormonal processes required for proper glucose regulation. Studies also show that people who gain weight later in life—such as when we adopt our lounge-chair lifestyles—are more apt to accumulate the weight in the area of the abdomen and thus increase the risk for diabetes than those who have been overweight since childhood.[11]

Researchers in the United States and Japan have reported that a hormone produced by fat cells may be a link between obesity and insulin resistance that is typically found in type 2 diabetes, according to Joan Stephenson, Ph.D. A protein known as adiponectin (Acp30) is reduced in laboratory mice and humans, suggesting a role in regulating energy balance. A deficiency in the protein may be involved in the obesity-dependent development of diabetes.[12] In two models with type 2 diabetes, researchers at the University of Tokyo reported that treating mice with Acp30 decreased insulin resistance. Insulin resistance was partially reversed in one group of animals by giving them Acp30 or leptin, which is another protein secreted by fat cells. At the Albert Einstein College of Medicine, Bronx, New York, researchers found that giving other strains of obese and diabetic mice injections of Acp30 also lowered their blood glucose levels.

Obesity and sedentary lifestyles have been associated with decreased insulin sensitivity and increased concentrations of blood insulin in the fasting state and after a glucose challenge.[13] The restriction of energy (calories) and vigorous exercise reduce glucose and insulin concentrations, according to clinical studies. Both of these lifestyle interventions provide a potent strategy that should be included as part of any program to reduce the risk of impaired glucose tolerance, insulin resistance, and diabetes in overweight and sedentary people.

Short-term studies have shown that weight loss in overweight and obese type 2 diabetics is associated with decreased insulin resistance, improved measures of glycemic control, and reduced blood pressure, according to J. Bruce Redmon, M.D., at the University of Minnesota at Minneapolis.[14] Long-term options to promote weight loss in type 2 diabetics include weight-reduction diets and very-low-caloric diets. Other approaches may include use of meal replacements, repetitive use of low-calorie diets, and weight-loss medications.

While diet and obesity are obviously related to diabetes, this complicated subject is not dealt with to any extent in this book. There are many books now available that go into detail about diet, menus, and so on. Since each diabetic is an individual, one's diet and lifestyle recommendations need to be reviewed by one's own physician. It is impossible to design a "one size fits all" approach to this complicated disease.

Metabolic Syndrome

The metabolic syndrome (previously called Syndrome X) is an important risk factor for cardiovascular disease and diabetes, according to Lena M. Thorn, M.D., at the Folkhalsan Institute of Genetics, in Helsinki, Finland. The syndrome is characterized by a clustering of independent risk factors, including impaired glucose regulation, central obesity, high levels of cholesterol and triglycerides, and high blood pressure.[15] Insulin resistance and chronic inflammation are also key features of the metabolic syndrome. The metabolic syndrome is a frequent finding in type 1 diabetes, especially in patients with advanced diabetic nephropathy (kidney disease) and poor glycemic control.

Data from the Third National Health and Nutrition Examination Survey suggest that approximately 20 percent of the U.S. adult population—up to 47 million people—meet the criteria for the metabolic syndrome, according to Justo Sierra-Johnson, M.D., of the Mayo Clinic, in Rochester, Minnesota. The criteria proposed by the third report of the National Cholesterol Education Program–Adult Treatment Panel III (ATP-III) require three or more of the following components: high waist circumference, high fasting glucose value, low HDL cholesterol level, high triglyceride level, and high blood pressure.[16]

The main elements that make up the syndrome include:

1. A waistline measurement greater than 39 inches in either men or women.

2. A ratio of total cholesterol to HDL ("good") cholesterol greater than 5:1.

3. Elevated triglyceride levels—usually about 150 mg/dl—associated with normal total cholesterol and high LDL ("bad") cholesterol levels, along with low HDL cholesterol.[17]

The metabolic syndrome puts a person at risk for developing diabetes, hardening of the arteries, and cardiovascular disease. Although the origin of the metabolic syndrome is essentially unknown, predisposing factors include aging, obesity, sedentary lifestyle, and genetics, according to Carlos Lorenzo, M.D., at the University of Texas Health Science Center, in San Antonio.[18] Certain high blood pressure medications, beta-blockers, diuretics, tobacco, alcohol, and a diet high in saturated fat may increase the risk of developing the syndrome.

Diabetes and all other degenerative diseases develop slowly, meaning that various degrees of pre-diabetes may exist for years. Diabetes is not an all-or-nothing disease and insulin resistance and the metabolic syndrome are common forms of pre-diabetes. "The early signs of diabetes are easy to overlook because the symptoms are often vague and ambiguous symptoms can indicate almost any disorder," according to Jack Challem, author of *Syndrome X*.[19] "It is much easier to prevent disease or to change the course of the illness before the damage becomes entrenched and irreversible. If you know that glucose intolerance and insulin resistance are potentially early signs of diabetes or heart disease, you can correct them before you become diabetic or have a heart attack."

The typical American diet—high in fat and refined carbohydrates and low in dietary fiber and nutrients—is a major factor in increasing the risk of insulin resistance. Smoking, lack of exercise, and excessive alcohol intake also contribute to the risk of the metabolic syndrome. Exercise reduces the risk of developing insulin resistance and associated conditions, such as cardiovascular disease and blood lipid abnormalities.

Studies have shown that physical activity can reduce the risk of diabetes by 50 percent. Further, every 500 kcal increase in leisure time physical activity is associated with a 6 percent reduction in the risk of developing diabetes.[20]

The key to preventing or reversing the metabolic syndrome is diet and exercise. With weight loss and less abdominal fat, there is improvement in insulin sensitivity. A diet low in refined carbohydrates and high in fiber helps offset this syndrome. In addition, regular physical activity can prevent insulin resistance and provide protection against the syndrome.[21]

NUTRIENTS BENEFICIAL FOR THE METABOLIC SYNDROME

- Alpha-lipoic acid—improves blood glucose control

- Arginine—promotes blood vessel health and improves insulin action; arginine may be beneficial as a stimulator of nitric oxide, which is known to mediate insulin's vasodilating effects on the endothelium

- Chromium—improves blood glucose control and insulin action; typical dose: 200 mcg per day

- Coenzyme Q_{10}—reduces elevated blood pressure, improves blood glucose control and enhances insulin action, as well as improving blood lipid profiles and reducing oxidative stress; typical dose: between 100 mg and 120 mg per day

- Magnesium—reduces blood pressure, improves blood glucose control, and improves insulin action; typical dose: 480 mg per day

- Omega-3 fatty acids—improve insulin action and improve blood lipid profiles

- Selenium—improves blood glucose control, improves insulin action and reduces oxidative stress

- Vanadium salt—improves blood glucose control and improve insulin action; typical dose: 100 mg per day, with an upper limit not to exceed 1,000 mg/day

- Vitamin C—promotes blood vessel health, reduces elevated blood pressure, improves blood glucose control, and improves insulin action; typical dose: 500 mg to 1,000 mg per day in divided doses

- Vitamin E—promotes blood vessel health, improves insulin action, and reduces oxidative stress; typical dose: between 100 IU and 1,200 IU per day.[22]

Hyperglycemia

If your blood glucose level is above 250 mg/dl or is at or above 180 mg/dl at the same time of day for three days in a row, you are considered to have hyperglycemia (high blood sugar), according to Robert H. Phillips, Ph.D., author of *Coping With Diabetes*. Elevated blood sugar levels may lead to diabetic ketoacidosis, which is generally associated with type 1 diabetes, or hyperglycemic hyperosmolar syndrome (elevated blood sugar), which is related to type 2 diabetes.[23] If high blood sugar levels last for several years, this can lead to diabetic complications such as damage to blood vessels and nerves. Warning signs of hyperglycemia include frequent urination, excessive thirst, frequent or excessive hunger, blurred vision, fatigue, and confused thinking.[24]

There are a number of causes of hyperglycemia, including eating the wrong foods, eating too much of the right foods, lack of exercise, psychological and emotional stress, illness or injury, and taking too much or too little medication. A number of popular drugs can elevate glucose levels (hyperglycemia) and thereby lead to diabetes, according to Beatriz Luna, Pharm.D., of Campbell University School of Pharmacy, in North Carolina. These drugs include beta-blockers, thiazide diuretics, corticosteroids, niacin, and Pentamidine.[25] Of interest are increasing reported cases of new-onset diabetes in patients receiving treatment with protease inhibitors or antipsychotic agents. Elevated blood glucose concentrations can have significant consequences, especially in high-risk populations, including impairment of white blood cell activity, which compromises the normal immunological response and the host's capacity to resist infection. In addition, hyperglycemia can impair the wound healing process.

Luna said that eighty-two patients treated with clozapine, a neuroleptic drug used to treat schizophrenia, were studied to determine the incidence of treatment-related impaired glucose tolerance and diabetes in patients without a prior diagnosis of diabetes. At the end of the five-year study, about 30 percent of the patients were diagnosed with type 2 diabetes. "Recent findings continue to support the theory that patients receiving beta-blocker treatment (for high blood pressure) may be at increased risk for developing hyperglycemia and subsequent diabetes mellitus," Luna added.[26]

While drug interactions may vary from person to person, there are a number of these medications that cause hyperglycemia, according to Seymour L. Alterman, M.D., and Donald A. Kullman, M.D. They include calcium channel blockers, isoniazid, nasal decongestants (epinephrine-like drugs), oral contraceptives, dilantin, rifampin, thiazide diuretics, and nicotinic acid.[27]

Although type 2 diabetes is often described as a disease of insulin resistance, it is hyperglycemia rather than high insulin levels that appears to be the primary defect, according to Matthew C. Riddle, M.D., of Oregon Health Sciences University, in Portland. When hyperglycemia is uncontrolled, it plays a significant role in driving disease progression.[28] When glucose is reduced, beta cell (beta cells in the pancreas produce insulin) responses to glucose and other stimuli become almost normal. At the same time, reductions in excess glucose in muscle and adipose tissues may improve insulin sensitivity—that is, bring it closer to a more normal state. Vigorous early treatment with insulin may allow enough recovery of insulin secretion and action to allow dietary or oral therapy to maintain control, at least for a time.

The progression of type 2 diabetes is driven by declining beta cell functions and increasing insulin resistance, states Dr. Riddle. The cause of the decline in beta cell function is unknown, but it seems to be related to accumulation of amyloid material (a waxy translucent substance) in the beta cell mass as well as a reduction in that mass. Declining rates of beta cell function appear to be a function of age. While the decline in rates of insulin secretion during the initial stages of diabetes may be due to some defect in the ability of beta cells to sense hyperglycemia, the progressive failure of beta cells is characteristic of the disease process.

Some experts, such as Derek LeRoith, Ph.D., of the National Institutes of Health, consider the defect in insulin secretion to be at least as important as insulin resistance. Blood sugar levels generally rise within 30 to 60 minutes after eating starchy foods. The levels then return to a baseline within 3 to 5 hours as starch is digested to glucose and absorbed. If the blood sugar level remains high, a pre-diabetic or a diabetic condition may result. This is because the pancreas may not synthesize enough insulin or the cellular mechanisms responding to insulin may be defective.[29] Sustained high blood sugar levels promote the bonding of glucose to proteins, including hemoglobin. Thus, the resulting proteins do not function normally and their gradual accumulation may contribute to the organ deterioration associated with uncontrolled diabetes.

Hyperglycemia not only defines diabetes, but it is the cause of its most characteristic symptoms and long-term complications. Diabetes is characterized by development of specific microvascular complications and by a high incidence of accelerated hardening of the arteries, according to Louis Monnier, M.D., of Lapeyronie Hospital, in Montpellier, France. However, as demonstrated by many studies, microvascular and macrovascular complications are mainly, or partly, dependent on hyperglycemia. There is a significant relationship between acute glucose swings and activation of oxidative stress. Controlling blood glucose reduces the incidence and progression of microvascular disease in diabetes. In the Diabetes Control and Complications Trial, researchers found an increase of hypoglycemia with intensive glycemic control therapies, but the participants rated their overall quality of life as improved.[30]

Too Much Sugar in the Diet

Since its first use in India around 400 B.C., sugar has become one of our most pervasive substances. In the United States alone, the average person consumes more than 150 pounds of sugar annually. Table sugar is obtained mostly from sugar cane and sugar beets, but various types of sugar are available, such as molasses, raw sugar, brown sugar, turbinado sugar, and others. Unfortunately, it is almost impossible to tell how much sugar we are consuming since it is used in so many foods and products. The body reacts to the metabolizing of sugar in a number of ways. If its effects were produced by a food additive, sugar would undoubtedly be banned from the marketplace. Many experts agree that sugar plays a significant role in several diseases of civilization, such as diabetes. Excess sugar intake can increase triglyceride levels in diabetics, contributing to the risk of heart disease. High sugar intake can also lead to overweight, another major problem for diabetics.

The historical case against sugar is laid out in a book by Surgeon-Captain T.L. Cleave, *The Saccharine Disease*. Cleave shows example after example of societies in which the addition of sugar to the diet was the starting point for the development of diabetes and of hardening of the arteries in the epidemic proportion now typical of a Western nation. Two striking examples in Cleave's global studies were Iceland, beginning in

1920, and the nomadic Yemenite Jews. Before sugar was introduced into these cultures, there was no diabetes or atherosclerosis. Two decades after their diets became similar to ours, because sugar was added, they began to develop nearly as high an incidence of these illnesses as we have today. In the U.S., the increased consumption of sugar and refined flour at the start of the 20th century translated into a dramatic increase in diabetes after 1915. This increase continued: from 1935 to 1968, the prevalence increased by 600 percent.[31]

At the end of World War I, statistics clearly showed that from 1914 to 1918, the mortality rates for diabetes had fallen sharply in Germany and only slightly less in England, the countries most affected by food rationing, according to Eberhard Kronhausen, Ed.D., in *Formula for Life*. The most pronounced food shortages were of fats, meats, and sugars, all known today to contribute to diabetes. The same thing happened during World War II, but still nobody made the connection.[32] Most people did not note the significance of another wartime dietary change—the milling of flour. In Denmark, high-fiber barley meal and rye meal further raised the fiber content of flour products during World War II. Consequently, the diet of some European countries during the war years was considerably lower in fats and much higher than usual in fiber. Both fat and fiber content in the diet are crucial factors in the cause and control of diabetes.

Types of Sugar

Chemists recognize more than 100 sweet substances that are described as "sugars," but only one is commonly called "sugar": sucrose ($C_{12}H_{22}O_{11}$), which is usually obtained in crystalline form from sugar cane or sugar beets. It is a disaccharide of the carbohydrate family, a chemical union of two monosaccharides, glucose (dextrose) and fructose (levulose). In addition to levulose and dextrose (corn sugar), other types of sugars include:

- Lactose or milk sugar, found in milk. It is usually made from whey and skim milk and is used mostly in pharmaceuticals.

- Maltose, or malt sugar, which is made from starch and yeast. It is often mixed with dextrose for infant foods, in bread-making, and for other foods.

- Corn syrup, a viscous liquid consisting of maltose, dextrin, dextrose, and other polysaccharides. It is often produce by heating corn starch with a dilute acid or by enzymatic action.

- Molasses, which consists of concentrates extracted from sugar plants, usually the thick liquid produced when the sugar is being refined. It also contains other substances that occur naturally in sugar cane and sugar beets. The highest grade, called edible molasses, is used as table syrup or in spice and fruit cakes, rye and whole-wheat breads, cookies, baked beans, gingerbread, candies, and other foods. It contains some minerals, primarily iron.

- Honey is an invert sugar with a small excess of levulose. It is made by an enzyme (honey invertase) from the nectar brought back to the hive by worker bees. The flavor and composition depend on the type of nectar (for example, orange blossom, sage, clover, or tupelo). Its constituents include levulose (27 to 44 percent), dextrose (22 to 41 percent), maltose (6 to 16 percent), sucrose (0.25 to 7.50 percent), higher sugars (0.13 to 13.0 percent), water (13 to 23 percent), and other substances (0.13 percent).

- Maple sugar and syrup come from the sap of the maple tree. Maple sugar is 90.69 percent sugar, 6.19 percent invert sugar, and 0.98 percent ash. Maple syrup is 95.12 percent sugar, 2.24 percent invert sugar, and 1 percent ash.

A Refined Lifestyle

Obesity and type 2 diabetes are occurring at epidemic rates in the United States, and these increases cannot be explained by the aging of the population alone, since similar increases are also being seen in U.S. children.[33] The types of carbohydrates in our foods has received particular attention as a culprit because they influence the digestion rate and blood sugar response. The glycemic index was developed to quantify these blood sugar responses caused by carbohydrates in different types of foods. Diets with a high glycemic index—sugar, bread, potatoes, rice, and so on—and low in fiber increase the risk of type 2 diabetes, especially in women with a sedentary lifestyle and a family history of diabetes. The quality of carbohydrates consumed is important in causing, or preventing, type 2 diabetes.[34]

Increasing intakes of refined carbohydrates such as corn syrup, which is found in many foods, along with decreasing amounts of dietary fiber have paralleled the increases in type 2 diabetes. Modern carbohydrates are considerably different from those consumed before the beginning of the 20th century and the U.S. food supply has become reliant on highly refined carbohydrates as significant sources of energy. The refining process has changed the composition and thus the quality of carbohydrates. For example, processing whole grains into white flour increases the caloric density by over 10 percent, while it reduces the amount of dietary fiber by 80 percent and the amount of dietary protein by almost 30 percent. Refining removes many of the main ingredients, leaving a dietary substance that is nearly pure starchy carbohydrate with fewer nutrients.[35]

Corn refining in the U.S. began in the middle of the 19th century with cornstarch. It was discovered that cornstarch could be made into glucose and soon the corn industry was manufacturing a product called "refined corn sugar." Corn syrup technology advanced in 1921 with the introduction of enzyme-hydrolyzed products, which meant that corn-based sweeteners could compete in some markets that had been the sole domain of the sugar industry. In the mid-1950s, the technology for commercially preparing low-conversion products such as maltodextrin syrup was developed. And the next step was the enzyme-catalyzed isomerization of glucose to fructose. The commercial production of high-fructose corn syrup began in 1967, at which time the fructose content of syrup was around 15 percent. With further modifications, a high-fructose corn syrup (HFCS) with a fructose content of 55 percent became the sweetener of choice for the soft drink and ice cream industries, and HFCS with a fructose content of 90 percent became a frequent choice for use in "natural" and "light" foods. By 2002, HFCS sweeteners represented over 56 percent of the U.S. nutritive sweetener market.[36]

A Threat to Health

John Pekkanen and Mathea Falco in a 1975 article in *The Atlantic*, called sugar "white gold." It is said to be addictive and many doctors and researchers believe that it poses a dire threat to our national health. One widely accepted and advertised value of sugar is as a supplier of quick energy, but energy can be obtained from many other foods that also supply minerals and vitamins at the same time. "Refined sugar is an additive, a sweetener, a filler, a texturizer, and a preservative, but it does not make us stronger or give us the sole source of quick energy," stated Pekkanen and Falco. "In fact, because of its effect on blood sugar levels, some researchers believe it may do quite the reverse."

The myth that we need sugar to survive has been discounted by many knowledgeable scientists and nutritionists. The late Roger J. Williams, Ph.D., of the University of Texas, at Austin, who discovered the B vitamin pantothenic acid, told me that it is generally accepted that sugar is not itself a nutritional requirement for the body. Various amino acids (proteins) and the glycerol from fats can be converted in the body to glucose. Glucose, of course, is the main fuel used by the brain and other tissues and it is regularly supplied in the blood for this purpose. If glucose is not supplied in the food, it is derived from the other sources and released continuously by the liver into the blood.

In reading information about diabetes, I am astonished at how many recipes call for sugar or sugar substitutes. The fact remains that the body

---

FOODS AND PRODUCTS THAT CONTAIN SUGAR

Sugar is a pervasive substance—here are some of its applications.

Alcoholic beverages, vitamin C, baby foods, bacon curing, baked beans, bakery products, bee feeding, beverage concentrates and bases, beverages, bread, candy, canned foods (fruits, fruit juices, vegetables, meats, soups, baby foods), catsup, cereal products (breakfast cereals, dry-mixed foods), chewing gum, chili sauce, chocolate, cider, citric acid, cocoa, condensed milk, condiments, confectionery, conserves, cordials, curing (fish, meat, and poultry), and dairy products (ice cream, ice cream mix, ices, sherbet, milk drinks, frozen custards, frozen eggs, sugar egg yolks, yogurt).

Desserts, dried fruits, drink mixes, drugs, edible dyestuffs, elixirs, emulsifiers, flavorings, flavoring extracts, flavoring syrups, folic acid, fountain syrups, freezing (eggs, fruits, vegetables), fruit butters, fruit nectars, gelatin desserts, glace fruits, grain mill products, ham curing, jam, jellies, liqueurs, lozenges, macaroni, malted milk mix, maraschino cherries, marmalades, mayonnaise, meat products, mince meat, and noodles.

Penicillin, pharmaceuticals, pickled fruits and vegetables, pickles, preserved fruits, puddings, preserved nuts, relishes, salad dressings, soft drinks, spaghetti, syrups, table syrups, tobacco products (including cigarettes), tomato sauces, water softeners, wieners, wines, and yeast culture.[37]

is perfectly capable of converting meat, cheese, fruits, vegetables, and other foods into glucose, so that sugar is not really necessary, except as an occasional treat. Whether or not sugar calories are called "empty," they are unaccompanied by nutrients. Moreover, they increase the requirement for certain vitamins such as thiamine (B_1), which are needed to metabolize carbohydrates, and they may increase the need for the trace mineral chromium as well. So, a greater burden is placed on other foods in the diet to show extraordinary "nutrient density" to compensate for the emptiness of the sugar calories.

You nearly have to be a Ph.D. to ascertain the sugar content on typical food nutrition labels, since sweeteners can be listed as sucrose, fructose, maltose, honey, dextrose, corn syrup, fruit juices, and on and on. A label is *supposed* to list the largest amount of sugar in the most prominent place, but when you add up the various sugars scattered throughout the label, some of the products, such as breakfast cereals, rightfully belong on the candy counter. When children are sent off to school each morning having eaten sugar-coated cereals, doughnuts, and other sweet foods, is it any wonder that their hyperactivity begins to surface about mid-morning? Candy bars, soft drinks, and other sweets taken later in the day ensure further unruly behavior.

The late Jean Mayer, M.D., of Tufts University. in Boston, once said, "Today, although it is a major component of the American diet, practicing nutritionists, especially those who work with children and the poor, consider sugar a menace to good nutrition. After reviewing the evidence, I believe it is adequate to show that the habitual consumption of large amounts of sugar is highly undesirable from the viewpoint of health and that sugar consumption should be reduced." Mayer said that we have more or less conquered most of the infectious diseases and nutritional deficiencies (scurvy, beriberi) only to fall prey to another set of ills, such as atherosclerotic diseases of the heart and blood vessels, cancer, diabetes, high blood pressure, obesity, and tooth decay.

Sugar's Effect in the Body

A large sugar intake means that huge amounts of rapidly digested and absorbed simple sugars (glucose and fructose) flood the body at intervals. This sudden glucose influx may represent a stress on the body such that the insulin-secreting islets of the pancreas in individuals who are genetically prone to diabetes cannot cope. A number of studies, while not totally conclusive, support the view that a large sugar intake promotes diabetes in susceptible people.

Preadolescent and adolescent boys are the nation's highest consumers of sugars and sweets at a time when, to lower triglycerides and blood cholesterol, sugar intake should be cut along with a considerable decrease in saturated fat and cholesterol. Unfortunately, some children find sugar as addictive as tobacco or alcohol and many of them get used to sweet desserts and snacks and feel deprived if these are not available.

Researchers at San Diego State University, in California, evaluated twenty-four San Diego county public middle schools, with children who were between eleven and thirteen years of age. Snacks purchased from student stores averaged 8.7 grams of fat and 23 grams of sugar. Overall, 88.5 percent of store inventory was high in fat and/or sugar. Sugar candy accounted for one-third of the sales.[38]

John Yudkin, M.D., the eminent English nutritionist, has said that there is no physiological need for sucrose. In fact, there is reason to believe that sugar (sucrose) plays a part in several diseases of civilization, such as dental caries, obesity, coronary thrombosis, and diabetes. He cites studies showing that sugar reduces the growth rate of animals in spite of consuming the same number of calories. It shortens the lifespan and accelerates protein deficiency, since sugar interferes with protein utilization. In addition, sugar increases the deposition of fat, increases the concentration of cholesterol and triglycerides in the blood, and reduces glucose tolerance, therefore, producing the diabetic condition. Sugar increases the amount of liver fat and produces pathological changes in the kidneys.

At the University of Michigan, Jerome W. Conn and I.E. Newburgh found that sugar levels were most balanced when blood sugar was produced from protein and not refined carbohydrates, reported R.O. Brennan, D.O., in *Nutrigenetics*. That's because protein takes longer to be digested, absorbed, and metabolized in the blood. He noted that the U.S. Department of Agriculture (USDA) had found that because protein takes longer, the bloodstream receives a greater supply of glucose.[39] "If Americans were getting enough protein and other nutrients, eating sugar (which lacks nutrients) would not cause as much damage as it does," Brennan stated. "[One] experiment showed that the sugar level remained relatively healthy and steady when glucose was eaten with high amounts of protein. Only alone, in snacks and desserts, do carbohydrates cause the large peaks and valleys in the blood sugar level."

William G. Crook, M.D., has said that sugars derived from cane, beet, or corn are "bad" carbohydrates, because they have been stripped of minerals, vitamins, and other nutrients. He added that the average American is consuming an estimated 150-plus pounds of caloric sugars each year and these calories replace those that could and should be obtained from good carbohydrates.[40]

"Sugar Disease"

In his book *Intelligent Medicine*, Ronald L. Hoffman, M.D., stated that one of the most common abuses, or perhaps *the* most common abuse, of the body in America today is the high-carbohydrate, sugar-laden diet that leads ultimately to some form of sugar disease—in its most damaging form, to diabetes. He added that you can get away with this kind of diet for twenty or thirty years or maybe even longer, but it will damage the system, whether or not the damage shows up right away.[41] "If you've never paid attention to your sugar consumption, perhaps now is the time to begin," Hoffman wrote. "Remember that sugar in its refined form, sucrose (table sugar) is not a naturally occurring food. It has to be refined through a chemical process from plant material, much as cocaine is refined from cocoa leaves or medicinal drugs are extracted from rain forest plants. In fact, sugar is more potent in the body than many drugs."

An individual may succumb to sugar cravings a million times in a lifetime, Hoffman said, generating a staggering over-production of insulin and leading to metabolic syndrome, which is a precursor of heart disease and diabetes. In fact, he added, the term *sugar disease* is a catch-all for a host of modern conditions that result form unbridled intake of sugar or refined carbohydrates. We can look at sugar disease as passing through three stages, from a milder form to more advanced and destructive forms: hyperglycemia, metabolic syndrome, and diabetes.

Statistics show that, since 1963, carbohydrate intakes have increased by about 126 grams per day, with high-fructose corn syrup constituting 10 percent of the total intakes. At the same time, diabetes has increased 47 percent.[42] During the past 200 years or so, the increased consumption of refined carbohydrate foods appears to have gone hand-in-hand with a reduced intake of traditional starchy foods, including truly whole-grain (pumpernickel) breads, cracked wheat (bulgur and tabouleh), dried peas, beans, and lentils. These foods are more slowly digested, have a lower glycemic index and, in general, are more nutritionally replete than are their currently consumed counterparts.

Writing on the editorial page, *New York Times* columnist Nicholas D. Kristof stated, "Our government needs to do much more to control potentially deadly substances—plutonium, anthrax, and high-fructose corn syrup."[43] He added that high-fructose corn syrup is found in everything from ketchup to pop to hot dog buns. Americans over the age of two get an average of 132 calories a day from high-fructose corn syrup.

His suggestion is to ban sugary drinks from schools, curb advertising for sugary drinks (especially when aimed at children), and impose a tax of 5 cents per fluid ounce on sugary drinks. An extra 100 calories a day adds about five pounds a year to one's weight. And for Americans, that amounts to an extra 750,000 tons of fat per year. "Most of the debate on our national health crisis has focused on financing, and indeed we need universal health care," Kristof concluded. "But it's equally important to change American's diet and exercise habits—and the first step to do that is to fight our addiction to sugary drinks."

THE GLYCEMIC INDEX (GI) OF TRADITIONAL AND CONTEMPORARY FOODS

Values are based on white bread with a GI of 100, rounded to the nearest 10 percent.

	Food	Glycemic Index
Traditional	Pumpernickel bread	80
	Bulgur	70
	Dried peas, beans, and lentils	40–60
	Parboiled rice	60
	Spaghetti	70
Contemporary	White bread	100
	White bagels	100
	Low-fiber, cold breakfast cereals	100–120
	Glutinous white rice	100
	Instant mashed potatoes	110

Does Cow's Milk Cause Diabetes?

The jury is still out as to whether or not cow's milk proteins are involved in type 1 diabetes. Researchers at the University of Florida, at Gainesville, suggest that diabetes may be induced by something in the environment. Evidence indicates that there is only one in every three pairs of identical twins affected by type 1 diabetes and that the incidence of childhood diabetes is increasing.[44] They refer to research that supports the long-held suspicion that proteins in cow's milk could be the key environmental factor in the disease. Breast-feeding may provide a protective influence against the risk of type 1 diabetes later in life, and increased frequencies of antibodies to cow's milk proteins in children with newly diagnosed type 1 diabetes have been reported. The frequency of type 1 diabetes parallels the frequency with which cow's milk is consumed around the world. However, it may be premature to eliminate cow's milk from the diets of growing children considered to be at risk for type 1 diabetes.

Type 1 diabetes is very likely to be initiated by foods containing diabetogens (substances that cause diabetes), such as wheat, soy, and, to a lesser degree, cow's milk given early in life, according to Canadian researchers. Type 1 diabetes may be prevented or delayed by avoiding these foods until weaning or even as late as adolescence.[45] In diabetic rodent models, wheat and soy are the major diabetogens in plant-based rodent diets. However, in diabetes-prone animals, cow's milk is a weaker diabetogen. Most diabetics require long-term food exposure to diabetogens after infancy, with the time around puberty being of special significance. The probability of preventing diabetes by avoiding only one dietary diabetogen in the first six months of life is small.

In an opposing view, researchers at the University of Helsinki, in Finland, reported that avoidance of cow's milk protein in early infancy could prevent type 1 diabetes in genetically susceptible infants. The development of type 1 diabetes may be related to genetic predisposition and the interaction of environmental factors, such as viruses, dietary factors, and toxins, which result in autoimmunity to beta cells, their destruction, and subsequent development of the disease. The researchers added that the indirect evidence from animal models and observations in human beings are sufficient to justify intervention trials to determine whether or not cow's milk protein is associated with type 1 diabetes.[46]

Another Finnish research team evaluated milk consumption with levels of cow's milk protein antibodies in 697 newly diagnosed diabetic children, 415 sibling control children, and 86 birthdate- and sex-matched controls. It was found that there were inverse correlations between the duration of breast-feeding or age when dairy products and antibodies were introduced and positive correlations between milk consumption and antibodies in the three populations studied.[47] High IgA antibody levels to cow's milk formula were associated with a greater risk of type 1 diabetes in both diabetic-population-control and diabetic-sibling-control pairs. The results indicated that young age introduction of dairy products and high milk consumption during childhood can increase the level of cow's milk antibodies. In addition, high IgA antibodies to cow's milk are associated with an increased risk of type 1 diabetes in susceptible children.

At the University of Tampere, in Finland, the same researchers reported that high milk consumption in childhood (more than 3 glasses per day) was associated with more frequent emergence of type 1 diabetes-associated autoantibodies than low consumption (less than 3 glasses per day).[48]

Two studies show the benefits of breast-feeding and confirm the theory that infants fed cow's milk formula in the first three months of life have an increased risk of developing type 1 diabetes. One study involved 90 percent of the infants who developed diabetes in New South Wales, Australia, over an eighteen-month period when compared to healthy controls. Infants fed exclusively breast milk for the first three months of life had a 34 percent lower risk of developing diabetes than those not breast-fed. Children fed cow's milk formula during the first three months of life were 52 percent more likely to develop diabetes than those not given cow's milk formula.[49]

A previous study found that bovine serum albumin, a protein in cow's milk, somewhat resembles a molecule on the surface of beta cells in the pancreas. This resemblance results in an autoimmune attack that causes beta cell destruction. In nine regions in Italy, it was reported that there was an 88 percent correlation between the amount of milk that children drank and their risk of developing diabetes.

Smoking

Cigarette smoking is the leading avoidable cause of mortality in the U.S., accounting for about 434,000 deaths annually.[50] A research team at Wake Forest University School of Medicine, in Winston-Salem, North Carolina, reported in *Diabetes Care* that, along with its other numerous threats to public health, smoking may be an independent risk factor for diabetes. Of current smokers in the study, ninety-six (25 percent) developed diabetes within five years compared with sixty volunteers (14 percent) who never smoked.[51] The researchers said their study "gives further credence to current recommendations against the adoption and maintenance of smoking, particularly for those who are at high risk of developing diabetes."

A study at the Birmingham Veterans Affairs Medical Center in Alabama has concluded that people exposed to second-hand smoke are more likely to develop diabetes. The study, headed by Thomas K. Houston, M.D., reached their findings after following the health of over 4,500 people over fifteen years. Some of the volunteers were smokers, some were non-smokers, and some had no exposure at all. The researchers found that about one-fifth of the smokers became glucose intolerant, a condition that leads to diabetes. This compared with only 12 percent who were not exposed to smoke. For non-smokers who were exposed to second-hand smoke, the figure was about 17 percent. One explanation is that smoking may redistribute body weight in a way that makes diabetes more likely. There was no evidence that smoking directly harmed the ability of the pancreas to produce insulin.[52]

A research team as the Veterans Affairs Medical Center in Palo Alto, California, reported that cigarette smoking is associated with elevated plasma triglycerides and decreases in plasma HDL ("good") cholesterol concentrations. In addition to increasing the risk of coronary artery disease, smoking increases glucose and fats in the blood.[53] The researchers found that smokers had significantly higher very-low-density lipoprotein (VLDL) cholesterol, triglycerides, and total cholesterol, and lower HDL than non-smokers. Chronic cigarette smokers have high insulin levels in the blood, as well as abnormal levels of fats in the blood, when compared with matched non-smokers.

Other Causes

Genetics

Although type 2 diabetes is on the rise due to poor diet and lifestyle choices, genetics play a significant role in many cases, according to Tracy Hampton, Ph.D. A research team from Iceland has identified a variant in a gene that is the most significant genetic risk factor for type 2 diabetes found to date. The researchers suggested that the population-attributable risk of this variant was 21 percent.[54] "That means that if you removed this one single variant from the population, you would get rid of 21 percent of all type 2 diabetes in society," said Kari Stefansson, M.D., cofounder of deCODE genetics, a pharmaceutical company in Reykjavik, Iceland.

Dr. Hampton added that a number of studies have confirmed a heritable predisposition to type 2 diabetes. One study in twins revealed a 37 percent concordance in dizygotic (fraternal) twins and a 50 percent to 90 percent in monozygotic (derived from a single egg) twins. In another study, families with a high risk of type 2 diabetes had an increased heritability of impaired beta cell function in the pancreas and features of insulin resistance syndrome.

The researchers studied 1,185 Icelandic people with type 2 diabetes and 931 unrelated population controls; 228 Danish type 2 diabetics and 539 controls; and 361 people in the U.S. with the disease and 530 controls. In addition, the researchers studied 228 small genetic variants along a region of chromosome 10 that they had previously shown may be linked to type 2 diabetes. "Combined results of all three populations showed that a version of one of these markers is present approximately 1.5 times more often in patients with diabetes than in controls," Dr. Hampton reported. "More than one-third of individuals in the study carried one copy of that at-risk variant and had a 45 percent increased risk of having type 2 diabetes compared with non-carriers; 7 percent carried two copies and had a 141 percent greater risk."

The genetic variant identified by Stefansson's team is located within a gene encoding a protein called transcription factor TCF71.2. While the role of this gene is in the development of type 2 diabetes is unknown, TCF71.2 is known to control the activity of a number of genes, including the proglucagon gene, which encodes the insulinotropic hormone glucagons-like peptide 1 (GLP-1). The latter, along with insulin, plays a role in blood glucose homeostasis.

Viruses

A number of researchers have implicated viruses as instigators of beta-cell damage in type 1 diabetes, especially enteroviruses, which are a group of viruses (such as poliomyelitis virus) that reside in the gastrointestinal tract but may also be associated with respiratory ailments, meningitis, and neurological disorders. Other viruses related to diabetes include mumps, measles, cytomegalovirus, and retroviruses.[55]

Loss of Sleep

Researchers at the University of Chicago report that the body's reaction to the loss of sleep resembles insulin resistance, the condition in which cells fail to effectively use the sugar-processing hormone. Insulin resistance produces high blood glucose concentrations that can lead to type 2 diabetes. A century ago, Americans averaged nine hours of sleep a night, compared to an average of less than seven hours today.[56] A research team headed by Bryce A. Mander, Ph.D., brought together thirteen people who were chronically short of sleep, averaging less than 6.5 hours nightly, and fourteen volunteers who typically slept more than 7.5 hours a night. For eight days, the recruits wore a wrist device that monitored nighttime movement and sleep patterns. On the last night, the volunteers left a saliva sample, slept through the night, and then skipped breakfast.

Before eating, the volunteers were given an intravenous dose of glucose to determine how each processed the sugar. Those who slept less during the preceding week needed to produce 50 percent more insulin to metabolize the glucose. In addition, insulin sensitivity (the measure of how well cells take up the hormone and use it to process sugars) was only about 60 percent as efficient in those getting less sleep as in the more rested individuals. Additional tests showed that the saliva of short-sleepers contained excess cortisol, a stress hormone.

CHAPTER 3

The Way Forward

Warning Signs of Diabetes

Answer the following questions—the more "yes" answers you have, the higher your risk for diabetes.[1]

Have you noticed increased thirst?	Yes/No
Has there been an increase in urination lately?	Yes/No
Have you experienced increased appetite?	Yes/No
Are you overweight?	Yes/No
Do you suffer with a dry or burning mouth?	Yes/No
Have you recently required a decided change in your prescription for eyeglasses?	Yes/No
Do you have tenderness of the gums?	Yes/No
Is there a history of diabetes in your family?	Yes/No
Have you lost considerable weight lately?	Yes/No
Have you ever been told that your blood sugar was suspiciously high?	Yes/No
Do you have periodontal disease?	Yes/No
Do you crave sweet foods and beverages?	Yes/No
For men, do you have a problem with impotency?	Yes/No
For women, do you suffer with vaginal itching or other signs of a possible infection?	Yes/No
For women, have you had a baby who weighed more than 9 pounds at birth?	Yes/No

Diagnosing Diabetes

Fasting Blood Glucose Test

The fasting blood glucose test can show if a person has diabetes. A blood sample is taken in the laboratory or doctor's office. The test is usually done in the morning before a person has eaten. The normal, non-diabetic range for blood glucose is from 70 to 100 mg/dl (milligrams per deciliter). If the level is over 140 mg/dl, it usually means the person has diabetes, except for newborns and some pregnant women.

Glucose Tolerance Test

The glucose tolerance test is given in a laboratory or doctor's office in the morning before the patient has eaten. A first sample of blood is taken and then the person drinks a liquid containing sugar. After one hour, a second blood sample is drawn, and after another hour, a third sample is taken. The idea is to see how well the body deals with the glucose in the body over time.

Blood Glucose Monitoring

This is a method of testing how much glucose is in the blood. A drop of blood, usually taken from the fingertip, is placed on the end of a testing strip, specially coated with a chemical that makes it change color according to how much glucose is in the blood. Telling whether the level of glucose is low, high, or normal can be determined by comparing the color on the end of the strip to a color chart that is printed on the side of the test strip container or by inserting the strip into a meter, which reads the strip and digitally displays the level of blood glucose. Blood testing is more accurate than urine testing in monitoring blood glucose levels since it shows the current level of glucose rather than what the level was an hour or so previously.

Interpreting the Tests

The fasting plasma glucose test is the preferred test for diagnosing type 1 and type 2 diabetes. However, a diagnosis of diabetes is made for any one of three positive tests, with a second positive test on a different day:

- A random plasma glucose value (taken any time of day) of 200 mg/dl or more, along with the presence of diabetes symptoms.

- A plasma glucose value of 126 mg/dl or more, after a person has fasted for eight hours.

- An oral glucose tolerance test plasma glucose value of 200 mg/dl or more in the blood sample, taken two hours after a person has consumed a drink containing 75 g of glucose dissolved in water. This test, taken in a lab or doctor's office, measures plasma glucose at timed intervals over a 3-hour period.

However, there are other methods for assessing glucose metabolism that may be below normal but not quite constituting diabetes. A person is considered to have *impaired fasting glucose* when fasting plasma glucose is 110 to 125 mg/dl. This is higher than normal but less than the level indicating diabetes. Approximately 13.4 million people in the United States (or about 7% of the population) have impaired fasting glucose. With *impaired glucose tolerance* (IGT), the blood glucose during the oral glucose tolerance test is higher than normal but not high enough for a diagnosis of diabetes. IGT is diagnosed when the glucose level is at 141–199 mg/dl two hours after a person is given a drink containing 75 g of glucose.

In patients with impaired glucose tolerance that was documented by a baseline glucose tolerance test, there is a greater chance that they could develop diabetes. In clinical studies, only 6% of those with normal glucose tolerance tests developed diabetes compared with 25% of those with impaired glucose tolerance. The researchers also found that a weight loss of 4.5 kilograms (10 pounds) reduced the risk of diabetes in both those with normal and abnormal glucose tolerance tests at the beginning of the study.[2]

Lifestyle Modifications

The American Diabetes Association, the North American Association for the Study of Obesity, and the American Society for Clinical Nutrition have recommended the following lifestyle modifications in the prevention and management of type 2 diabetes. Weight loss is recommended for all overweight (a BMI of 25.0 to 29.9) people. Obese adults who have or who are at risk of developing type 2 diabetes should not have a BMI greater than 30. The main approach for reducing weight loss is a reduction in energy intake and an increase in physical activity.

- A moderate decrease in caloric intake—500 to 1,000 kcal per day—will bring a slow, but progressive weight loss of 1 to 2 pounds a week. For most patients, weight loss diets should supply around 1,000 to 1,200 kcal per day for women and 1,200 to 1,600 kcal per day for men. Overweight and obese patients with diabetes are encouraged to adopt the dietary recommendations known to reduce the risk of coronary heart disease, such as eating more fruits, vegetables, and grains, cutting down on saturated fat, limiting salt intake, cutting down on alcohol consumption, and eating more fiber-rich foods. In conjunction with a reduction in calories, this diet is likely to result in moderate weight loss as well as improvements in cardiovascular disease risk factors. Dietary choices should be tailored to each person, allowing for individual food preferences and ways of reducing caloric intake.

- Regular, moderate-intensity physical activity enhances long-term weight maintenance. Regular activity also improves insulin sensitivity, glycemic control, and selected risk factors for cardiovascular disease such as high blood pressure and abnormal amounts of fats in the blood. Increased aerobic fitness decreases the risk of coronary heart disease. Where possible, the duration and frequency of physical activity should increase to thirty to forty-five minutes of moderate aerobic activity three to five days weekly. Greater activity levels of around one hour per day of walking or thirty minutes per day of vigorous (jogging) activity may be needed to achieve successful long-term weight loss.

Natural Treatment Options for Diabetes

People with diabetes should see a doctor who helps them learn to manage their diabetes and monitors their control. An endocrinologist is one type of doctor who may specialize in diabetes care. Also, those with diabetes often see ophthalmologists for eye examinations, podiatrists for routine foot care, dietitians, and diabetes educators to help teach the skills of day-to-day diabetes management.[3]

As explained throughout this book, numerous vitamins, minerals, herbs, and other natural nutrients can help to prevent or control diabetes. If your doctor is not familiar with the literature, ask him or her to read the papers detailed in the endnotes. As for diet and recipes, I do not dwell on these subjects, leaving them to be answered by the patient's doctor or health care provider. My goal is to lead doctors and patients alike to the vast literature supporting a nutritional approach to diabetes.

In Part Two, we'll examine some of the proven dietary strategies and supplements for treating and preventing diabetes. We'll cover the importance of the glycemic index and fiber for a healthier diet as well as a range of supplements, including vitamin A and the carotenoids, B-complex vitamins, vitamins C, D, and E, minerals, and herbs, as well as a look at the benefits of exercise. Part Three looks at natural options for alleviating some of the complications resulting from diabetes, such as cardiovascular disease, eye problems, foot problems, kidney disease, thyroid imbalances, and impotence.

PART TWO

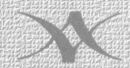

Therapies for Diabetes

CHAPTER 4

Why a Healthful Diet Is Important

Eating a healthy diet may be critical in reducing your risk for developing diabetes. A research team at the Harvard School of Public Health, in Boston, headed by Frank B. Hu, M.D., tracked the eating habits of more than 42,000 men, forty to seventy-five years old, over a twelve-year period and found proof that the typical Western diet increases the chances of developing diabetes. Further, they said that a diet high in red meat, processed meat, high-fat dairy products, refined grains, and sweets increases the risk of developing type 2 diabetes. The risk is worse for those with a sedentary lifestyle.[1]

The researchers, whose complete study appeared in the February 2002 issue of *Annals of Internal Medicine,* divided the volunteers into two groups based on their eating habits: those who followed a Western-type diet and those who followed a "prudent" diet characterized by a high consumption of fruit, vegetables, whole grains, fish, and poultry. During the study, 1,321 new cases of type 2 diabetes were diagnosed. Men with the so-called worst diets were 16 percent more likely to develop diabetes than were men with the best diets.

Studies on the Best Diets for Diabetics

While evaluating 9,665 volunteers for about twenty years, researchers found that 1,018 had developed diabetes. The participants ranged in age from twenty-five to seventy-four. It was found that the mean daily intake of fruits and vegetables, and the percentage of those consuming five or more fruits and vegetables daily, was lower among those who developed diabetes when compared to those who did not get the disease.[2]

Another study compared seven patients with type 2 diabetes who were vegans to four diabetics on a low-fat diet. The researchers found that blood glucose levels decreased an average of 28 percent in the vegan group, but only 12 percent in the low-fat controls. The vegans lost more weight (an average of 16 pounds) than the low-fat group, which lost about 8 pounds. One of the vegans was able to wean himself off hypoglycemic drugs and three others were able to reduce their dosages.[3]

At the Weimar Institute, in California, Milton O. Crane, M.D., and colleagues studied twenty-one patients, average age sixty-four, with type 2 diabetes and systemic distal polyneuropathy (a nerve disorder). The volunteers were placed on a low-fat (10 to 15 percent fat), high-fiber, total vegetarian diet of unrefined foods and an exercise program for twenty-five days. This brought a complete resolution of systemic distal polyneuropathy pain in seventeen patients in 4–16 days. Weight loss averaged 4.9 kilograms during the study and fasting blood glucose levels were 35 percent lower on average in eleven patients. Five patients no longer needed hypoglycemic drugs.[4] The researchers added that serum triglycerides and total cholesterol had decreased 25 and 13.6, respectively, within two weeks. In a follow-up of seventeen patients for up to four years, it was found that 71 percent remained on the diet and exercise program. The research team added that a total vegetarian diet is simple and economical and can benefit some patients with type 2 diabetes.

At the Kerala Agriculture University, in India, researchers evaluated the effect of a food on blood sugar levels in twenty type 2 diabetics, who consumed meals containing 60 percent carbohydrate, 20 percent protein, and 20 percent fat. It was found that the wheat-based meals showed the lowest glycemic response, followed by ragi, a type of millet cultivated in India. The researchers said that the low glycemic response to wheat may be attributed to the high amylose content (27 percent), a component of starch.[5]

One study that chronicled the relationship between diet and the risk of type 2 diabetes involved more than 84,360 women in the United States. During the six years of follow-up, 702 women were diagnosed with diabetes. The researchers found that body mass index (BMI), a measure of obesity, was a powerful indicator for getting the disease. After allowing for BMI, previous weight change, and alcohol intake, the researchers found no association between intakes of energy, protein, sucrose, carbohydrate, or fiber and the risk of developing diabetes. The researchers concluded that the prevention of obesity is more likely to reduce the incidence of type 2 diabetes than any modification of intake of specific nutrients.[6]

Getting the Right Kinds of Fats

At the University of Vermont, at Burlington, Nancy F. Sheard, Sc.D., R.D., stated that the dietary formula most frequently prescribed for diabetics is 15 to 20 percent of calories from protein, less than 30 percent from fat, and 50 to 60 percent from carbohydrates. However, recent studies have shown that such a diet may increase triglycerides (the major class of fats in the diet, which is often associated with type 2 diabetes), lower HDL ("good") cholesterol, increase hypoglycemia, and increase insulin levels in some people.[7] Sheard added that type 2 diabetics often have lower amounts of fats, glucose, and insulin when following an increased monounsaturated fatty acid diet compared to the traditional high-carbohydrate, low-fat diet. Vegetable oils such as olive and canola are typical monounsaturated fats. Her data support the hypothesis that substituting monounsaturated fat for carbohydrates improves blood glucose, triglyceride, and insulin concentrations while not adversely affecting LDL ("bad") and HDL cholesterol.

After analyzing a meta-analysis (a complication of many studies) comparing a low saturated fat, high-carbohydrate diet and a high monounsaturated fat diet for diabetics, researchers at the University of Texas Southwestern Medical Center, in Dallas, reported that a diet rich in monounsaturated fat may be beneficial for both type 1 and type 2 diabetics who are trying to maintain or lose weight. Further, high monounsaturated fats helped to control blood sugar levels. A high monounsaturated fat diet reduced triglycerides and VLDL (very-low-density) cholesterol by 19 percent and 22.6 percent, respectively.[8]

In another study, twelve patients with type 2 diabetes had serum total cholesterol levels of 235 mg/dl and triglycerides of 180 mg/dl. The volunteers were given home-prepared meals in which olive oil was the main edible fat, accounting for 8 to 25 percent of daily energy expenditures in the low-fat and high-fat diets, respectively. The researchers said that a diet high in total and monounsaturated fat is a good alternative diet to the traditional low-fat diet that has been used for patients with type 2 diabetes.[9] In this study at least, the traditional low-fat, high-carbohydrate diabetic diet and a diet enriched with monounsaturated fatty acids, given for six weeks, had similar effects on body weight, glucose metabolism, and lipids in diabetic volunteers who had fair glycemic control and no significant dyslipidemia (abnormal levels of fats in the blood) at the beginning of the study. High blood pressure and dyslipidemia are associated with abnormalities in insulin metabolism that are independent of body weight.

In a study reported in the *American Journal of Clinical Nutrition,* ninety-one type 2 diabetics were given either about 10 percent of their energy from a low glycemic index breakfast cereal or oil or margarine containing monounsaturated fatty acids (MUFAs) for six months. Those given the cereals consumed about 10 percent more energy from carbohydrates than did those in the MUFA group.[10] HDL cholesterol increased about 10 percent in the MUFA group when compared with those who were given either the high or low glycemic index cereals. Also, the ratio of total to HDL cholesterol was higher in the volunteers who consumed the high glycemic index cereal than in the MUFA group when measured at three months, but not after six months. The researchers added that a 10 percent increase in carbohydrate intake associated with breakfast cereal consumption had no adverse effects on control of blood sugar levels or blood fats in type 2 diabetics. The increase in plasma insulin and the reduction of free fatty acids associated with high carbohydrate intake may reduce the rate of progression of diabetes, the researchers said.

A high monounsaturated fat and low-carbohydrate diet has clinical and metabolic benefits for type 2 diabetics, according to researchers at the University of Naples, in Italy. Ten type 2 diabetics, with a mean age of fifty-two, randomly received either a high monounsaturated fat and low-carbohydrate diet (40 percent carbs, 40 percent fat, 20 percent protein, 24 g fiber) or a low monounsaturated fat and high-carbohydrate diet (60 percent carbs, 20 percent fat, 20 percent protein, 24 g fiber) for fifteen days. The participants were then switched to the alternate diet. The research team found that with the high monounsaturated fat and low-carbohydrate diet, there was a decrease in glucose and blood insulin levels following a meal, along with lower triglyceride levels.[11]

Researchers in Denmark studied twelve type 2 diabetics, who were given 300 milligrams (mg) of mashed potato in combination with either olive oil (40 or 80 grams) or butter (50 or 100 grams). The research team found that blood glucose levels after potatoes with 100 g of butter were significantly lower than that after the other meals. Insulin levels increased with 50 and 100 g of butter, but the addition of 40 or 80 g of olive oil had no effect.[12] The researchers also reported that triglyceride levels went up with the fat content of the meals, regardless of the type of fat. However, it was found that butter increased insulin levels more than olive oil and that large amounts of butter increased fatty acid and triglyceride concentrations.

SPECIFIC FOODS AND DIABETES RISK

Caffeine—Countries with the highest coffee consumption per capita had the highest incidence of type 1 diabetes, according to researchers at the National Public Health Institute, in Helsinki, Finland. Finland has the highest incidence of type 1 diabetes in the world, and incidence has increased during recent years as has the consumption of coffee.[13] According to the Diabetes Epidemiologic Research International Study Group, caffeine, the most widely used psychotropic agent, could be a risk factor in utero for type 1 diabetes. Its half-life is prolonged in pregnancy and is known to cross the placenta into the fetus. The report added that pregnant women who consume large amounts of coffee have an increased risk of spontaneous abortions, premature deliveries, and giving birth to infants with low birth weights. The study group added that these results are only a hypothesis and must be interpreted with caution.

Blueberries—Anthocyanins, which are natural components found in blueberries and European bilberries, give the berries their color. They also have a high antioxidant capacity. Of the forty different fruits and vegetables that researchers tested, blueberries contained the highest antioxidant capacity. The berries are said to reduce eye strain, control diabetes, and improve circulation.[14]

Mushrooms—Researchers in Japan gave 1 g per day of maitake mushroom (*Grifola frondosa*) to genetically diabetic mice. The mushroom therapy brought a reduction in blood glucose, insulin, and triglycerides in the mushroom-treated animals.[15]

Trans-Fats—The Center for Nutrition Information, in Washington, D.C., reported that there is considerable evidence that vegetable fat may enhance the risk of chronic disease when it is converted by hydrogenation to harmful trans-fatty acids. A good example is margarine. Diseases that may be affected by these fats are diabetes, coronary artery disease, and cancer, as well as reproduction.[16]

The Glycemic Index: What It Reveals About Blood Sugar

Developed by David Jenkins in 1981, the glycemic index (GI) measures the rise in blood sugar after eating a certain food compared to the blood sugar rise caused by glucose. Glucose (blood sugar) was assigned a glycemic index of 100 as a baseline measurement.[17] Any carbohydrate will cause a rise in blood sugar, and foods with a high glycemic index (meaning they raise it fast) include processed breakfast cereals, breads, root vegetables (yams, sweet potatoes, potatoes, and carrots), and most canned foods.

The magnitude of blood glucose response depends on the type of food and the form in which it is consumed. For example, spaghetti produces a smaller rise in blood glucose than wholemeal or white bread, since the glycemic index for pasta is only 40 percent of white bread and roughly 60 percent that of wholemeal bread. Pureed vegetables and fruits provide a more pronounced glucose response than do whole or cut-up vegetables and fruits. A whole apple produces a lot less of a blood glucose

GLYCEMIC INDEX OF SELECTED FOODS

All values are given in comparison to sucrose with a glycemic index of 100. The higher the value, the greater the impact on blood sugar.[18]

Breads		Muesli	66	Banana	53
French	95	Bran Chex	58	Pineapple	52
Wholemeal	72	All Bran	42	Orange	43
White	70			Apple	36
Barley	65	Potatoes		Peach	28
Rye	65	Various kinds	80–100		
Sourdough	57	Dairy Foods		Rice	
Pumpernickel	41	Ice cream, full fat	61	Low amylose,	
Heavy mixed grain	30–45	Yogurt, low fat,		white or brown	70–90
		fruit-flavored	33	High amylose,	
Breakfast Cereals		Milk, skim	32	Basmati, etc.	50–60
Cornflakes	84	Milk, full fat	27	Legumes	
Cheerios	83			Baked beans, canned	48
Rice Krispies	82	Fruits		Lentils	28
Cream of Wheat	66	Watermelon	72	Soybeans	18

response and has a lower glycemic index than apple puree. Apples, oranges, and grapefruit, because of their fiber content, have a lower glycemic index than juices made from these fruits. Cooked fruits and vegetables produce higher blood glucose response than do raw apples or carrots.[19]

A study evaluated the role of the glycemic index in diabetes and found that in 11 medium- to long-term studies, all but one showed positive findings with regard to the relationship between the absorption values reflected in the glycemic index and diabetes, according to researchers at the University of Sydney, in Australia. A low GI diet reduced glyco-sylated hemoglobin by 9 percent, fructosamine by 8 percent, urinary C-peptides by 20 percent, and day-long blood glucose by 16 percent. Gly-cosylation refers to the joining of glucose (sugar) to the hemoglobin pro-tein in red blood cells. The fructosamine test measures the glycation of a protein in the blood that has a shorter half-life than hemoglobin. C-pep-tide levels indicate how much insulin the body is making. On average, cholesterol was reduced by 6 percent and triglycerides by 9 percent.[20]

The researchers also found low glycemic index diets to be very "user friendly." Of forty-four foods evaluated, there was often no difference in glycemic index values between sweetened and non-sweetened foods. For example, the GI of tropical fruits ranged from mango at 51 to watermel-on at 72; breakfast cereals from 43 to 90; beverages from orange juice at 53 to an orange soft drink at 68; and dried fruits from apricots at 30 to sultanas (seedless grapes) at 61. Dairy products with added sugar had a higher glycemic index than those without. Fat reduces the glycemic response to foods.

"In subjects with type 1 and type 2 diabetes, low glycemic index diets, in comparison with high GI diets of similar nutrient composition, lead to improvements in glucose and lipid metabolism," according to Janette Brand-Miller, Ph.D., and Kay Foster-Powell, B.Sc.[21] "The GI of the diet may be the most important dietary factor in preventing type 2 diabetes. Two large-scale prospective studies . . . showed that diets with a high glycemic load increase the risk of developing type 2 diabetes after con-trolling for known risk factors such as age and body mass index."

Foods with a low glycemic index are said to be beneficial in relation to insulin resistance, according to Elin M. Ostman and colleagues at Lund University, in Sweden. Originally, the index was introduced to classify carbohydrate foods according to their effect on how much glucose was in the blood following a meal. Data now suggest that a diet with a low GI improves blood glucose control, the blood lipid profile, and blood clotting activity, suggesting a therapeutic role in the treatment of disease related to insulin resistance. Epidemiologic studies also suggest that such a diet may reduce the risk of type 2 diabetes and heart attack.[22] "In dietary recommendations from the Food and Agricultural Organization and the World Health Organization, an increased consumption of low glycemic index foods is strongly advocated," stated the researchers. "Pasta, legumes, and products based on whole cereal grains are examples of commercially available low glycemic index foods. Unfortunately, most breakfast cereals and conventional bread products belong to the group of foods that elicit high metabolic responses. It is known that the use of whole cereal grains and sourdough fermentation in breadmaking produces bread products with lower glycemic indexes."

In the Swedish study, lactic acid in fermented milk products (such as yogurt) did not lower the glycemic and insulinemic indexes. The latter refers to the amount of insulin circulating in the blood. In spite of low glycemic indexes of 15 to 30, all of the milk products produced high insulinemic indexes of 90 to 98, which were not significantly different from the insulinemic index of the bread that was studied. Also, the addition of yogurt and pickled cucumber to a breakfast with a high glycemic index bread significantly lowered the after-eating levels of glycemia and insulinemia (abnormal amounts of insulin in the blood) compared with the reference meal. In contrast, the addition of regular milk and fresh cucumber had no favorable effect on the metabolic responses.

In a six-year study involving more than 65,000 women, it was found that those who consumed diets high in carbohydrates from white bread, potatoes, white rice, and pasta had 2.5 times the risk for type 2 diabetes than participants who ate a diet rich in high-fiber foods, such as whole-wheat bread and whole-grain pasta, according to Walter Willett, Ph.D., of the Harvard School of Public Health.[23] He adds that low-fiber carbohydrates, such as pasta, behave like white sugar during digestion and that fiber helps to reduce the rate of carbohydrate absorption. Enriched white flour is nutritionally stripped of its nutrients: of the fifteen key nutrients in white flour, including vitamin E, only five equal or surpass levels found in whole-wheat flour. Unground whole wheat is even better than ground whole wheat. Dr. Willett said in studying the blood glucose levels in sixteen adults with diabetes, who had eaten breads made with varying ratios of whole grains and millet flours, the higher proportion of whole grains (unmilled grains), the lower the blood glucose. People should eat as many whole grains (in a coarse form) as possible and if the first word in the ingredient list is not "whole," other grains should be selected, according to Dr. Willett.

In another study of the glycemic index, sixty-two commonly eaten foods and sugars were given individually to groups of 5–10 healthy, fasting volunteers. Blood glucose levels were monitored over two hours. The largest rises in glucose were seen with vegetables, about 70 percent, and lower increases were found with breakfast cereals (65 percent), cereals and biscuits (60 percent), fruit (50 percent), dairy products (35 percent), and dried legumes (31 percent). There were obviously great variations within food groups and there was a significant negative relationship between fat and protein and after-meal glucose rise, but not with fiber or sugar content.[24]

It was found that the sugars glucose, maltose, and sucrose produced large increases in blood sugar levels, whereas fructose (fruit sugar) is metabolized without insulin and causes minimal increases, even in diabetics. Foods that are high in sticky fiber or foods that are resistant to forming a jelly-like consistency show slower rates of digestion and absorption. These foods may be called low glycemic index foods. In a study of forty-four foods containing simple sugars, there was no difference in the GI between the sweetened and unsweetened products.

At the University of Toronto, in Canada, researchers said that it is generally thought that foods high in viscous fiber or anti-nutrients result in slower rates of digestion and absorption and that these are low glycemic index foods. Increased meal frequency reduces after-dinner insulin and glucose responses in those with type 2 diabetes and in non-diabetic volunteers, and it lowers serum concentrations of LDL ("bad") cholesterol and lipoprotein-b. Increased meal frequency may also slow small intestinal absorption in diabetes, hyperlipidemia, and obesity, the researchers said. Eating foods that are low in the glycemic index, along with eating smaller portions more frequently, can lower the glycemic response.[25] Lipoprotein-b is a single protein found in LDL cholesterol, which allows LDL to attach itself to cells. LDL cholesterol is associated with cardiovascular disease by way of oxidation and free radical damage. When LDL becomes oxidized, it can clog arteries and lead to cardiovascular disease.[26]

Potatoes have a high glycemic value, regardless of variety, cooking methods, and maturity, reported a research team from the University of Sydney. New potatoes have a low glycemic index, probably due to differences in their starch content as compared to mature potatoes. In their study, the glycemic values ranged from 65 for canned new potatoes to 101 for boiled potatoes. The average size of the tuber was found to correlate with the glycemic index.[27]

At the King Fahd Central Hospital, in Gizan, Saudi Arabia, researchers evaluated the glycemic index for eleven common foods that were consumed by fifty-five Indian volunteers with type 2 diabetes. It was found that the GI was low (13 to 26) for Bengal gram, banana, apple, ground nuts, and milk; the GI was high (72 to 95) for wheat chapatti, millet bread, and potato; and rice, sago, and white bread registered intermediate GI values (55 to 64). Foods with a low glycemic index resulted in a low insulin response.[28]

Researchers studied the effect of extruded rice noodles on digestibility and glycemic response in healthy volunteers and type 2 diabetics. The extrusion process which reduced the starch digestibility by 15 percent, also lowered the glycemic index in healthy volunteers consuming the foods by 36 percent. In the diabetics, the reduction of GI was about 24 percent. The researchers suggested that the low glycemic response to high amylose and rice noodles suggests that these foods may be beneficial to diabetics (and non-diabetics). Amylose is a component of starch characterized by its glucose content.[29]

One study evaluated the glycemic index of twenty-eight carbohydrate foods in forty-seven healthy subjects compared with twelve type 2 diabetics. Carbohydrates rich in soluble fiber had the lowest GI, but other factors were involved. For example, a low GI is registered in foods that are rich in fat as well as carbohydrate or when fructose contributes significantly to the total carbohydrate content. Thus, fruits high in glucose, such as grapes, have a higher glycemic index than fructose itself.[30] Whole grains have a lower GI than when the cereal is extensively processed and the cellular structure altered. Whole fruits have a lower glycemic index than pureed forms, in spite of a similar content of total sugars.

Eight healthy volunteers were studied for the glycemic index and insulin response from twelve rice products at the University of Sydney. The products were brown and white versions of three commercial varieties of rice, waxy rice, a converted rice, a quick-cooking brown rice, puffed rice cakes, rice pasta, and rice bran. The glycemic indexes of the products ranged from 64 to 93 with glucose as the standard at 100. The high-amylose rice gave a lower glycemic and insulin index than the normal-amylose and waxy-rice varieties. As might be expected, the converted rice and most of the other rice products had high glycemic indexes. Insulin indices correlated positively with the GI. Many rice products should be classified as high GI foods, the researchers stated. However, the high-amylose rice varieties may have a potential value in low glycemic diets.[31]

Using the Glycemic Index

The simplest way to consume a moderately high-carbohydrate, but low glycemic index diet is to follow the 2005 Dietary Guidelines for Americans and to incorporate the recommendations of the World Health Organization/Food and Agriculture Organization—the GI should be used to compare foods of similar composition within food groups, according to

SUPPLEMENTS FOR BLOOD SUGAR CONTROL

A variety of supplements may contribute to sugar control and prevention or management of diabetic complications, according to Michael Janson, M.D., author of *Dr. Janson's New Vitamin Revolution.*[32] His supplement recommendations include:

- Bilberry: 100 mg, twice daily
- Bioflavonoid mix: 1,000 mg, twice daily
- Chromium: 200 mcg, twice in the morning and twice in the afternoon
- Coenzyme Q_{10}: 200 mg, once daily
- *Ginkgo biloba:* 60 mg extract, once in the morning and once in the afternoon
- Gamma-linolenic acid from borage oil: 240 mg, once daily
- Alpha-lipoic acid: 333 mg, once in the morning and twice in the afternoon
- Magnesium aspartate: 200 mg, once in the morning and once in the afternoon

Alan W. Barclay, BSC, and colleagues at the University of Sydney. By choosing the lower GI options within a food group (breads, breakfast cereals, etc.), an individual automatically chooses those with a lower GI. Since most fruits and vegetables, other than potatoes, are not major contributors to carbohydrate intake, their GI should not be the basis for restriction. "The evidence, as it stands, suggests that for preventing type 2 diabetes, we ought to encourage low GI carbohydrate foods but not those that simply have low 'net carbs,' low GI, or produce a low glycemic response."[33]

A diet with a low GI can be achieved in several ways: by replacing energy from carbohydrates with energy from protein, by replacing energy from carbohydrates with energy from fat, by replacing a high GI source of carbohydrate with a low GI source, or a combination of all these approaches, according to Janette C. Brand-Miller of the University of Sydney.[34] "Whether each of these strategies equally prevents the development of diabetes is unknown," she states. "A high carbohydrate intake from low GI sources may well be superior in terms of increasing fat oxidation and improving overall glucose disposition. If this is the

EARLY WARNINGS ABOUT REFINED CARBOHYDRATES

Neil Stamford Painter, M.D., and colleagues in Great Britain were among the first to explain that low-fiber diets and too much white sugar and refined carbohydrates in the diet were responsible for increases in diabetes, heart disease, obesity, and other common health problems.[35] Denis P. Burkitt, M.D., another British researcher, wrote as early as the 1960s that highly refined starches and sugars were responsible for diabetes, coronary heart disease, varicose veins, gallstones, ulcerative colitis, colon cancer, and other health problems.

Surgeon Captain T.L. Cleave of the Royal Navy, author of *The Saccharine Disease*, spent a lifetime collecting evidence showing that the refining of carbohydrates and, in particular, the eating of purified sugar, was responsible for diabetes, coronary thrombosis, and other disorders. He explained that the removal of fiber from sugar cane and sugar beets concentrates sugar in a form that fools the appetite, so that the mechanism that regulates our intake of calories is bypassed. Cleave added that refined sugar is the cause of diabetes, because of the unnatural strain imposed on the pancreas, and this is, in turn, the cause of coronary heart disease because of the striking association of diabetes to that disorder.

case, it might explain why the quality of carbohydrate (i.e., GI) more often shows a significant association with disease risk (diabetes, heart disease, and cancer) than does the carbohydrate content or glycemic load of the diet." Like the GI, the glycemic load classifies carbohydrate-containing foods according to their effects on after-meal glucose concentrations. Brand-Miller goes on to say that ample research supports the view that after-meal glycemia should be minimized, even when fasting glucose concentrations are normal.

Fiber

On average, Americans consume only about one serving of whole grains daily. Compared with refined-grain foods, whole-grain foods contain larger amounts of micronutrients that may convey significant health advantages. In addition, whole-grain foods have been studied in relation to the development of diabetes, heart disease, stroke, cancer, and in death. While various beneficial constituents of whole grains—fiber, magnesium, zinc, and vitamin E—have been identified, the underlying mechanisms linking diet to some of the observed health advantages remain unclear. However, dietary behaviors characterized by higher intakes of whole grains may be associated with increased insulin sensitivity.[36] Greater insulin sensitivity, or lower insulin resistance, may be one underlying factor leading to the health benefits associated with whole-grain intake, including a reduced risk of developing diabetes.

The Importance of Whole Grains

The quality and quantity of dietary fiber determines whether or not it will influence impaired fasting glucose and impaired glucose tolerance, stated Daniela Saes Sartorelli and colleagues at the University of San Paulo, in Brazil. Their findings are consistent with those of the Melbourne Collaborative Cohort Study, in which the highest intake of white bread was associated with a 37 percent increase in the risk of diabetes. They added that in the Framingham Offspring Cohort Study, fiber from cereals (mostly whole grains) was inversely related to the metabolic syndrome and insulin resistance, whereas total dietary fiber in fruits, vegetables, and legumes were not associated, emphasizing the importance of the type of dietary fiber on insulin action and degree of insulin resistance.[37]

A research team from Simmons College, in Boston, Massachusetts, reported that, in men, a diet high in whole grains is associated with a reduced risk of type 2 diabetes that may be mediated by cereal fiber. Earlier studies revealed an inverse association between whole-grain intake and type 2 diabetes in women.[38] "Other epidemiologic studies . . . showed an inverse association between dietary fiber and type 2 diabetes and a positive association with glycemic load," the researchers said. "In addition to the influence of fiber and glycemic load on postprandial (after meal) glucose and insulin response, whole grains may also reduce the risk of type 2 diabetes through the action of such nutrients as vitamin E and magnesium." The researchers found that a higher whole-grain intake was associated with a lower risk of type 2 diabetes in men, especially in non-obese men. Given the current overall low intake of whole grains, efforts should be made to increase the consumption of whole-grain products. This has the potential to substantially reduce the incidence of type 2 diabetes and possibly other chronic diseases when sustained over time.

Whole-grain foods are a rich source of antioxidants, such as vitamin E and selenium, as well as other vitamins, trace minerals, phenolic acids, lignins and phytoestrogens. Other trace minerals such as copper, zinc, and manganese are found in the outer layer of grains. Also, phytic acid, considered an anti-nutrient, may also function as an antioxidant. Whole grains are a potent source of numerous antioxidant compounds, which may help to inhibit oxidative damage.[39]

Types of Fiber

Fiber, also called roughage or bulk, consists of a mixture of various non-starch, complex carbohydrate and noncarbohydrate materials. This breaks down to cellulose, hemicellulose, pectin, maculage, gums, algal materials, and lignin. Insoluble fiber, which includes cellulose and lignin, swell in water, increasing stool weight and stool frequency. These substances help to prevent constipation, colonic inflammation, and hemorrhoids by softening stools and speeding up transit time of waste through the intestines. While cellulose is not digested, colon bacteria break down 40 to 80 percent of it. Lignin, which may lower cholesterol levels, is not degraded and passes through the system unchanged.[40] Dietary fiber reduces the speed at which carbohydrates are converted into glucose and it can reduce cholesterol and triglyceride levels, which contribute to heart attacks and strokes.

Bran, which is derived from the outer husk of wheat and other grains, is the most common insoluble fiber. Bran contains cellulose and other materials that slow the rise of blood sugar following a meal and may help to prevent precancerous polyps in the colon. Good sources of insoluble fiber include the skins of vegetables and fruits, whole grains (excluding white flour), high-fiber cereals, dried beans, broccoli, bulgur wheat, and bran.

Soluble fiber swells in water and forms a glue-like gel. It consists of non-cellulose carbohydrates, such as pectins, gums, algalpolysaccharides, and some types of hemicellulose. Soluble fiber slows starch digestion and glucose uptake, thus lowering the amount of insulin needed to process blood glucose after a meal. This, of course, may help those with diabetes. Oat bran is thought to effectively lower blood sugar levels. Reliable sources of soluble fiber include fruits, cooked dried beans, chickpeas, barley, lentils, navy beans, squash, carrots, barley, oat bran, rice bran, guar gum, glucomannan, and pectin.

Over the years, researchers have suggested that an increase in dietary fiber might inhibit the absorption of minerals and contribute to the development of mineral deficiencies. This concern is unfounded, according to a study at the Beltsville Human Nutrition Research Center and the University of Maryland. Volunteers were given a basic diet alone or supplemented with the insoluble fiber cellulose or a soluble fiber (locust bean gum or karaya gum) at a concentration of 7.5 grams of fiber per 1,000 calories. The insoluble fiber had an adverse effect on manganese absorption, but it did not affect the absorption of calcium, magnesium, iron, copper, or zinc. The soluble gum fibers did not affect mineral absorption, while karaya gum improved the absorption of all minerals.[41]

The Benefits of Fiber

Diets that are rich in whole-grain foods have been linked to a lower prevalence of the metabolic syndrome, which has been linked with an increasing risk of both type 2 diabetes and cardiovascular disease, according to Nadine R. Sahyouan and colleagues at the University of Maryland.[42] "Recent estimates indicate that the prevalence of the metabolic syndrome is increasing in the United States, with an estimated 40 percent of men and 51 percent of women in their sixties," the researchers said. "The cause of the syndrome is largely unknown, but presumably represents a complex interaction between genetic, metabolic, and environmental factors, which includes diet. Whole-grain foods may confer protection through potential effects on weight gain or through direct effects of whole grain or its constituents on insulin sensitivity and other components of the metabolic syndrome."

They added that whole-grain products may bring a reduced risk for cancer, type 2 diabetes, and cardiovascular disease. In contrast, refined grains do not appear to offer protection and, in fact, may predispose some people to chronic disease. Whole-grain foods provide fiber, vitamins, minerals, and other unmeasured constituents that are removed during the refining process. In spite of being nutritionally inferior, most grain products consumed in the U.S. are refined, with the average older American consuming five servings of refined grains per day and less than one serving of whole grains daily. Around three servings a day of whole grains are recommended.

A consumption of grain products with a high content of whole-grain flour, milled from all edible components of grain, has been inversely associated with mortality from diabetes and ischemic heart disease in several population studies, reported researchers at the Harvard School of Public Health. However, in these studies, the intake of refined flour, which consists mostly of the starchy endosperm, was not a contributing factor.[43] "It has been hypothesized that the observed health benefits of whole-grain intake may be attributable to the synergistic effects of dietary fiber and micronutrients found in whole-grain foods," the researchers said. "The bran and germ are rich in fiber, vitamins, minerals, and phytoestrogens." The lower risk of disease in those ingesting whole-grain products and bran may be mediated through effects on glycemic control, blood fats, or inflammation. Various studies have shown that the consumption of foods with a high whole-grain content is associated with improved insulin sensitivity and lower concentrations of serum triglycerides and total and LDL cholesterol.

Previous studies have suggested that fiber may lower cholesterol, inhibit oxidation of fats, increase insulin sensitivity, and improve homocysteine levels (a risk factor for cardiovascular disease).[44] When damaged by free radicals, fats and cholesterol form toxic compounds known as lipid peroxides and oxidized cholesterol, which can damage artery walls and speed the progression of hardening of the arteries. The diabetic has two to three times the risk of dying prematurely from hardening of the arteries than a non-diabetic.[45]

Type 2 diabetes is associated with low-grade systemic inflammation and accelerated rates of hardening of the arteries. The inflammatory process seems to play a pivotal role in the development of hardening of the arteries and is thought to be responsible for the increased cardiovascular complications among diabetics. Consumption of whole grains and fiber is associated with lower inflammatory markers among diabetics, supporting the recommendation that people with type 2 diabetes should eat more whole-grain products and maintain a low glycemic index diet.[46]

The consumption of two to three servings of whole grains daily has significant benefit in the prevention of cardiovascular disease in diabetics. Recommending that an individual incorporate moderate amounts of whole grains, including dark bread, whole-grain breakfast cereals, popcorn, cooked oatmeal, or brown rice in their diet may have important implications in the prevention of Western diseases. In a study involving thirteen type 2 diabetics, the volunteers were given two diets, each for six weeks. One of the diets, recommended by the American Diabetes Association (ADA), contained 24 grams of total fiber (8 g of soluble fiber and 16 g of insoluble fiber), and the other was a high-fiber diet containing 50 grams of total fiber (25 g of soluble fiber and 25 g of insoluble fiber). In week six of the high-fiber diet as compared to week six of the ADA diet, mean after-eating blood glucose levels were 13 mg/dl lower and mean daily urinary glucose excretion was 1.3 g lower. In all, the high-fiber diet reduced total blood cholesterol concentrations by 6.7 percent, triglycerides by 10.2 percent, and very-low-density lipoprotein cholesterol by 12.5 percent.[47]

Sources of Fiber

Oats

At the Beltsville Human Nutrition Research Center, in Maryland, researchers evaluated the effect of beta-glucan in oats on twenty-three volunteers (sixteen females and seven males) between the ages of thirty-eight and sixty-one who had moderately high cholesterol levels. The participants consumed oat extract with either 1 percent or 10 percent soluble beta-glucans added and were consumed in a five-week crossover study. The reactions of glucose were reduced by both extracts in both men and women, while the reactions of insulin did not vary between men and women but were lower after oat extracts were eaten. The researchers stated that oat extracts could be substituted for fat energy with minimal changes in overall food selection to improve the diets of those at risk for heart disease and diabetes. Oats may have a beneficial effect on high blood sugar factors.[48]

At the University of Alberta, in Canada, researchers studied eight type 2 diabetics, with a mean age of forty-five, during a 24-week crossover study. Four of the men ate high-fiber, oat bran concentrate bread at the beginning, while four others were given white bread. After twelve weeks, the volunteers switched diets. Mean dietary fiber intake was 19 grams per day in the white bread group, compared with 34 grams per day in the oat bran group. The researchers found that mean glycemic and insulin responses were lower for the oat bran group than for the white bread group. It was also found that the oat bran group had a lower total cholesterol and LDL cholesterol.[49]

Oat gum is as effective, if not better, than guar gum in lowering after-meal glucose and insulin levels, reported a research team from the University of Ottawa, in Canada. In the study, glucose and insulin response to consuming 14.5 grams of oat gum with 50 grams of a glucose drink were compared to responses from consuming guar gum with glucose or from glucose alone. Healthy volunteers were given test meals after a twelve-hour fast, while their blood samples were recorded before, during, and after the test.[50] Reductions in after-eating glucose and insulin levels were similar for both guar gum and oat gum. Oat gum is a soluble fiber from oats, and about 80 percent of the gum is beta-D-glucan or beta-glucan. This sticky fiber consists of about 4 percent of rolled oats and 7 to 10 percent of oat bran. The researchers said that oat gum is potentially helpful in stabilizing after-meal glucose and insulin levels.

Guar Gum

Guar gum is a vegetable gum derived from the Indian cluster bean. Guar gum reduced after-meal blood glucose, insulin requirements, and total blood cholesterol in type 1 diabetics, according to a research team in Finland. During the study, nine type 1 diabetics ate a regular diet plus a 5 gram placebo four times a day before meals for four weeks. The volunteers were then given a guar gum supplement diet for four weeks, taken in 5 g doses four times daily before eating. Following four weeks of guar gum therapy, blood glucose response to a test meal was significantly reduced when compared to the placebo diet. Insulin sensitivity was unchanged, but the average daily insulin dose was slightly lower (by 5 percent) after the guar gum supplementation. This was attributed to the smaller after-meal glucose rise. Blood levels of total cholesterol fell 21 percent following the guar gum period with a similar reduction in LDL cholesterol; there was no change in HDL cholesterol. The researchers said that, because diabetics have an increased risk for heart disease, the cholesterol-lowering effect of guar gum can contribute to a long-term positive prognosis in type 1 diabetics.[51]

Guar gum can be consumed for an extended period by type 2 diabetics without compromising mineral balance, according to researchers at the Beltsville Human Nutrition Research Center and Sinai Hospital in Baltimore, Maryland. They added that guar gum is an effective aid to glycemic control and its use might have a role in the treatment of type 2 diabetes.[52] However, guar gum seems to interfere with selenium utilization, according to researchers at the University of Nebraska at Lincoln. Also, overall selenium balance and glutathione peroxidase activity decreased when guar gum was eaten. Glutathione peroxidase, which requires selenium as a co-factor, is an antioxidant that inactivates dangerous free radicals. These effects were found regardless of how much selenium was in the diet.[53]

At the Helsinki University Hospital, seventeen type 1 diabetics were randomly assigned 5 g of granulated guar gum or a placebo, four times daily before meals and in the evening snack, for six weeks. Patients getting the guar gum had a significant reduction in glucose, LDL cholesterol (20 percent), and the LDL to HDL ratio (28 percent). The placebo group recorded no changes.[54]

Psyllium

The addition of psyllium (*Plantago psyllium*) to a traditional diet for those with diabetes is safe and well tolerated and improves glycemic and lipid control in men with type 2 diabetes and moderate cholesterol levels, according to James W. Anderson, M.D. After two weeks of dietary stabilization, thirty-four men with type 2 diabetes and mild-to-moderate cholesterol levels were randomly assigned to receive 5.1 grams of psyllium or a placebo twice daily for eight weeks. The research team reported that there were significant improvements in glucose and lipid values compared to the volunteers getting the placebo. For example, serum total cholesterol and LDL cholesterol concentrations were down 8.9 percent and 13 percent, respectively, in the psyllium group compared to controls.[55]

In another study, it was found that psyllium reduces after-meal glucose and insulin levels in type 2 diabetics, regardless of whether their disease is controlled by diet or requires oral hypoglycemic drugs. In the study, eighteen type 2 diabetics consumed psyllium or a placebo before breakfast and dinner. Fasting glucose levels were recorded prior to the morning supplement and meal. Psyllium was not consumed during the lunch meal, so that residual or second-meal effects could be measured. The research team reported that maximum after-eating glucose elevation decreased 14 percent at breakfast and 20 percent at dinner in the fiber-supplemented group compared to controls. In addition, after-meal blood insulin levels after breakfast dropped 12 percent. Second-meal effects after lunch brought a 31 percent reduction in glucose in the psyllium group.[56]

Barley

In Iraq, barley bread is a common treatment for diabetes, since it modulates the glycemic response to carbohydrate ingestion, slows weight loss, and reduces excessive water consumption. One of the advantages of barley is that it contains about 5.69 mcg of chromium (a mineral of benefit to diabetics) per gram.[57]

High–Complex Carbohydrate, High-Fiber Diet

A high–complex carbohydrate, high-fiber diet, advocated by James W. Anderson, M.D., can significantly lower blood fats and reduce the risk of cardiovascular disease; reduce fasting blood sugar, glycosylated hemoglobin, and blood lipids; help maintain desirable body weight; and reduce insulin and oral hypoglycemic medications (or eliminate them entirely). This diet includes 60 percent of calories as complex carbohydrates with 35 grams of dietary fiber per 1,000 kcal. The diet has been shown to improve glycemic control and reduce insulin requirements by 30 to 40 percent for type 1 diabetics, and 75 to 100 percent for type 2 diabetics. In most cases, insulin has been discontinued after 10–21 days of dietary treatment in type 2 diabetics. In addition, serum cholesterol levels were reduced 30 percent for type 1 diabetics and 24 percent for type 2 diabetics. Dr. Anderson has found water-soluble fibers are especially effective, such as those from oat bran, oatmeal, oat bran muffins, beans, psyllium, and soy fiber.[58]

The high–complex carbohydrate, high-fiber diet includes 50 to 60 percent of calories from carbohydrates (two-thirds of which are complex carbohydrates), 15 to 20 percent protein (minimum of 45 g per day), 20 to 25 percent fat (less than 10 percent saturated fat), 200 mg or less of cholesterol daily, 40–50 g of total dietary fiber (25 g per 1,000 kcal), and 10–15 g of soluble fiber daily.

Fiber Supplements

In a study at the University of Minnesota, at Minneapolis, researchers evaluated the effects of 10 grams or 20 grams per day of a fiber supplement compared to a look-alike supplement. They found that total cholesterol, LDL cholesterol, and the ratio of LDL to HDL cholesterol were significantly reduced in those in both fiber groups compared to the volunteers who took a placebo. However, the fiber supplement had no effect

POPCORN FOR FIBER?

While popcorn is considered a good source of fiber, a large order of popcorn at some of the large theater chains has more than a day's worth of fat and two day's worth of artery-clogging fat, according to the Center for Science in the Public Interest, in Washington, D.C. And that is *without* butter. With the butter-flavored topping, the heart-unhealthy fat is equal to nine McDonald's Quarter Pounders.[59] It is said that seven out of ten movie theaters use coconut oil, which is about 80 percent saturated fat, to pop their popcorn. Some use partially hydrogenated soybean oil, which contributes both saturated and trans-fatty acids. Trans-fats are thought to elevate cholesterol levels. If the theaters use partially hydrogenated canola shortening, not canola oil, this could also be unhealthy.

on HDL cholesterol or triglycerides. The fiber supplement contained guar gum, pectin, soy, pea, and corn bran.[60] Note: Patients with diverticulitis, ulcerative colitis, and Crohn's disease should not take fiber supplements without medical supervision. High levels of fiber can impede the absorption of iron, calcium, zinc, copper, and other minerals in these patients.

CHAPTER 5

Vitamin A and the Carotenoids

Vitamin A

Also known as retinol, axerophthol, biosterol, anti-infective vitamin, and other names, vitamin A was discovered in 1912 by Elmer V. McCollum and Marguerite Davis at the University of Wisconsin. They had determined that something in butter fat or egg yolk fat made the difference between moderate success in the nutrition of young rats on certain diets and prompt nutritive failure.[1] This something turned out to be vitamin A and this theory was confirmed several months later by Thomas Burr Osborne and Lafayette Benedict Mendel at Yale University.

Vitamin A is available from such animal sources as milk, butter, eggs, liver, and fish liver oils. However, it can be formed in the liver of humans and animals from beta-carotene (provitamin A). Experiments show that carotene, found in green- and yellow-colored fruits and vegetables, is utilized less effectively than vitamin A; however, individuals differ in their ability to convert carotene into vitamin A.

Vitamin A is essential for the health of eyes, skin, teeth, gums, and mucous membranes. Those who have difficulty seeing at night and when they enter a darkened room or who are bothered by an oncoming car headlight at night are said to have "night blindness"—they are probably deficient in vitamin A. This is also true for those who are bothered by the glare of sunlight during the day.

Clinical Studies on Vitamin A

At the Massachusetts Eye and Ear Infirmary, in Boston, researchers found that 15,000 IU per day of vitamin A had a beneficial effect in dealing with retinitis pigmentosa. The study involved 601 patients ranging in age from 18 to 49, who were diagnosed with the eye disorder.[2]

In the first National Health and Nutrition Examination Survey, which collected data between 1971 and 1972, the frequency of consumption of fruits and vegetables rich in vitamin A in those forty-five years of age or older was inversely related to age-related macular degeneration.[3] In studying 2,900 people between the ages of 49 and 97, higher intakes of vitamin A, protein, vitamins B_3, B_1, and B_2 were associated with a reduced risk for nuclear cataract.[4]

Since free-radical formation is a common biological occurrence, an organism must be able to defend itself against this form of cellular damage. Vitamins play a significant role in these defenses. For example, vitamins A and E have been shown to absorb free radicals, and vitamin C, which is present in circulating blood, is part of the first line of defense against free radicals. Because of their capacity to defend the body against the oxygen free radicals, vitamins A, E, and C have been termed *antioxidants*.[5]

Vitamin A, along with beta-carotene, is of particular importance to diabetics, since they not only pick up infections easily but also have very poor wound-healing abilities, according to Eberhard Kronhausen, author of *Formula for Life*.[6] "Vitamin A has definitely been shown by researchers at Albert Einstein College of Medicine in New York to be of help with regard to diabetic animals," the authors stated. "It is not yet known whether these benefits also apply to humans, but indications are that they may."

Taking Vitamin A

The daily requirement for vitamin A, a fat-soluble vitamin, is given in retinol equivalents (RE): 1 RE is defined as 1 microgram (mcg) of retinol or 6 mcg of beta-carotene. The vitamin is also listed in international units (IU), with 1 IU of vitamin A activity equal to 0.3 mcg of retinol or 0.6 mcg of beta-carotene. The Recommended Dietary Allowance (RDA) of vitamin A for men, ages twenty-five to fifty, is 1,000 mcg of retinol (RE); it is 800 mcg (RE) for non-pregnant women.

Pregnant women should not take vitamin A without a doctor's recommendation, since amounts above 10,000 IU (3,000 RE) are thought to cause birth defects.[7] Prior to the RE designation by the National Research

Council, the RDA for vitamin A for most adults was 5,000 IU. Researchers reported that 4,500 RE (or 15,000 IU) per day of vitamin A caused no toxic manifestations in young and middle-aged adults with retinitis pigmentosa during a twelve-year follow-up.[8]

Beta-Carotene and the Carotenoids

Carotenoids are naturally occurring compounds that are abundant in plants. While 500 to 600 carotenoids have been identified, only a small number of them are found in appreciable quantities in human blood and tissues. The major carotenoids are alpha-carotene, beta-carotene, lutein, zeaxanthin, cryptoxanthin, and lycopene.[9] Carotenoids have diverse biological functions and despite their similarities in structure, they play very different roles. Certain carotenoids are precursors of vitamin A and can be metabolically converted into the vitamin. Beta-carotene has the highest potential vitamin A activity; other provitamin A carotenoids are alpha-carotene and cryptoxanthin.

"Carotenoids function as chain-breaking antioxidants, protecting cells and other body components from free radical attack," according to Sharon Landvik, M.S., R.D. "Oxidative damage resulting from free radical attack has been linked to the onset of premature aging, cancer, atherosclerosis, cataracts, age-related macular degeneration, and an array of degenerative diseases."[10] Free radicals, which are dangerous molecules that sometimes contain oxygen, can multiply by chain reactions, making them even more devious.

Lutein and zeaxanthin are the only carotenoids found in the macular region of the retina. They are linked to normal function of the macula, which is responsible for sharp and detailed vision. The two carotenoids are thought to serve as filters for harmful blue light in the macula and as scavengers of singlet oxygen in retinal tissues. (Singlet oxygen, a higher energy form of oxygen, can react with atmospheric pollutants to cause smog formation, thus providing harmful biological effects.)

Clinical Studies on Carotenoids

Physicians have long suggested that diet is a principal risk factor for type 2 diabetes and that a high intake of refined carbohydrates and sugar is associated with an increased risk of getting the disease. Researchers studied blood levels of various carotenoids in 1,665 volunteers, ranging in age from 40 to 74, and it was found that the highest beta-carotene levels were in those with normal glucose tolerance. However, levels declined progressively among those with impaired glucose tolerance and diabetes. Further, people with impaired glucose tolerance had beta-carotene levels 13 percent below normal and those with newly diagnosed diabetes had beta-carotene levels 20 percent below normal.[11] While the study did not demonstrate a protective effect of beta-carotene, the findings were consistent with existing research which shows that antioxidants may protect against insulin-damaging free radicals and, therefore, reduce the risk of developing diabetes.

In a study involving 106 type 2 diabetics and 201 matched controls, those with diabetes had lower serum levels of beta-carotene and vitamin E. High levels of the two nutrients were associated with a reduced risk for type 2 diabetes, but this association disappeared after adjusting for cardiovascular risk factors.[12]

Beta-carotene, as an antioxidant, may reduce the risk of certain diseases, such as heart disease. Researchers studied disease and dietary patterns in 12,733 men and women who participated in the ongoing Atherosclerosis Risk in Communities Study. It was found that, in both men and women, carotenoid-rich foods were associated with a substantially lower prevalence of cholesterol deposits in the carotid artery, a major blood vessel. Women eating beta-carotene-rich diets benefited more than men.[13]

A study reported in the *American Journal of Clinical Nutrition* found that in fifty-six men with cardiovascular disease, ages thirty to sixty-nine, the visceral fat at the L1 and L4 vertebra was much greater in cardiovascular disease patients with diabetes than in the controls. It was also reported that the cardiovascular disease patients had higher blood levels of homocysteine (a risk factor for cardiovascular disease) and lower blood levels of superoxide dismutase (SOD), an antioxidant that destroys harmful free radicals, than controls. Blood levels of lycopene and beta-carotene were lowest in the patients with diabetes.[14]

Beta-carotene and other carotenoids, which are fat-soluble antioxidants, prevent free-radical damage to fats (lipid peroxidation), which contributes to cell damage leading to heart disease. In one study, nine women were put on a very low-carotenoid diet and/or given beta-carotene and mixed carotenoid supplements. It was found that women consuming low levels of carotenoids had high blood levels of malondi-alhyde-thiobarbituric acid (MDA-TBA), which is an established signal for lipid peroxidation. When the women were given supplements of beta-carotene and mixed carotenoids, the MDA-TBA levels decreased.[15]

A research team at Erasmus University Medical School, in Rotterdam, the Netherlands, reviewed evidence that antioxidants provide protection against ischemic heart disease and decided to test this suggestion on a group of elderly volunteers, ranging in age from fifty-five to ninety-five.[16] The researchers reported that high dietary intakes of beta-carotene provided protection against heart disease, which can be a complication of diabetes.

Food Sources of Carotenoids

The richest dietary sources of carotenoids are fruits and vegetables.

- Apricots, cantaloupe, carrots, leafy green vegetables, pumpkin, sweet potato, and winter squash are good sources of beta-carotene.

- Carrots and pumpkins are good sources of alpha-carotene.

- Lutein and zeaxanthin are found in leafy green vegetables, pumpkin, and red pepper.

- Guava, pink grapefruit, tomatoes and tomato products, and watermelon are rich in lycopene.

- Cryptoxanthin is found in mangoes, nectarines, oranges, papaya, peaches, and tangerines.[17]

Taking Carotenoids

Currently, there is no official recommended dietary intake for carotenoids. Based on dietary guidelines of government agencies for optimal intake of fruits and vegetables to help prevent chronic disease, it appears that a daily intake of 6 milligrams (mg) of beta-carotene could be recommended. The Alliance for Aging Research has recommended 10–30 mg per day of beta-carotene for optimal health, especially in older people. In the United States, the amount of carotenoids supplied by the average diet is estimated at 1.5 mg per day of beta-carotene.

The preferred form of carotenoid supplements are those derived from algae, such as *Dunaliella salina*, or whole-food concentrates. An average adult may opt to take 10,000–25,000 IU daily for preventive care. For protection against cancer and macular degeneration, Robert Atkins, M.D., bolstered *D. salina*'s carotenoids with additional lycopene, lutein, and zeaxanthin.[18]

Carotene supplements are available over the counter, and some vitamin A supplements also contain beta-carotene. The only common side effect associated with high intakes of carotenoids (30 mg daily or more) from supplements or carotenoid-rich foods is yellowing of the skin, which is harmless and goes away when the amount of carotenoid is reduced.[19]

CHAPTER 6

The B-Complex Vitamins

The eight members of the B-complex family, and three vitamin B "cousins," play significant roles in preventing or treating diabetes. Some work directly to help type 1 and type 2 diabetics, while others deal with life-threatening problems for diabetics, such as heart attack and stroke.

- Vitamin B_1 (thiamine) is a co-factor in many enzyme systems and plays an active role in carbohydrate metabolism.

- Vitamin B_2 (riboflavin) is also necessary for carbohydrate metabolism and it becomes deficient when people are under severe stress.[1]

- Vitamin B_3 (niacin, niacinamide, and nicotinic acid) helps to lower cholesterol levels and protects against hardening of the arteries. It is necessary for energy, growth, nerve function, healthy skin, and gastrointestinal function. Another form of B_3, inositol hexaniacinate, is even more effective in many applications and it doesn't cause flushing. The vitamin should be used with caution by diabetics, since it can deteriorate glycemic control.[2]

- Vitamin B_6 (pyridoxine) is needed for amino acid (protein) metabolism, hemoglobin formation, nerve impulses, and hormone synthesis. It is being used to treat high homocysteine levels and neuropathy (nerve damage). In a double-blind trial using vitamin B_6 at 200 milligrams (mg) per day in eight patients with diabetic mononeuropathy (nerve damage), it was found that the vitamin is associated with improvements in motor and sensory activity in the median nerve and sensory activity in the ulnar nerve (in the upper arm). In addition, vitamin B_6 may be considered an alternative form of therapy with diabetics who have failed to respond to other forms of traditional therapy for carpal tunnel syndrome (a painful nerve condition in the wrist).[3]

- Vitamin B_{12} (cobalamin) plays an important role in hemoglobin synthesis and lowering of homocysteine levels. A deficiency in the vitamin may result in altered glycosylated hemoglobin (amount of glucose in the blood). When vitamin B_{12} therapy is given along with iron, hemoglobin A_{1C} levels have been shown to decrease after three weeks. It does not appear that this reduction in hemoglobin A_{1C} improves glycemic control; instead, improved glycemic control indicates an increase in the red blood cell population. Most of the hemoglobin (the oxygen-carrying component in red blood cells) exists in a form known as hemoglobin A. A small amount is converted into hemoglobin A_{1C} or glycosylated hemoglobin.[4]

- Folic acid is needed in amino acid metabolism and nucleic acid synthesis. A deficiency in folic acid can result in anemia, gastrointestinal lesions, poor growth, and glossitis (inflammation of the tongue). It is instrumental in lowering homocysteine levels and in preventing cardiovascular disease.

- Biotin is needed for the production of fatty acids and the conversion of food into energy. Biotin may help to prevent diabetic neuropathy and it is used to treat low blood sugar.

- Pantothenic acid aids in the production of energy from fat, protein, and carbohydrates; one form of the vitamin, pantethine, helps to lower cholesterol and triglyceride levels.

- Choline and inositol, although associated with the B complex, are not officially vitamins, but they may help diabetics. Para-aminobenzoic acid (PABA) is the third vitamin B cousin.

Since the members of this complex are water-soluble, they should be taken in supplement form in divided doses during the day, because large amounts pass out of the body during the day in urine and feces.

Vitamin B_1

In *Body, Mind, and the B Vitamins*, Ruth Adams and I reported on the case of a 3-year-old girl who suffered from diabetes and deafness and who later developed pernicious anemia. Doctors at Duke University, in North Carolina, gave her vitamin B_{12} and folic acid, the usual treatment for this anemia, but it did not help. However, she began to improve after they gave her a high-potency multivitamin supplement. She returned home without any supplements and her condition worsened and her insulin requirements also increased. Again admitted to the hospital, the girl was given large amounts of each of the vitamins in the multivitamin tablet. Her insulin requirements lessened with large amounts of vitamin B_1. She was sent home once again without supplements and again she relapsed. Finally, the doctors gave her 20 mg per day of vitamin B_1 and sent her home with instructions for her family to continue this treatment. The child had no more relapses.[5]

Why did B_1 make the difference? The doctors concluded that the child had a defect in a single B_1-dependent enzyme and that dietary amounts were insufficient to keep her from developing anemia. The doctors could not tell whether or not B_1 affected her diabetes, deafness, or other health problems, but they feared that their treatment came too late to reverse the damage that had already been done.

A research team from the University of Michigan, in Ann Arbor, reported that a vitamin B_1 deficiency may occur in a large number of patients with congestive heart failure and that a dietary deficiency in the vitamin may contribute to an increased risk. They found a B_1 deficiency in eight patients and a risk for dietary thiamine deficiency in ten out of thirty-eight patients. Those with congestive heart failure frequently experience cardiac cachexia, a type of malnutrition. Previous studies have shown that a B_1 deficiency may be the result of increased urinary losses in association with loop therapy for congestive heart failure.[6]

Taking Vitamin B_1

Food sources of B_1 include Brazil nuts, enriched bread, soybeans, brewer's yeast, dried whey, wheat germ, turkey, broccoli, cabbage, kidney, salmon, brown rice, cashews, sunflower seeds, chicken, liver, peas, lentils, mushrooms, eggs, flounder, chickpeas, and cauliflower.

Is vitamin B_1 safe? According to the Council for Responsible Nutrition, thiamine is nontoxic and has a long history as an oral supplement without adverse effects. It is safe at intakes up to 50 mg and perhaps as high as 200 mg per day. There are no reports of adverse effects by taking B_1 supplements, even at dosages of several hundred milligrams.[7]

Vitamin B₂

Formerly known as vitamin G, chemical research on riboflavin or vitamin B_2 started in 1879, but its function and importance in nutrition were not realized until 1932, when Otto Warburg and W. Christian in Germany studied a yellow enzyme in yeast and were able to split it into a protein and a pigment (flavin).[8] Deficiency in vitamin B_2 may result in soreness and redness of the tongue and lips, atrophy of papillae (small bumps) on the surface of the tongue, and cracks at the corners of the mouth. In vitamin B_2 deficiency, dermatitis of the scrotum may also spread to other areas of the body. Another complication is disturbances in the blood vessels in the eye.

Riboflavin is excreted when protein in the body is broken down and it is retained when protein is being accumulated. Thus, in acute starvation, uncontrolled diabetes, and other conditions associated with negative nitrogen balance, excretion in the urine does not adequately reflect body stores of the vitamin.

In 1941, government statistics showed that many Americans were not getting sufficient amounts of vitamins B_1, B_2, B_3, and iron, so the Food and Nutrition Board proposed that the four nutrients be added to flour and bread—to build strong bodies during World War II. The government then ruled that this "enrichment" program should be utilized by the Army and Navy as well as the general public. However, B_2 was not available in adequate amounts until the end of 1943.[9]

Taking Vitamin B₂

Riboflavin or B_2 is widely distributed in foods of plant and animal origin. Some of the best food sources are milk, meat, liver, heart, kidney, cheese, eggs, leafy green vegetables, and whole-grain cereals and bread.

Is vitamin B_2 safe? There are no reports of adverse effects from orally consumed riboflavin. Although the data are sparse at very high intakes, there is sufficient evidence to suggest that oral intakes of 200 mg per day are safe.[10]

Fiber products, such as Metamucil, are used as bulk laxatives to lower cholesterol, to improve blood sugar in diabetics, and for weight reduction, according to Sheldon Saul Hendler, M.D., Ph.D. However, long-term use of these products can negatively affect vitamin B_2, as well as zinc, iron, manganese, copper, and beta-carotene.[11] When researchers evaluated 368 gluten-free products, they found that many do not provide the same levels of B_1, B_2, B_3 as enriched wheat flour products. Those who consume a gluten-free diet could be deficient in one or more of the three vitamins, so celiac disease patients on a gluten-free diet should be checked for B vitamin deficiencies.[12]

Vitamin B_3

Vitamin B_3 (niacin) is a "cluster" that includes nicotinic acid and nicotinamide, both of which are natural forms of the vitamin with equal niacin activity. In the body, both forms are active as nicotinamide adenine dinucleotide (NAD) and nicotinamide adenine dinucleotide phosphate (NADP)—they serve as coenzymes, often in conjunction with B_1 and B_2 coenzymes to produce energy within cells.[13] NAD and NADP function in many important enzyme systems necessary for cell respiration and they are involved in the release of energy from carbohydrates, proteins, and fats. In addition, the two coenzymes are involved in the synthesis of fatty acids, protein, and DNA. However, for these processes to occur, they require three B vitamins: B_6, pantothenic acid, and biotin.

According to researchers at the University of Bristol, in England, nicotinamide is being used as a potential way of preventing type 1 diabetes in high-risk, first-degree relatives. Long-term nicotinamide use appears to be highly favorable and this may be an excellent treatment for diabetes prevention. Further, high-dose nicotinamide can protect beta cells in the pancreas in response to a range of toxic and immune stimuli in animal and test-tube models, suggesting that the vitamin may react as a free-radical scavenger.

For type 1 diabetes, doses have ranged from 200 mg per day to 30 mg/kg (equivalent to 3.5 g daily) for twelve months. To prevent type 1 diabetes in high-risk groups, doses ranged from 1 g to 3 g daily, from four months to four years. The researchers added that the vitamin has been used at pharmacological doses for many years with a low incidence of side effects or toxicity. However, it was found that, at very high doses, there is reversible hepatoxicity (toxic damage to the liver) in both animal and human studies, and minor abnormalities of liver enzymes have surfaced with dosages used for diabetes prevention. Most maximum doses are about 3.5 g per day, but some researchers have used doses as high as 6 g per day.[14]

Nicotinic acid has been known as a cholesterol-lowering agent since 1955, according to Jeffrey L. Probstfield, M.D., of the Fred Hutchinson Cancer Research Center, in Seattle, Washington. Daily doses between 2 g and 12 g can have a major effect in lowering LDL ("bad") cholesterol. The dosage is generally 3 g daily or less, since larger doses can cause flushing and itching in susceptible people. Excess amounts can also cause gastrointestinal complaints, high amounts of glucose in the blood, injury to the liver, a buildup of uric acid, and gout. Some of these side effects can be minimized by taking the supplement with food, and gradually increasing or decreasing the dose. Sustained-release dosages, which are also available over the counter, have been shown to reduce symptoms, but they are also related to liver damage and reduce efficiency in increasing HDL ("good") cholesterol levels.[15]

While there is a recorded 26 percent reduction in LDL cholesterol with lovastatin, LDL can also be reduced by up to 23 percent with nicotinic acid. The vitamin was more effective than the drug in increasing HDL cholesterol and apolipoprotein-a1 levels, as well as decreasing triglycerides and lipoprotein-a levels. Dr. Probstfield also said that nicotinic acid would be useful for type 2 diabetics with cholesterol, triglyceride, and other fat abnormalities, except that it must be used with caution because it can affect blood glucose control. It may be useful to start with a low dose of 100–125 mg three times daily, which may produce fewer symptoms and better patient compliance, with a slow buildup to higher doses. The flushing can be reduced by taking the vitamin during or after meals.

By keeping lipid levels normal, vitamin B_3 should protect diabetics against the most dangerous chronic side effect—hardening of the arteries, according to Abram Hoffer, M.D., Ph.D., author of *Orthomolecular Medicine for Physicians*. The vitamin may also have an effect on glucose levels in the blood, on glucose tolerance, and on insulin requirements. Insulin requirements may be increased or decreased. Dr. Hoffer said that some researchers concluded that niacinamide given to young type 1 diabetics produced a remission of the disease. Their double-blind experiment involved sixteen newly diagnosed type 1 diabetics, ranging in age from ten to thirty-five. After one week of intensive insulin, the volunteers were started on 3 g per day of niacinamide or a placebo. If insulin was needed after six months, the vitamin was discontinued. "Our results and those found from animal experiments indicate that, in type 1 diabetes, niacinamide slows down destruction of beta-cells and enhances their regeneration, thus extending remission time," the researchers stated. Beta-cells in the pancreas make and release insulin. Of the 16 treated volunteers, three reached two-year remissions.[16]

Researchers at the University of Massachusetts, at Amherst, reported that niacinamide may prevent the onset of type 1 diabetes. Doses of up to 3,000 mg per day were said to be nontoxic. The vitamin's role is thought to be involved in DNA damage repair processes or in providing protection against free-radical damage. The researchers added that both vitamin C and vitamin E may prevent high blood sugar levels and that vitamin E, given at 100 IU per day, can greatly lower glycosylated hemoglobin levels (amount of glucose in the blood). Further, red blood cell lipid peroxidation is associated with glycosylated hemoglobin levels and vitamin E can correct this abnormality. Also, 126 mg per day of sodium vanadate (vanadium) has been shown to lower insulin requirements and plasma cholesterol levels in type 1 diabetics.[17]

At the Center for Human Nutrition in Dallas, Texas, thirteen type 2 diabetics were given 1.5 g of nicotinic acid, three times daily, or a placebo for eight weeks. The researchers found that the niacin supplement reduced cholesterol by 24 percent, triglycerides by 45 percent, very-low-density lipoprotein (VLDLs) by 58 percent, and LDL cholesterol by 15 percent, with a 34 percent increase in HDL cholesterol. The vitamin therapy altered blood sugar control, with a 16 percent increase in plasma glucose, 21 percent increase in glycosylated hemoglobin levels, and increased glycosuria (glucose in urine). There was also an increase in uric acid, which is a potent antioxidant. However, the researchers did not recommend this therapy for first-time type 2 diabetics with elevated cholesterol.[18]

Nicotinamide may protect beta-cells in type 1 diabetes, while nicotinic acid may help with insulin resistance in type 2 diabetes. Type 2 diabetics often produce sufficient insulin but their bodies do not regulate the insulin, causing insulin resistance. In four case studies, it was reported that 250–750 mg per day of niacin benefited patients with diabetes, high blood pressure, congestive heart failure, and circulatory problems. Beta-cell injury is thought to be associated with low nicotinamide adenine dinucleotide (NAD) and adenosine triphosphate (ATP) levels, which results in oxidative injury and organ failure. NAD levels are known to be low in diabetics. Antioxidants, plus vitamin B_3, which is an NAD precursor, may prevent this condition.[19]

John P. Cleary, M.D., of Madison, Wisconsin, said that in the early 1940s, nicotinamide was used to reduce insulin requirements in treating diabetes, but following World War II, there was not much interest in vitamin B_3 for treating the disease. However, low NAD may impair the enzyme NaKATPase, which can cause impaired glucose transport, and insulin may not be able to correct this defect. Type 1 diabetics utilize nicotinamide, which inhibits the loss of NAD in the beta-cells and subsequent loss of insulin production. A dose of 25 mg/kg of body weight per day of nicotinamide is recommended to correct the problem. Dr. Cleary added that 100–200 mg daily of nicotinamide in the early onset of diabetes may also be useful. For type 2 diabetics, 500 mg per day of nicotinic acid is recommended. Larger amounts are not recommended, since some patients may experience liver dysfunction, glucose intolerance, hyperuricemia (large amounts of uric acid in the blood), and flushing.[20]

At the University of Rome and the University Cattolica in Rome, Italy, researchers reported that type 1 diabetics might benefit from taking nicotinamide. This therapy brought a partial remission of diabetes, indicated by reduced insulin need, in 32 percent of twenty-two volunteers given 200 mg daily of the B vitamin for one year. A control group of thirteen patients who were given only insulin had a 7.5 percent partial remission rate. Total remission (no insulin needed) was reported in three patients getting the vitamin but not in the controls.[21] Researchers in California gave fifty-six type 1 diabetics 25 mg/kg of nicotinamide or a placebo for twelve months. Their data showed that the vitamin can be added to insulin in these patients to prevent beta-cell destruction.[22]

A combination of niacinamide and vitamin E may be beneficial in future trials of insulin-dependent diabetes (type 1) at the beginning of the disease, according to a research team at St. Bartholomew's Hospital Medical College, in London, England. These observations were made following a study of eighty-four type 1 diabetics, ranging in age from five to thirty-five. Forty-two of the volunteers were given 15 mg/kg body weight per day of vitamin E for one year and the other forty-two received niacinamide for one year at 25 mg/kg of body weight per day. Glycosylated hemoglobin and insulin were similar in both groups and all were getting 3–4 insulin injections daily. In patients under the age of fifteen who were getting vitamin E, there was an increased need for insulin compared to the niacin-treated patients one year after diagnosis. The researchers added that the two vitamins have similar effects in protecting beta-cell function in patients recently diagnosed with type 1 diabetes.[23]

Lipid-modifying doses of timed-release vitamin B_3 can be used safely in patients with stable, controlled type 2 diabetes, according to Marshall B. Elam, Ph.D., M.D., of the University of Tennessee, at Memphis. Niacin may be considered an alternative to statin drugs or fibrates, two of the most common lipid-lowering drugs, in those with diabetes in whom these drugs are not tolerated or fail to sufficiently correct high levels of triglycerides or low levels of HDL cholesterol. The study involved 468 participants, including 125 with diabetes, who had diagnosed peripheral arterial disease. The volunteers were selected to receive either 3,000 mg per day of niacin (64 with diabetes and 173 without the disease) or placebo (61 with diabetes and 170 without diabetes) for up to 60 weeks. Niacin significantly increased HDL cholesterol by 29 percent in both groups and decreased triglycerides by 23 percent and 28 percent, respectively. Low-density lipoprotein cholesterol dropped as well.[24]

Taking Vitamin B₃

Food sources of B_3 include liver and kidney, lean meat, poultry, fish, rabbit, mushrooms, nuts, milk and cheese, eggs, and enriched cereals.

The optimum dose of niacin varies from 3 g to 6 g per day in three divided doses, according to Abram Hoffer, M.D., Ph.D. This can begin suddenly or by starting with smaller doses and gradually increasing them. Few people will not have pronounced vasodilation (flush) beginning in the forehead and extending downward, but most will flush very little after a period of days or weeks.[25] If the flush remains a problem, the niacin may need to be discontinued. It may then be replaced by a niacin derivative such as inositol niacinate, if the beneficial vascular effect is essential, or by niacinamide if it is not. Few people will flush with niacinamide. The flush can also be moderated by taking aspirin (1 tablet) before each dose of niacin for a few days, or by using antihistamines or tranquilizers.

The safest form of niacin is inositol hexaniacinate, according to Michael T. Murray, N.D. This form has been used in Europe to lower cholesterol levels and to improve blood flow. It yields slightly better results than niacin and is better tolerated during long-term use. In one study, 153 patients treated with inositol hexaniacinate at dosages ranging from 600 mg to 1,800 mg per day experienced no side effects.[26] Patients who experience the niacin flush can take inositol hexaniacinate, which seems to slow the release of niacin and is less likely to cause flushing.

Vitamin B$_6$

Found in foods in three forms—pyridoxine, pyridoxal, and pyridoxamine—this B vitamin is rapidly absorbed from the upper part of the small intestine and is present in many body tissues, with high concentrations in the liver.[27] Vitamin B$_6$ in its coenzyme forms, usually as pyridoxal phosphate but sometimes as pyridoxamine phosphate, is involved in a large number of physiologic functions, especially in protein (nitrogen) metabolism and, to a lesser extent, in carbohydrate and fat metabolism. It is an essential part of phosphorylase, the enzyme that brings about the conversion of glycogen to glucose-1-phosphate in muscle and liver. It also takes part in fat metabolism and is believed to be involved in the metabolism of unsaturated linoleic acid into another fatty acid called arachidonic acid.

John M. Ellis, M.D., has reported that vitamin B$_6$ deficiency is common in both type 1 and type 2 diabetes. In 1989, Dr. Ellis and colleagues began an intensive study of twenty-one diabetics, all but one taking 100–300 mg per day of vitamin B$_6$. "We can conclude from our studies that every diabetic at every stage should be given a therapeutic dose of 100 to 300 mg per day of B$_6$," Dr. Ellis stated. "A quick response to vitamin B$_6$ is not so evident in the late stages of diabetic retinopathy and nephropathy. However, it is in the prevention of these catastrophic conditions the vitamin becomes important. The rheumatic improvements seen within three months of beginning treatment with vitamin B$_6$ signal the long-term prevention of diabetic retinopathy and nephropathy."[28] The biochemistries and cellular activities in the different bodily tissues, including those of the eye, are responsive for a number of enzymatic activities, many of which require vitamin B_6 and affect the collagen in the vitreous, retina, and matrix of the retina. This explains why one result of a long-term vitamin B_6 deficiency is the leakage of serum and lipids, including cholesterol, into the vitreous and retina. Ellis's study reveals the beneficial effects of vitamin B_6 in treating diabetes and its complications.

Diabetes is a condition in which blood glucose levels are high and vitamin B_6 levels are low in the body, according to Chandra Mohan, Ph.D. If vitamin B_6 levels are low, the insulin response is reduced and the circulating levels of insulin are lower, which leads to further increases in blood glucose levels. When there is a B_6 deficiency, storage of glycogen in the liver is impaired, leading potentially to hypoglycemia. A reduced level of B_6 with an increased amount of blood glucose and uncontrolled hyperglycemia, can lead to damage to the eyes, kidneys, and nervous and vascular systems over time. Also, reduced amounts of B_6 can cause problems with amino acid (protein) transport and perhaps protein synthesis. Inefficient protein synthesis is a major problem with diabetics, since it requires insulin. In addition, diabetics have a high rate of protein breakdown due to the needs of amino acids for gluconeogenesis processing (the synthesis of glucose from non-carbohydrates, such as protein or fat).[29] Dr. Mohan recommends taking about 2 g daily of vitamin B_6, the so-called Recommended Dietary Allowance (RDA), but taking two to three times the RDA is not going to cause complications.

Vitamin B_6 has been used with some success in treating gestational diabetes, the type of the disease that sometimes accompanies pregnancy, reports Alan Gaby, M.D. In addition, B_6 can improve the abnormal glucose tolerance that develops in some women who take birth control pills. It seems that B_6 is related to xanthurenic acid (XA), a byproduct of the metabolism of the amino acid tryptophan. Vitamin B_6–deficient patients have abnormalities in tryptophan metabolism that leads to the production of excess XA, which can bind to insulin and inactivate it.[30]

Dr. Gaby discusses the work of Charles L. Jones, D.P.M., a podiatrist, and Virginia Gonzalez, M.D., who studied ten type 1 diabetics with symptoms of peripheral neuropathy. The patients excreted more XA than did other diabetics without neuropathy, suggesting that a B_6 deficiency was more pronounced with neuropathy. When the researchers gave each patient 50 mg of B_6, three times daily, for six weeks, XA excretion became normal, suggesting that B_6 deficiency had been corrected. Most of the patients noticed some relief of pain and paresthesia (tickling sensation) in about 10 days. "Seven of the patients continued on B_6 supplements and did well," Dr. Gaby added. "The other three stopped taking the vitamin and noticed a recurrence of their symptoms about three weeks later. When they resumed taking B_6, their symptoms also disappeared. Two patients also had a marked improvement in their blood sugar measurements, which had been chronically elevated (275 and 315 mg/100 ml, respectively) and difficult to control. After B_6 therapy, their glucose levels fell to 195 and 200 mg/100 ml, respectively, and remained there as long as they continued taking B_6."[31]

Researchers at Kaiser Permanente Medical Center, in Hayward, California, also found that vitamin B_6 may be an effective therapy in the treatment of diabetic neuropathies. Volunteers who reported chronic, painful diabetic neuropathies were given 160 mg daily of B_6 and then monitored monthly afterward. The researchers said that pain consistently decreased and activity increased with B_6 supplements. Also, complaints of pain decreased and mood increased. The researchers also found that hypoglycemic drugs, such as insulin or oral medications, were reduced with the supplement. No adverse side effects were recorded.[32]

Taking Vitamin B₆

Food sources include liver and kidney, fish, lean meat, soybeans, poultry, brown rice, nuts, bananas, avocados, and whole grains.

Is vitamin B_6 safe? Pyroxidine produces no reliably identified adverse effects at intakes up to 200 mg per day, reported the Council for Responsible Nutrition. Daily intakes of 2,000–6,000 mg have caused a distinct pattern of sensory neuropathy, which slowly and perhaps incompletely regresses after the megadoses are stopped. An intake of 500 mg daily carries some risk of neurotoxicity. The validity of the single report in the literature of adverse effects at daily intakes near 100 mg remains controversial.[33]

Vitamin B₁₂

Like other members of the B-complex, vitamin B_{12} is not a single substance but consists of a number of closely related compounds with similar activity. The term *cobalamin* is applied to these substances since they contain the mineral cobalt, and the vitamin is called "cyanocobalamin" for the cyanide ion in the molecule. Other compounds include hydroxo-cobalamin and nitrocobalamin.[34] Vitamin B_{12} is involved in the synthesis of nucleoproteins and it has a close association with folic acid in stimulating blood regeneration. Pernicious anemia is the most important disease due to B_{12} deficiency. The deficiency is due not necessarily to a dietary deficiency, but to a failure of absorption of the vitamin from the intestinal tract in the absence of intrinsic factor in the gastric juice. Intrinsic factor is a substance produced by gastrointestinal mucosa that facilitates the absorption of B_{12}.

A research team at the Tokyo Metropolitan Geriatric Hospital, in Japan, evaluated homocysteine plasma levels in fifty-two type 2 diabetic patients with microangiopathy, eighty-four diabetic patients without the condition, and fifty-seven nondiabetic controls. Microangiopathy refers to blood clots in the small blood vessels. It was found that total plasma homocysteine levels were higher in the patients who had microangiopathy than in those who did not. Further, high levels of homocysteine were clearly associated with the presence of diabetic microangiopathy. However, when the patients were given 1,000 mcg per day of methylcobalamin (B_{12}) for three weeks, plasma levels of homocysteine in ten diabetics were significantly reduced.[35]

Vitamin B_{12} supplements have been used with some success in treating diabetic neuropathy, according to Michael T. Murray, N.D., in *Diabetes and Hypoglycemia*. It is not apparent if the success is due to the correction of a deficiency or the normalization of the deranged B_{12} metabolism seen in diabetics. Clinically, he added, diabetic neuropathy is similar to that of classical B_{12} deficiency. A typical symptom of B_{12} deficiency is megaloblastic anemia, which is characterized by abnormal red blood cells in the bone marrow.[36]

Diabetic neuropathy, a common factor in the disease, has an unknown etiology, most likely related to faulty diet and inadequate exercise. It is theorized that changes in the nerve bundles, as a result of faulty metabolism of carbohydrates, cause tissue swelling and therefore pain. The two pathologic changes seem to be ischemia to the nerve and/or accumulation of certain metabolites of sugar within the cells that result from inadequate insulin.[37]

A researcher in Louisiana reported on an elderly man with mild diabetes who was unable to open his right eyelid and was diagnosed with peripheral neuropathy. Following vitamin B_{12} therapy for six weeks, the eyelid became perfectly normal. The researcher, Vincent F. Chicola, M.D., began adding 0.25 cc of B_{12} to the protocol for patients on insulin and he has found no further problem with peripheral neuropathy.[38]

Is a vegetarian diet effective in alleviating diabetes? Since 1980, Milton Crane, M.D., of the Weimar Institute, in California, has been using the lacto-ovo-vegetarian diet in his practice. He initially began prescribing the diet in 1946, realizing that a more restrictive diet—excluding milk, meat, eggs, and refined foods (sugars, refined cereals, free fats, shortening or margarine)—was very effective for diabetes, high blood pressure, and coronary artery disease. He said that 80 percent of the patients with systemic, distal diabetic neuropathy have relief of pain in four to seventeen days.[39] In addition, one-third of type 2 diabetics and 10 percent of type 1 diabetics can be maintained with a fasting glucose level below 120 mg/dl with this therapy.

It may take up to ten years for evidence of a B_{12} deficiency to become symptomatically evident. Since many vegetarians are deficient in vitamin B_{12}, Dr. Crane recommended a B_{12} supplement. "There are no foods that are consistently eaten that contain B_{12} naturally or which have been supplemented by B_{12}. The increasing concern over cleanliness in our society to avoid infectious diseases decreases the number of bacteria that would produce B_{12} in foods. I believe strongly that it does not make sense to wait for vitamin B_{12} levels to go down before taking a supplement." He added that when B_{12} is taken orally in adequate amounts, the intrinsic factor is the initial limiting factor and the intestinal wall is the second limiting factor. If excess B_{12} is absorbed, the excess is readily disposed in the urine. He said that three sea vegetables—arame, wakame, and Kombu—may be good sources of B_{12} for the strict vegetarian, but studies are needed to confirm this.[40]

Taking Vitamin B_{12}

Vitamin B_{12} is available in animal foods such as liver and kidney, muscle meats, milk, cheese, fish, and eggs. There is no known B_{12} in fruits and vegetables.

Is vitamin B_{12} safe? No toxic effects of vitamin B_{12} have been reported in man or animals at any level of oral intake, according to the Council for Responsible Nutrition. There is a case of cobalamin-induced acne in association with an unspecified dosage given by injection twice weekly and a single case of contact dermatitis has been found in the literature. There is sufficient experience with intakes up to 3,000 mcg (3 mg) to establish the safety of this amount.[41]

Folic Acid

This B vitamin is sometimes referred to as folacin, pteroylmoboglutamic acid, and anti-anemia factor. The importance of folacin for the manufacture of blood cells apparently resides in its function in the formation of purines and pyrimidines.[42] Folic acid stimulates the formation of blood cells in certain anemias (megaloblastic anemia, for example), which are characterized by oversized red blood cells and the accumulation in the bone marrow of immature red blood cells called megaloblasts. Bone marrow is the organ that manufactures blood cells, but it can't complete the process without folic acid. Vitamin B_{12} is also required for the formation of blood cells and is effective in the treatment of a number of anemias (specifically, pernicious anemia). Folic acid is also related to vitamin C and the amino acid tyrosine. In addition to the anemias, folic acid deficiency causes diarrhea, inflammation of the tongue, and sprue (celiac disease and the malabsorption of nutrients).

Folic acid is instrumental in decreasing plasma concentrations of homocysteine. An amino acid, homocysteine is a natural product of the synthesis and breakdown of protein. While it is normally processed by the body, it can build up in the bloodstream and increase the risk of stroke, heart attack, and blood clots in the legs and lungs. Diabetes may be a risk factor for increased levels of homocysteine and for cardiovascular disease.

Since the causes of abnormal homocysteine levels are multifaceted and vitamin supplements can lower homocysteine, it would be prudent to include folic acid, B_6, and B_{12} in a supplement intended to lower homocysteine in those with abnormal levels of the amino acid. Researchers found that supplementing a group of volunteers with folic acid, B_6, and B_{12}—in doses 2.5 to 10 times the Recommended Dietary Allowance (RDA)—lowered homocysteine levels by about 32 percent.[43] According to researchers in the Netherlands, a dose of 250 mg per day of folic acid decreased homocysteine levels significantly in an eight-week, placebo-controlled study involving 144 healthy women, ranging in age from eighteen to forty.[44]

Researchers in Canada evaluated 5,506 men and women, ranging in age from thirty-five to seventy-nine, and found 165 coronary heart disease deaths among the group. They reported that there was a statistically significant association between the blood levels of folic acid and the risk of coronary heart disease. The lower the folate levels, the higher the risk.[45]

Researchers at the University of Pretoria in South Africa evaluated folic acid, B_{12}, and B_6 levels in 44 healthy men with moderately elevated levels of homocysteine and compared them with 274 controls without elevated levels. The research team found lower levels of folic acid, B_{12}, and B_6 in the group with high homocysteine. In a placebo-controlled follow-up study, a daily vitamin containing 10 mg of B_6, 1 mg of folic acid, and 400 mcg of B_{12} normalized homocysteine levels within six weeks. The authors said that an increased risk of premature hardening of the arteries due to raised homocysteine levels should be easy to prevent with the B vitamins.[46]

Researchers at the University of Calgary, in Alberta, Canada, evaluated 1,171 patients for blood levels of folic acid. Patients were sixty-five years of age or older. Those with the lowest amounts of the B vitamin in their blood were associated with an increased risk of stroke.[47]

Taking Folic Acid

Food sources of folic acid include beef liver, lima beans, spinach, cottage cheese, kidney, peanuts, filberts, walnuts, potatoes, endive, asparagus, turnip greens, lentils, cowpeas, collards, cabbage, sweet corn, lettuce, chard, beet greens, and whole-grain bread.

Is folic acid safe? Three concerns have been identified as possible adverse effects from taking too much folic acid:

- The masking of pernicious anemia, thereby permitting the neurologic disease of vitamin B_{12} deficiency to progress unchecked

- The disruption of zinc function by folic acid

- The antagonisms of medications, especially antifolate agents

However, the evidence is weak that folic acid has adverse effects by these or any other mechanisms.[48]

Biotin

Biotin is a sulfur-containing vitamin absorbed primarily from the upper part of the small intestine. The vitamin plays a significant role in the metabolism of carbohydrates, fats, and proteins.[49] A great deal of biotin is synthesized by intestinal bacteria, since 3–6 times more biotin is excreted in the urine and feces than is ingested. A number of variables affect the microbial synthesis of biotin in the intestines, including the carbohydrate sources of the diet (starch, glucose, sucrose, etc.), along with the presence of other B vitamins and the concurrent use of antimicrobial drugs and antibiotics. The vitamin is closely related to folic acid, pantothenic acid, and B_{12}.

Diabetics tend to be low in B vitamins, perhaps because diabetes uses up B vitamins and poorly controlled diabetes causes these water-soluble nutrients to be excreted in the urine, according to Mary Dan Eades, M.D. For example, some people may benefit from taking biotin in amounts up to 15 mg a day, she stated. A study by Japanese researchers reported that biotin helps cells in muscle tissue to use sugar more effectively.[50]

Biotin, at up to 2,000 mcg three times daily, may help diabetes-related neuropathy, reports Ralph Golan, M.D. The vitamin has successfully reversed symptoms of peripheral neuropathy. The recommended dose is 10 mg per day intramuscularly for six weeks, followed by 5 mg per day orally. The 10 mg per day dosage can be also taken orally, according to Dr. Golan.[51]

Because research showed biotin's ability to produce significant improvement in glucose readings, Robert C. Atkins, M.D., incorporated mega-biotin therapy into his routine. Concerning other nutrients, he said that one of the most promising is pyridoxine alpha-ketoglutarate (PAK): studies in Italy showed that this compound significantly reduced the sugar elevations in both type 1 and type 2 diabetics. Similarly, Japanese researchers demonstrated improvement in diabetic parameters using coenzyme Q_{10}.[52]

Taking Biotin

Food sources of biotin include cheese, wheat germ, brewer's yeast, nuts and peanut butter, eggs, chocolate, sardines, salmon, cauliflower, mush-rooms, and chicken. However, avidin, a protein found in raw egg white, binds biotin and prevents its absorption; cooking inactivates the protein.

Is biotin safe? No toxic effects of oral biotin have been reported in humans or animals.[53]

Pantothenic Acid

Present in all cells, pantothenic acid plays a significant role in energy pro-duction from fat, carbohydrates, and protein. It forms the core of coen-zyme A (coA), the enzyme helper that carries fatty acids throughout the metabolism, which includes fat synthesis and fat degradation. Coenzyme A helps to synthesize compounds such as citric acid and most fats, including cholesterol, steroid hormones, and ketone bodies. Ketones are substances formed by the liver when the digestion of fats is com-promised, which occurs in diabetes. CoA is also required for the synthe-sis of acetylcholine, a chemical needed for nerve transmission, and it is involved in the synthesis of heme for the formation of hemoglobin. Some research has indicated that pantethine helps in preventing the clumping of proteins in the eye that causes cataracts.[54]

Pantethine, a molecule of pantothenic acid, may help to lower choles-terol and triglyceride levels. It may be easier to convert pantethine (rather than pantothenic acid) to coA, thus pantethine may be more effec-tive therapeutically in certain instances.[55]

For hypoglycemia, Ralph Golan, M.D., recommends pantothenic acid —or calcium pantothenate—to boost the adrenal glands. Extra amounts may be needed for those who have not responded to B-complex supple-ments for chronic fatigue and characteristic low blood sugar symptoms within one month. He recommends taking 500 mg, one to three times daily, with meals for up to three months, then gradually reducing the dosage.[56]

Francisco Coronel, M.D., of San Carlos University Hospital, in Madrid, Spain, found that of 92 kidney transplant patients studied, 29.3 percent suffered from excess fats in the blood. Pantethine was administered in doses of 900 mg per day and after two months of treatment, there was a significant decrease in total cholesterol, triglycerides, very-low-density lipoprotein cholesterol, LDL cholesterol, and the total-to-HDL cholesterol ratio. These readings continued to be reduced at four and six months.[57]

Three of the transplant recipients stopped the pantothenic acid due to gastric irritation.

Because diabetes increases the risk for cardiovascular disease, pantothenic acid or pantethine may prove beneficial. The escalation of the two most dangerous blood fats—LDL cholesterol and triglycerides—stops dead in its tracks when confronted by pantethine, according to Robert C. Atkins, M.D. In one study, a daily dose of 900 mg of pantethine led to a 32 percent drop in triglycerides, a 19 percent drop in total cholesterol, and a 21 percent drop in LDL cholesterol. At the same time, HDL

A SUPPLEMENT PROGRAM FOR HYPOGLYCEMIA

To treat hypoglycemia, Ralph Golan, M.D., recommends the following supplements:

- Chromium (200 to 300 mcg, three times daily)
- Biotin
- B-complex (25–50 mg of each, three times daily)
- Pantothenic acid (500 mg, one to three times daily)
- Niacin (500 to 1,000 mg, twice daily)
- Vitamin C (up to 1,000 mg, three times daily)
- Brewer's yeast (1/2 tsp, daily)
- Calcium and magnesium (1,000 mg per day)
- Magnesium (500 mg per day)
- An amino acid cocktail containing glutamine, 5-hydroxytryptophan, and tyrosine

"For hypoglycemia, approximately 1,000 mcg, three times daily, of biotin with meals will enhance glucose utilization, generally improve low blood sugar symptoms, as well as tend to reduce sugar cravings," states Dr. Golan. "Biotin is largely synthesized by friendly intestinal bacteria and if you have used antibiotics (which kill these bacteria), this vitamin is particularly important to use. Once your condition has stabilized, 300 mcg per day should suffice."

Because several of the B-complex vitamins are crucial to the utilization of carbohydrates and the release of energy, a deficiency of these vitamins can contribute to hypoglycemia. For example, biotin is a critical co-factor for glucokinase, an enzyme that is involved in the initial step of glucose utilization by the cells.[58]

cholesterol rose by 23 percent.[59] Dr. Atkins found more than half a dozen similar accounts in the medical literature and all of them documented dramatic improvements in supplement takers' blood fats, even when the lipid abnormality was due to other illnesses.

Pantethine protects the heart and arteries in other ways, according to Dr. Atkins. It encourages the production of enzymes that help break down fats and helps vitamin E's action against cholesterol buildup. In addition, pantethine is one of the few nutrients that increases the amount of clot-busting omega-3 fatty acids and reduces clot-promoting fats in cell membranes. By generating more coenzyme A, pantethine enhances metabolism in the heart muscle, strengthens the force of its contractions, and slows the rate at which it beats.[60]

Pantethine has significant lipid-lowering characteristics while pantothenic acid has little value in lowering cholesterol and triglyceride levels, according to Michael T. Murray, N.D. A dose of 900 mg per day of pantethine significantly reduced serum triglyceride and cholesterol levels while increasing HDL cholesterol. These effects are especially impressive, since it has virtually no toxicity when compared to conventional lipid-lowering drugs, Dr. Murray stated. Pantethine's mode of action is due to its ability to inhibit cholesterol synthesis and accelerate the utilization of fat as an energy source. There appears to be no toxicity or side effects from pantethine.[61]

Because pantothenic acid is closely related to lipid metabolism, it may be of help to obese patients, according to Li-Hung Leung, M.D., of Central Hospital, in Hong Kong. The B vitamin may be beneficial in its ability to mobilize fatty acids and convert them to fully utilized energy. In the study, involving sixty males and sixty females between the ages of fifteen and fifty-five who were on a 1,000-calorie-a-day diet, 10 g of pantothenic acid was given in four divided doses. The average weight loss was 1.2 kg (2.6 lbs) per week. Ketones in the urine were monitored and found absent in most instances. To maintain body weight after reaching a desired goal, Dr. Leung recommended 2–3 g of pantothenic acid daily, which allows the body to freely mobilize fat for energy.[62]

Taking Pantothenic Acid

Food sources include liver, beans, peas, whole grains, wheat germ, brewer's yeast, dark green leafy vegetables, nuts, peanuts, and eggs.

How safe is pantothenic acid? Toxicity of oral pantothenic acid is extremely low, and no cases have been reported in humans. Intakes as high as 10 g per day in humans have been tolerated without adverse effects.[63]

Choline

A constituent of lecithin, choline is necessary for the prevention of fatty livers, the transmitting of nerve impulses, and the metabolism of fat. Choline is a lipotropic agent, meaning that it has an affinity for fat. In this role, the substance prevents the abnormal accumulation of fat in the liver by promoting its transport as lecithin or by increasing the utilization of fatty acids in the liver.[64] Without choline, fatty deposits build up inside the liver, blocking its hundreds of functions and throwing the whole body into a state of ill health.

Although associated with the B-complex, choline is not officially a B vitamin. Of the various related compounds that can replace choline, the primary one is betaine, which derives its name from the Latin word *beta* meaning "beet" which is a rich source. Thus, choline can be replaced by betaine in preventing fatty liver in some species. The amino acid methionine and vitamin B_{12} can also spare choline in certain species.

Patients who have induced choline deficiency have developed liver dysfunction, such as fatty liver, which is also seen in choline-deficient animals, according to Steven H. Zeisel, M.D., Ph.D., of the University of North Carolina, at Chapel Hill. The fatty liver occurs in choline deficiency because phosphatidylcholine (PC) synthesis is needed for the production of very-low-density lipoprotein cholesterol secretion. This could ultimately lead to liver cancer.[65]

"Fatty liver" is common in diabetes, according to Adelle Davis, probably because choline and inositol are so readily lost in urine. Biopsies of the livers of diabetic patients taken before and six weeks after they had adhered to a diet particularly high in protein and the B vitamins, and supplemented with choline, inositol, and vitamin B_{12}, showed that even the more serious cases were corrected in this time period. Vitamin C, vitamin E, and the sulfur-containing amino acids in eggs are also particularly valuable in correcting fatty liver. Fifty-one out of 102 people with fatty livers, recognized as a choline deficiency, had high blood urea and albumin in the urine, showing mild nephrosis (kidney disease). These conditions quickly disappeared when choline was given with an adequate diet, Davis stated. In a study involving forty-eight people, their blood pressure fell to normal and albumin cleared from the urine when choline was taken.[66]

A combination of choline, phosphatidylcholine, and lecithin fights heart disease in a variety of ways, according to Robert C. Atkins, M.D. While PC brings only a modest reduction in total cholesterol, it improves the ratio between good and bad cholesterol. PC serves as the main source of choline, which is essential for the formation of acetylcholine, an important neurotransmitter. And choline is essential for our bodies to make lecithin.[67]

Researchers at Rush Medical College and Presbyterian–St. Luke's Medical Center, in Chicago, reported that those with untreated high levels of homocysteine develop premature vascular disease, thrombosis, and thromboembolism, which bring on strokes and coronary occlusion. Vitamins B_6 and B_{12} are useful in lowering homocysteine levels. In addition, a restriction of choline in the diet along with folic acid deficiency increases the severity of high homocysteine levels. Betaine supplementation effectively corrects most types of high homocysteine, the researchers said.[68]

Even though the mechanism of high homocysteine (hyperhomocysteinemia) is unknown, small amounts of folic acid and sometimes B_6, choline, or betaine, can return levels of homocysteine to normal. These substances are innocuous in the absence of pernicious anemia. It might be prudent that those with hardening of the arteries, or family members, be screened for the presence of homocysteinemia and be treated on an individual basis as is the case for other risk factors.[69]

Taking Choline

Food sources of choline include egg yolk, brewer's yeast, liver, soybeans, potatoes, cabbage, wheat germ, rice bran and polish, buttermilk, dried skimmed milk, hominy, turnips, wheat flour, whole grains, and blackstrap molasses.

Inositol

Widely distributed in foods and closely related to glucose, inositol has been known as a chemical compound since 1850. It was initially referred to as "muscle sugar" because it is largely stored in the brain, heart muscle, and skeletal muscle. In animal cells, it occurs as a component of phospholipids, substances containing phosphorus, fatty acids, and nitrogenous bases. Clinical interest in inositol is focused on impairment of growth and development, nerve function, diabetes mellitus, renal disease, and respiratory distress syndrome. Small amounts are normally excreted in the urine; however, diabetics excrete rather large amounts. While associated with the B-complex, inositol has not been officially named a B vitamin.[70]

Inositol escapes freely from the nerve cells of diabetics, according to Robert C. Atkins, M.D. This loss may be partly responsible for diabetic neuropathy, the painful destruction of nerves in the arms and legs following years of poor blood sugar control. Dr. Atkins used inositol in his diabetes treatment protocol, ever since reading an impressive study in 1978 in which 1 g per day eased pain and improved nerve function in a group of patients with neuropathy. Vitamin C may help head off the loss of inositol.[71]

Inositol deficiency can be an important factor in some of the underlying complications of chronic diabetes. If either inositol or choline is undersupplied, lecithin cannot be produced in adequate amounts, reports Adelle Davis. When patients recovering from heart attacks receive 2,000 mg of choline and 750 mg of inositol daily, the size of cholesterol particles and the amount of fat in the blood quickly decreases. Two months later, the blood cholesterols dropped to normal.[72] The antioxidant function of inositol hexaphosphate (IP-6) makes it ideal for controlling the damage done to the heart muscle (myocardium) during heart attacks.[73]

Researchers at the University of Birmingham, in England, reported that diabetes is associated with a reduction in serum magnesium levels. The magnesium ion is a positive effector of inositol transport and is capable of promoting a 2.5-fold increase in the affinity for the transporter for inositol. In fact, magnesium reduction in diabetes may cause reductions in inositol transport in diabetic patients by as much as twofold.[74]

Taking Inositol

Food sources of inositol include kidney, brain, brewer's yeast, liver, wheat germ, citrus fruits, and blackstrap molasses. Bruce J. Holub, Ph.D., found that adults consume about 1 g per day of inositol in animal products and plant sources, especially inositol hexaphosphate or phytic acid. Inositol is found in high amounts in breast milk.[75]

CHAPTER 7

Vitamin C

Type 2 diabetes is often caused or aggravated by a deficiency of certain vitamins and other essential nutrients in millions of cells in the pancreas, liver, and the blood vessel walls, as well as other organs in those with a genetic predisposition to diabetic disorders, according to Matthias Rath, M.D. Optimum intake of vitamins and other nutrients can help prevent the onset of adult diabetes and correct, at least in part, existing diabetes and its complications.[1] Clinical studies indicate that in diabetic patients, vitamin C (ascorbic acid) not only contributes to prevention of cardiovascular complications, it also helps to normalize the imbalance in glucose metabolism, according to Dr. Rath.

Clinical Studies on Vitamin C

A study by Professor R. Pfleger and colleagues at the University of Vienna showed that diabetic patients taking 300–500 milligrams (mg) per day of vitamin C significantly improved glucose balance. Blood sugar levels could be lowered on average by 30 percent and daily insulin requirements by 27 percent; sugar excretion in the urine could almost be eliminated. "It is amazing that this study was published in 1937 in a leading European journal for internal medicine," states Dr. Rath. "If the results of this important study had been followed up and documented in medical textbooks, millions of lives would have been saved and cardiovascular disease would no longer threaten diabetic patients."

The consumption of vitamin C above the Recommended Dietary Allowance (RDA) of 60 mg per day may provide important health benefits for those with type 1 diabetes, researchers reported in the *Journal of the American College of Nutrition*. It has been known that vitamin C levels are lower in diabetics than in those without the disease. The vitamin normalizes red blood cell sorbitol concentrations in those with type 1 diabetes. Sorbitol is a sugar alcohol that is produced in the body during the conversion to glucose.[2]

In a study at the University of Massachusetts at Amherst, fifty-eight adults, nineteen to thirty-four years of age, were given either 100 mg or 600 mg of vitamin C per day. Nine of the volunteers were type 1 diabetics and eleven of the participants were non-diabetics. It was found that red blood cell sorbitol levels were significantly higher in the type 1 patients. Either dose of the vitamin normalized the sorbitol levels in the type 1 diabetics within thirty days.[3] Because of vitamin C's low toxicity, the researchers suggest that it is superior to pharmaceutical aldose reductase inhibitors, which block an enzyme that results in the accumulation of sugar byproducts. The researchers added that there appears to be no advantage in the larger doses of the vitamin, since 100 mg daily effectively normalizes red blood cell sorbitol levels.

A research team at the University of Washington, in Seattle, reported that supplementing the diet of diabetics with vitamin C might protect them against the oxidative damage of LDL ("bad") cholesterol, thus reducing their risk of developing hardening of the arteries. In the study, susceptibility to low-density lipoprotein oxidation relative to vitamin C and vitamin E was measured in twenty-five type 2 diabetics and twenty-two healthy controls. The results found that vitamin C levels were low in the diabetics, while vitamin E levels were higher when compared to controls. Vitamin C can assist against vitamin E depletion, but when vitamin C levels are low, diabetics must depend on available stores of vitamin E.[4]

Supplementation with antioxidant vitamins significantly reduced the susceptibility of LDL cholesterol to oxidation, reported James W. Anderson, M.D., of the Veterans Affairs Medical Center, in Lexington, Kentucky. In the study of forty men, twenty non-diabetics and twenty type 2 diabetics were given a placebo for eight weeks, followed by twelve weeks of antioxidant supplements, including 24 mg per day of beta-carotene, 1,000 mg of vitamin C mg per day, and 800 international units (IU) of vitamin E per day, followed by eight weeks of placebo. Dr. Anderson and colleagues reported that LDL cholesterol in diabetics was more susceptible to oxidation and its resultant harm than LDL in non-diabetics.[5]

At Mahidol University, in Bangkok, Thailand, researchers found that elderly diabetics either do not consume or absorb sufficient amounts of vitamin C or the chronic manifestations of their disease alter the vitamin's status. The research team evaluated twenty-six elderly diabetics and twenty-three healthy controls. They found that healthy controls had significantly higher levels of vitamin C in their blood than did the diabetics. There was no difference between the groups in the amount of vitamin B_1, vitamin A, and vitamin E in their circulating blood.[6]

At the University of Sydney, in Australia, researchers evaluated twenty diabetics who were randomized to receive either 500 mg of vitamin C or a placebo, twice daily, for twelve months. The research team reported that the vitamin C therapy increased blood levels of vitamin C and reduced albumin excretion rate after nine months. Albumin is a protein and above normal levels may be a sign of kidney disease, especially for diabetics who have had the disease for a long time. Vitamin C supplements given to diabetics may have long-term benefits in slowing the progression of diabetic complications.[7]

An increased intake of vitamin C lessens the risk of developing heart disease, according to researchers at the Harvard School of Medicine, in Boston. The study evaluated 87,245 female nurses, between the ages of thirty-four and fifty-nine, who were symptom-free when the study began in 1980. The women reported on their vitamin C intake via questionnaires. During eight years, there were 437 heart attacks and 115 coronary deaths. In tabulating the results of the study, the researchers reported that those with the highest intake of vitamin C were better protected from heart disease than those with low intakes of the vitamin.[8] This could be vital to diabetics, who are at greater risk of developing cardiovascular disease.

Supplementing with vitamin C might be a useful therapy in the treatment of high blood pressure, according to researchers at the Human Nutrition Research Center, in Beltsville, Maryland. During the study, twenty volunteers, twelve of whom were borderline hypertensives, supplemented their regular diet with 1,000 mg per day of vitamin C or a placebo for two 6-week periods. The test group was not deficient in the vitamin. The vitamin was associated with a significant reduction in systolic (beating) blood pressure and pulse pressure, but it had no effect on diastolic (resting) blood pressure, total blood cholesterol, HDL cholesterol, or total triglyceride levels.[9]

Results of studies have indicated that diabetes is associated with oxidative stress and reduced levels of antioxidants, according to Maryam Sadat Farvid, Ph.D., and colleagues at Shaheed Beheshri University of Medical Sciences, in Tehran, Iran. In addition, levels of vitamin C in the blood were found to be significantly lower in diabetics when compared to controls in most other studies. Based on the researchers' results, it was suspected that diabetics have significant defects in antioxidant protection, which may enhance their susceptibility to oxidative stress. Vitamins C and E and and other antioxidants such as magnesium and zinc may improve kidney function in type 2 diabetics.[10]

Researchers studied the value of vitamins C and E in fruits and supplements and the risk of diabetic retinopathy. They found no support for using the vitamin in foods combined with supplements, but admitted that the observed association between risk and retinopathy and supplement use may reflect non-dietary factors or a possible benefit of supplementation.[11] It should be noted that megadoses of the vitamins might be needed to reach proven results.

Low blood levels of vitamin C have been reported in diabetics, according to Kenzo Iino, M.D., and colleagues at Fukuoka University, in Japan. They added that nephropathy can develop in diabetics and decreased kidney function and high blood pressure could reportedly accelerate hardening of the arteries in patients with type 2 diabetes. In their study, low blood levels of vitamin C in type 2 diabetics were closely associated with kidney dysfunction and low-grade inflammation.[12]

Taking Vitamin C

Food sources of vitamin C include citrus fruits, cantaloupe, guavas, gooseberries, peppers, papaya, black currants, strawberries, green leafy vegetables, and tomatoes and tomato juice.

How safe is vitamin C? Very large daily doses of vitamin C have been taken over many years, and only minor undesirable effects have been attribute to this water-soluble vitamin. Placebo-controlled clinical trials that utilized doses up to 10,000 mg per day for over a year reported no adverse effects.[13]

CHAPTER 8

Vitamin D

The importance of vitamin D lies in its role of regulating the minerals calcium and phosphorus. In the absence of vitamin D, mineralization of bone matrix is impaired, which results in rickets in children and osteomalacia in adults. Rickets, a bone disorder, has been known since 500 B.C. and it was first described in detail more than 300 years ago. The word *rickets* comes from the Old English word *wrikken*, which means "bent" or "twisted."[1] Because vitamin D is fat-soluble, small amounts are stored in body fats for later use. There are about ten sterol compounds with vitamin D activity, but only two vitamin D precursors are commonly found in foods—ergocalciferol (vitamin D_2 or calciferol) and cholecalciferol (vitamin D_3).

Vitamin D has a dual role as vitamin and hormone. Like other hormones, the vitamin's active metabolites are produced in the liver and kidneys, but have their effects on other tissues, such as the intestinal mucosa and bone tissue.[2] Vitamin D deficiency is related to increased parathyroid hormone secretion, increased bone loss, osteoporosis, and mild osteomalacia. The parathyroid glands release parathyroid hormone, which increases blood levels of calcium and magnesium, two minerals essential for bone health.

The "Sunshine Vitamin"

Vitamin D is unique among the vitamins in that it can be formed in the body by exposure of the skin to ultraviolet (UV) rays from the sun. Hence, it is known as the "sunshine vitamin."[3] Vitamin D can be obtained from sunlight through the conversion of 7-dehydrocholesterol to provitamin D, which is then converted to vitamin D. Also, vitamin D from food sources or from the skin is converted to 25-hydroxyvitamin D in the liver and 1,25-dihydroxyvitamin D (the active hormone) in the kidneys.[4] Blood levels of 25-hydroxyvitamin D decrease with age but increase slightly with sunlight exposure and vitamin D intake in foods and supplements. In the Framingham Heart Study, 14 percent of women and 6 percent of men had low serum 25-hydroxyvitamin D stores. In 290 people with a mean age of 62, poor vitamin D intake (66 percent of those with low 25-hydroxyvitamin D amounts had estimated vitamin D intakes that were less than adequate for their age group) and remaining indoors contributed to low 25-hydroxyvitamin D amounts in their blood.

Vitamin D's activation in the skin is restricted by skin pigments and keratin, which screens UV light. Smog, fog, smoke, clothing, screens, and most glass screen the UV light and, therefore, interfere with vitamin D formation.[5] An often-asked question is whether or not sunscreens inhibit the formation of vitamin D from the sun. In evaluating vitamin D levels and the use of sunscreen in more than 113 individuals, 40 years of age or over, researchers at the University of Melbourne, in Australia, reported that over an Australian summer sufficient sunlight is probably received through both the sunscreen and the lack of total skin coverage. This assures adequate vitamin D production in those who are advised to use sunscreen regularly.[6]

After reviewing 117 studies on vitamin D from 1971 to 1990, a research team at St. Michael's Hospital, in Dublin, Ireland, reported that vitamin D fortification or supplementation is necessary to maintain optimal amounts of this vitamin in the elderly. The researchers said that while exposure to summer sun is critical in providing vitamin D, oral intake combined with either fortified foods or supplements is essential for maintaining proper tissue stores of the vitamin. Vitamin D intakes are, of course, lower during winter months, when the elderly wear clothes that prevent the formation of vitamin D through their skin.[7]

Clinical Studies on Vitamin D

A vitamin D deficiency may contribute to type 1 diabetes in childhood.[8] Researchers in Sweden reported that vitamin D supplementation was associated with a reduced risk of type 1 diabetes. They added that most European studies indicate a positive effect for vitamin D supplementation for infants, so they theorized that vitamin D may contribute to immune modulation and protect or arrest an ongoing immune process begun in susceptible children by early environmental exposures.[9] In another study, children receiving vitamin D supplements from the age of one year onward had an 80 percent decreased risk of developing type 1 diabetes.[10]

Low levels of vitamin D may be a significant risk factor for glucose intolerance, according to researchers at the Royal London School of Medicine and Dentistry, in London. The study evaluated 142 elderly Dutchmen, ranging in age from 70 to 88. It was found that the one-hour glucose tolerance test was inversely associated with blood concentrations of 25-hydroxyvitamin D. With the exclusion of newly diagnosed diabetics, total insulin concentration during the glucose test was inversely associated with the concentration of vitamin D.[11]

Vitamin D is needed by the islet cells in the pancreas to secrete insulin normally. This may be because it helps to ensure an adequate supply of calcium upon which many enzymes related to insulin secretion and release are dependent. Vitamin D is directly related to the capacity to secrete insulin and inversely to glucose tolerance. The researchers also found that vitamin D status relates inversely to insulin sensitivity. In animal studies, there is considerable evidence that vitamin D supplements can improve insulin secretion in the pancreas's islets. Further, vitamin D supplements given to humans over a considerable time can improve insulin secretion and glucose tolerance in those who have osteomalacia (softening of the bones), since these patients are severely deficient in vitamin D.[12]

Using data from the Keys Epidemiological Seven Countries Studies, David S. Grimes, M.D., and associates at the Royal Infirmary, in Blackburn, England, recorded blood cholesterol levels and compared them to the recorded hours of sunshine at 136 locations in the United Kingdom. A sunlight deficiency can increase blood cholesterol by allowing squalene (a precursor of sterols, such as cholesterol) metabolism to synthesize cholesterol instead of vitamin D, which would happen with greater sun exposure. Increased amounts of cholesterol in the blood during the winter were confirmed by this study to be due to reduced sunlight exposure. Sunlight may influence our susceptibility to various diseases, such as coronary artery disease. For example, there is a clear relationship between cholesterol and the latitude where one resides: cholesterol levels rise with increasing distance from the equator. Dr. Grimes suggests that vitamin D slows the progression of heart disease.[13]

In studying 173 volunteers at high and moderate risk for coronary artery disease, vitamin D levels (specifically, 1,25-dihydroxyvitamin D) were inversely related to the extent of vascular calcification. Vitamin D is also important in bone mineralization, which may explain the association between osteoporosis and vascular calcification (calcium deposits in blood vessels). Vascular calcification is found in more than 90 percent of patients with coronary heart disease.[14]

Arthur A. Knapp, M.D., a New York ophthalmologist, has treated some eye conditions of elderly people with massive doses of vitamin D. He believes that myopia, or shortsightedness, is not just an eye condition, but rather a manifestation of vitamin D deficiency. He gave a group of patients vitamin D and calcium supplements for 5–28 months and found a decrease in the nearsightedness in over one-third of them, with a definite halt in the process in another 17 percent.[15] Dr. Knapp said that a lack of vitamin D and calcium may be related to the formation of cataracts. A drug used to decrease blood calcium in several diseases occasionally produces cataracts. Diabetics are known to suffer from a calcium imbalance and they develop cataracts more often than non-diabetics.

A number of studies suggest that circulating concentrations of vitamin D may be inversely related to the prevalence of diabetes, to the concentration of glucose, and to insulin resistance, reported researchers from the U.S. Centers for Disease Control and Prevention, in Atlanta, Georgia. In addition, a vitamin D deficiency may be related to the metabolic syndrome, a compilation of health conditions related to diabetes. "Because of the close interrelationships between vitamin D, parathyroid hormone, calcium, and phosphate, untangling the contributions of each of these factors on insulin resistance and glucose homeostasis (balance) is important in developing possible future approaches in the prevention of insulin resistance, the metabolic syndrome, and diabetes," stated Earl S. Ford, M.D., MPH, the lead researcher.[16]

Accumulating research suggests that low 25-hydroxyvitamin D_3 concentrations may be inversely associated with type 2 diabetes, metabolic syndrome, insulin resistance, and cardiovascular disease, reported Massimo Cigolini, M.D., and colleagues at the Hospital of Arzignano, in Venice, Italy. Since C-reactive protein and fibrinogen levels increase the risk for cardiovascular disease (CVD), these findings could help explain the CVD excess typically observed during winter months, a period in which vitamin D status tends to be poor, and suggest a rationale for vitamin D supplementation in the prevention of CVD, especially in the elderly. "Low vitamin D_3 concentrations result in elevations of parathyroid hormone, which has been linked to insulin resistance," Dr. Cigolini stated.[17]

David J. Di Cesar, M.D., and colleagues at the State University of New York, in Syracuse, reported that vitamin D deficiency is more common in type 2 diabetes than in type 1 diabetes, unrelated to age, sex, or insulin treatment. "Despite most type 2 diabetics being prescribed a daily multivitamin, usually containing 400 IU of vitamin D, the percent who were deficient remained unchanged," Dr. Di Cesar said. "Further studies are needed to better understand the causes and clinical significance of the observed hypovitaminosis D and to investigate response to vitamin D replacement therapy."[18]

Taking Vitamin D

The main food sources of vitamin D are fatty fish, egg yolks, liver, cream, butter, cheese, fortified milk, fortified cereals, fortified bread, and fortified margarine.

According to Robert D. Utiger, M.D., adults probably need 800–1,000 international units (IU) per day of the vitamin. This can be given as a single capsule of 5,000 IU or at a dose of 100,000 IU every four to six months. He said that the amount of the vitamin in supplemental multivitamins and calcium supplements should be increased substantially and that all adults should be advised to take supplements of the vitamin.[19]

How safe is vitamin D? For adults, vitamin D intakes of less than 2,000 IU (50 mcg) cause no known risk and there is sufficient evidence to establish the safety of intakes up to 800 IU (20 mcg). In most adults, daily intake in excess of 50,000 IU (1.25 mg) is needed to produce toxicity, but much less may cause adverse effects in persons with certain diseases or idiopathic hypercalcemia (too much calcium in the blood). In children, dietary vitamin D intakes as low as 2,000–4,000 IU (50 to 100 mcg) per day have led to adverse effects. The majority of dietary supplements that include vitamin D contain 400 IU (10 mcg), an amount known to be safe and recommended by many scientific authorities.[20]

CHAPTER 9

Vitamin E

itamin E is a potent antioxidant that protects diabetics and others from serious health problems. Antioxidants are natural substances that inhibit the formation of free radicals, which can lead to serious illnesses. An antioxidant prevents substances from combining with oxygen (oxidation) to form free radicals. Although oxygen is an essential element, it can combine with various substances to become harmful to the body.

Clinical Studies on Vitamin E

Diabetics are especially susceptible to blood clots, according to Robert C. Atkins, M.D. In addition to ridding the blood of harmful fats and improving circulation, vitamin E also thins the blood naturally. "Thinning the blood is actually a misnomer," Dr. Atkins stated. "Actually, blood tends to form clots through the process of platelet clumping. A clot that lodges in an artery can impede blood flow, causing a heart attack or, if the brain is affected, a stroke. When volunteers in a 1996 study took 400 IU of vitamin E daily, along with aspirin, they suffered fewer transient ischemic attacks (TIAs). These mini-strokes interrupt blood flow to the brain only briefly but often portend a more serious stroke."[1] Blood platelets in diabetics contain less vitamin E than platelets of non-diabetics, according to Dr. Atkins.

When vitamin E levels are low, the risk of acquiring type 2 diabetes rises by a ratio of nearly four to one. In one study, type 1 diabetics, when given 100 international units (IU) per day of vitamin E for three months, significantly reduced the tissue damage from high blood sugar, a process called glycation, as well as the accumulation of triglycerides, a diabetes-related heart disease risk factor.[2]

It has been suggested that accelerated glycosylation and free radical–generated oxidative reactions may be the reason hyperglycemia (high blood sugar) causes diabetic complications. Vitamin E supplementation may, therefore, benefit diabetics due to its antioxidant activity and its inhibiting of protein glycosylation by normalizing blood platelet activity.[3] For example, protein glycosylation has been slowed with the addition of 600–1,200 IU per day of vitamin E in diabetic patients. Vitamin E is involved in the production of prostacylin, a potent vasodilator and inhibitor of platelet aggregation. In one study, 900 IU per day of vitamin E for four months reduced oxidative stress and improved insulin action in fifteen patients with type 2 diabetes compared with ten controls. In a related study, twenty-five elderly diabetics given 900 IU per day of vitamin E for three months showed significant declines in plasma levels of hemoglobin A_{1C} (glycosylated hemoglobin), triglycerides, total cholesterol, low-density lipoprotein (LDL) cholesterol, and apolipoprotein-b (a risk factor for ischemic heart disease).[4]

Glycosylated hemoglobin forms when sugar becomes attached to hemoglobin molecules, the iron-containing pigment in red blood cells. The more glucose (sugar) in the blood, the more hemoglobin becomes glycosylated. The hemoglobin molecules remain glycosylated until the blood cells die, which is normally about three months. Blood glucose levels are monitored with the glycosylated hemoglobin test, which measures the amounts of hemoglobin A_{1C}.[5] Usually only a small amount of hemoglobin is glycosylated, but in poorly controlled diabetes, the level of hemoglobin A_{1C} is much higher, perhaps 9 percent to 12 percent more. A high reading suggests that blood glucose has been elevated over the previous month or six weeks. If the reading is in the normal range, it usually means that blood glucose has been normal during that same period. Constant self-monitoring, along with periodic measurements of hemoglobin A_{1C}, is important in achieving overall control of diabetes.[6]

Daniel Baker, Pharm.D., reported that glycosylated proteins and hemoglobin A_{1C} decreased significantly in a group of diabetics given vitamin E. Those receiving 1,200 mg daily of the vitamin had the greatest reductions. These findings suggest that the vitamin may be useful in preventing diabetic complications, including cataracts.[7] At the LSU Medical Center, in Shreveport, Louisiana, Sushil K. Jain, Ph.D., supplemented thirty-five diabetic patients with either 100 IU per day of vitamin E or a placebo for three months. Results of this double-blind study showed that vitamin E lowered glycosylated hemoglobin, glucose, and triglycerides, but it did not have any effect on red blood cell indices in type 1 diabetics.[8]

Vitamin E supplements are useful therapy for reducing oxidative stress and improving insulin activity in type 2 diabetics, according to researchers at the University of Naples and the University of Udine in Italy. The study involved giving ten healthy controls and 15 type 2 diabetics 900 mg daily of vitamin E for four months.[9]

Paolo Pozzilli, M.D., and his research team at St. Bartholomew's Hospital Medical College, in London, have found that vitamin E and nicotinamide (vitamin B_3) are both likely to be effective in preserving beta-cell function in recent type 1 diabetics up to one year after diagnosis. Beta cells in the pancreas make and release insulin. Both vitamins have few adverse side effects, and because they may act at different levels in the process leading to beta-cell destruction, a combination of the two nutrients may be considered for future trials.[10] As soon as a type 1 diabetic is diagnosed, the researchers recommend that nicotinamide therapy be given. Vitamin E may also be beneficial, but before both vitamins are given, a trial using the two together must be performed. The suggested vitamin E dose is 15 mg/kg body weight, while the B_3 dose is 25 mg/kg body weight.

Diabetics suffer oxidative stress related to glucose levels. Since vitamin E is an antioxidant and free-radical scavenger, it can reduce oxidative stress and curb the blood-clotting effect of thromboxane B_2, a substance formed from endoperoxides that cause the constriction of vascular and bronchial smooth muscle and promote blood coagulation. In the study, researchers evaluated 85 diabetics and 85 healthy controls, measuring their levels of isoprostane, thromboxane B_2, and glucose. Isoprostane is a byproduct of free-radical reactions and increased levels suggest oxidative stress. Ten of the diabetics were given 600 IU per day of vitamin E for two weeks. It was found that diabetics had higher levels of both isoprostane and thromboxane B_2 when compared to healthy controls. Results showed that the volunteers who were taking vitamin E had declines of 37 percent in isoprostane levels and 43 percent in thrombox-ane B$_2$ levels.[11]

In a study of twenty-nine diabetics (mean age of 12.4 years) and twen-ty-one non-diabetics (mean age of 10.9 years), the red blood cells of dia-betic patients had 21 percent higher malondialdehyde (which suggests fatty acid oxidation) and 15 percent lower glutathione (an antioxidant) concentrations than in the healthy volunteers. The volunteers were given 100 IU per day of vitamin E or a placebo for three months. Vitamin E supplements increased glutathione concentrations (by 9 percent), and lowered malondialdehyde (by 23 percent) and hemoglobin A$_{1C}$ (by 16 percent) in the red blood cells of the diabetics.[12]

Vitamin E and Cardiovascular Disease in Diabetics

Diabetics develop cardiovascular disease at an earlier age than do non-diabetics. In one study, researchers measured free radical and inflamma-tory activity in seventy-five volunteers: twenty-five type 2 diabetics with cardiovascular disease, twenty-five type 2 diabetics without this compli-cation, and twenty-five healthy controls. The markers for inflammation included elevated levels of interleukin-lb and white blood cell stickiness, which contributes to inflammation. Following three months of supple-mentation with 1,200 IU per day of vitamin E, the diabetics were meas-ured for free radical and inflammatory activity. All diabetics had higher levels of free radicals and indicators of inflammation when compared to the controls. However, the vitamin not only reduced levels of free-radi-cal oxidation of cholesterol among all volunteers, but also reduced indi-cators of inflammation in all three groups. The researchers added that excess inflammation is regarded as a leading risk factor for cardiovascu-lar disease and that vitamin E is a safe and inexpensive means of con-trolling inflammation in many people, especially diabetics.[13]

Antioxidants, such as vitamin E, can reduce the risk of developing ischemic stroke. In one study, male smokers, ranging in age from fifty to sixty-nine, took either 50 IU of vitamin E, 20 mg of beta-carotene (pro-vitamin A), both vitamins, or a placebo daily for three years. Vitamin E decreased the likelihood of ischemic stroke among those with high blood pressure and diabetes, without elevating the risk of subarachnoid hemor-rhage. Beta-carotene supplements seemed to increase the risk of ischemic stroke among men with greater alcohol intake.[14]

It has been known for some time that the body's production of prostaglandin E2 (PGE2) increases with age and apparently contributes to the age-associated increase in coronary artery disease. PGE2 is produced by COX-2, an enzyme that plays an important role in promoting inflammation. Peroxynitrite, a type of free radical, increases the production of PGE2, but in a study using laboratory mice, vitamin E quenched peroxynitrite and reduced COX-2 activity. Therefore, the research team said, vitamin E appears to reduce the risk of heart disease by preventing the oxidation of cholesterol, by reducing the risk of blood clots, and by reducing the production of inflammatory PGE2.[15]

Many diabetics experience cardiac autonomic neuropathy, which is thought to result in an unbalanced communication inside the body's nervous system, perhaps related to low levels of antioxidants in the body. Researchers asked fifty type 2 diabetics to take 600 mg per day of vitamin E (equivalent to 600 IU) or a placebo for four weeks. Those taking vitamin E noted improvements in heart rates as well as decreased blood levels of insulin and glycosylated hemoglobin. The lower levels of insulin suggested a more efficient use of glucose, while the lower glycosylated hemoglobin indicated better control of diabetes.[16]

Inflammation of blood vessels is considered a major risk factor in heart disease and C-reactive protein is emerging as a measure of such inflammation. However, vitamin E supplements can reduce some of the signs of inflammation. Researchers took measurements of C-reactive protein and interleukin-6 (another indicator of inflammation) in seventy-two patients. The study involved three groups: diabetics with cardiovascular disease, diabetics without cardiovascular disease, and healthy volunteers. Initial measurements revealed that the diabetics with cardiovascular disease had elevated C-reactive protein levels. The volunteers were then given 1,200 IU per day of natural vitamin E (d-alpha tocopherol) for three months. Following vitamin E therapy, people in all three groups benefited from a 30 percent reduction in C-reactive protein levels and a reduction in interleukin-6 levels. These changes might reduce the risk of cardiovascular disease.[17]

Free-radical damage (oxidation) to LDL cholesterol and very-low-density (VLDL) cholesterol is thought to be a key factor in the development of coronary artery disease. Researchers divided forty-four type 1 diabetics into two groups: one group was given 750 IU per day of natu-

ral vitamin E for one year, and the other group received a placebo for six
months followed by 750 IU per day of vitamin E for another six months.
All the diabetics' blood showed that, after vitamin E supplementation,
LDL and VLDL cholesterol were far more resistant to oxidation and there
were fewer indicators of free-radical damage. There was no improvement when volunteers received a look-alike pill. Natural vitamin E
appears ro reduce free-radical damage to LDL and VLDL cholesterol
among diabetics, a change that in turn might reduce the risk of heart disease. Because the improvement in lipoprotein oxidizability is reversible,
lifelong supplementation with vitamin E should be considered in patients
with type 1 diabetes, the researchers said.[18]

Three prominent vitamin E researchers analyzed data from five clinical trials of vitamin E and heart disease. Four of the studies showed that
vitamin E supplements, in dosages ranging from 50 IU to 800 IU per day,
had significant benefits in reducing the risk of heart attacks in those with
pre-existing heart disease. For example, one study found that the risk of
non-fatal heart attack was lowered by 38 percent; in another study, the
reduction was 77 percent.[19]

Vitamin E and Other Diabetic Complications

Age-related macular degeneration is probably due to increased levels of
oxidative stress, according to Jeffrey Blumberg, Ph.D., of Tufts University, USDA Human Nutrition Research Center on Aging, in Boston. An
increase in vitamin E supplementation, carotenoids, vitamin C, and selenium can significantly lower the risk of this eye problem.[20]

In an eight-month, double-blind study involving thirty-six type 1 diabetics and nine non-diabetics, ranging in age from eighteen to forty-five,
the test group was given 1,800 IU per day of vitamin E or a placebo for
four months and then the volunteers' protocols were reversed for an
additional four months. The researchers found that the vitamin normalized retinal function and improved kidney function in type 1 diabetics
who had had the disease for a short time. The research team added that
vitamin E may be beneficial in reducing the risk of diabetic retinopathy
(eye disease) and nephropathy (kidney disease).[21]

At a small hospital in Pennsylvania, a nurse reported on the case of a
59-year-old woman with diabetes who was admitted with ulceration of
her right foot. She had not received any medication prior to admittance.

The doctors immediately gave her insulin and 800 IU per day of natural vitamin E. Then, they packed the ulcerated area with cotton saturated with vitamin E. Two months later, all wounds had healed.[22]

Vitamin E may have value in treating gangrene, a complication of diabetes that often requires having a foot or leg amputated. A.J. DeLiz, M.D., of New York, treated twenty schizophrenic patients, all of whom were suffering from circulatory problems in their feet and legs. All were diabetic and three of them had gangrene. He began by giving the patients 20 capsules (100 IU) daily of vitamin E and later increased the dosage to 40 capsules. Four months later, all of the patients were without leg pains.[23]

A Hungarian physician reported "spectacular" results using vitamin E to treat ten cases of thrombosis of the arteries, sixteen cases of thrombophlebitis, and twelve cases of Buerger's disease (inflammation of blood vessels). He gave the vitamin in large doses, up to 24,000 IU daily. Not all cases were successful, but a patient who had had a leg ulcer for twenty years was completely healed after six weeks with vitamin E supplements plus vitamin E rubbed on the skin.[24] Another case involved a 53-year-old diabetic who had a perforating ulcer on his foot. It was dark purple, the color of a gangrenous foot. On 375 IU per day of vitamin E, he healed completely in seventy-one days, and within several months, his insulin requirements had decreased to about a third of what it had been and he returned to work.[25]

The prevalence of type 2 diabetes in the Korean population has steadily increased in recent years and currently over 8 percent of the population are affected, reported Sunmin Park and Soo Bong Choi, of Hoseo University and Kon-Kuk University Chungjoo-Si. Vitamin E acts as a free-radical scavenger to reduce oxidative stress and their study was to determine whether or not the vitamin could reduce oxidative stress in non-obese patients with type 2 diabetes. They found that oxidative stress persisted after glycemic control with continuous subcutaneous insulin infusion (CSII) alone in the Korean diabetics. However, daily supplementation with 200 mg of vitamin E plus CSII formed a remarkable defense against free radicals and lipid peroxides. "Vitamin E supplementation may be beneficial in improving the complications of diabetes associated with increased oxidative stress in patients with type 2 diabetes treated with CSII," they stated.[26]

Taking Vitamin E

Food sources of vitamin E include salad and cooking oils, green leafy vegetables, butter, lobster, salmon, shrimp, tuna, nuts, avocados, eggs, oatmeal, liver, heart, kidney, wheat germ, and wheat germ oil.

How safe is vitamin E? The lack of toxicity of this fat-soluble vitamin has been consistently reported for twenty years in the research literature. The only reported contraindication concerns possibly decreased blood coagulation. However, studies with the vitamin have shown no changes in platelet aggregation or adhesion with daily vitamin intakes as high as 1,200 IU (800 mg).

There is a report of prolonged bleeding time during chronic warfarin therapy (an anticoagulant) in a patient taking 1,200 IU per day of the vitamin. However, in another study, neither 800 IU nor 1,200 IU was found to influence prothrombin times in patients on warfarin therapy. It has also been reported that a vitamin E intake of 900 IU per day does not affect coagulation activity in persons not taking anticoagulant drugs.[27]

When taking large amounts of vitamin E, diabetics should consult with their physician, since megadoses can raise blood pressure in susceptible individuals. It's best to begin with lower doses and gradually increase as needed. When taking vitamin E and selenium, take one in the morning and the other in the evening for better results.

In giving dosages for vitamin E, researchers use both international units and milligrams. For the record, 1.49 IU of vitamin E is equivalent to 1 mg of natural-source vitamin E (d-alpha tocopherol).

CHAPTER 10

Minerals of Importance to Diabetics

Chromium

Chromium is a critical component of glucose tolerance factor (GTF), which contains niacin, glycine, glutamic acid, cysteine, and chromium. GTF is a compound that helps insulin to transport glucose from the blood to the cells. Chromium may also facilitate the binding of insulin to the cell membrane. Animal studies have found that a deficiency in chromium brings glucose intolerance.[1]

Walter Mertz, Ph.D., stated that thirty-five years of research has shown that chromium plays a significant role in the progression of glucose intolerance and the increased risk of developing diabetes and cardiovascular disease. In thirteen of fifteen studies evaluating chromium supplementation's effect on glucose tolerance, benefits were shown by maintaining glucose levels that produced less insulin. He added that monitoring the effects of glucose tolerance is the only way to discover if there is a chromium deficiency. A chromium deficiency results in insulin resistance, which can therefore improve with chromium supplementation. Marginal deficiencies of chromium are common in the United States and other countries and this is a major cause of insulin resistance in many populations. Insulin resistance is a significant risk factor for cardiovascular disease and may be a more important factor than low-density lipoprotein (LDL) cholesterol.[2]

Type 2 diabetics tend to be deficient in chromium, either as a cause or result of their condition. Since chromium potentiates insulin's action, diabetics can benefit from chromium supplementation.[3]

Clinical Studies on Chromium

Richard A. Anderson, Ph.D., found in a double-blind study involving twenty-nine type 2 diabetics that 1,000 micrograms (mcg) per day of chromium improved insulin sensitivity without significant changes in body fat. Also, in 48 type 1 diabetics and 114 type 2 diabetics, type 1 diabetics reduced their insulin dosage by 30 percent and their blood sugar variations were considerably smaller after 10 days of supplemental chromium picolinate at 200 mcg per day.[4] The dosage of 200 mcg of chromium picolinate three times daily reduced glycosylated hemoglobin (hemoglobin A_{1C}; a measure of glucose in the blood) from 11.3 percent to 7.9 percent after three months of supplementation in a 28-year-old woman who had had type 1 diabetes for eighteen years. In another study, which involved supplementation with 250 mcg of chromium chloride daily, twenty-five diabetics with hardening of the arteries saw improvements in high-density lipoprotein (HDL) cholesterol and triglycerides following six months of supplementation.

Dr. Anderson states that, in studies that have shown no beneficial effects using chromium, the dosages were usually 200 mcg or less, which is not adequate for those with diabetes, especially if the chromium is in a form with low absorption. In another study, thirty women with gestational diabetes, between twenty and twenty-four weeks of gestation, were divided into three groups. Each was given 4 mcg or 8 mcg of chromium per kilogram of body weight or a placebo for eight weeks. Chromium supplements enhanced glucose tolerance and lowered hyperglycemia (high levels of glucose in the blood); the higher dosage was the most beneficial. Steroid-induced diabetes was held in check in 47 of 50 volunteers who were given 200 mcg of chromium picolinate three times a day. Secondary diabetes, which is relatively rare, occurs when steroids and other medications damage the pancreas.[5]

In a double-blind study involving chromium picolinate, eleven diabetics who were not taking insulin were given 200 mcg per day of chromium or a placebo for forty-two days. While on the mineral, the volunteers' fasting blood glucose, glycosylated hemoglobin, total cholesterol, and low-density lipoprotein (LDL) cholesterol dropped considerably. Eight of the eleven patients reported a positive response to the mineral. Their blood glucose range decreased by 24 percent, glycosylated hemoglobin dropped by 19 percent, total cholesterol went down 13 percent, and LDL cholesterol dropped 11 percent.[6]

In a study in Beijing, China, 188 volunteers with type 2 diabetes, between the ages of thirty-five and fifty-five, were given either a placebo, low-dose chromium (200 mcg per day), or high-dose chromium (1,000 mcg per day) for four months. The researchers reported that hemoglobin A_{1C} values went down significantly in the high-dose group at two months and in both supplemented groups at four months, when compared to controls. Fasting blood glucose was lower in the high-dose group, but not significantly in the low-dose and placebo groups. The researchers also found that fasting insulin amounts fell significantly in the chromium-supplemented volunteers, as did the two-hour oral glucose tolerance insulin values.[7]

In another study, Chinese volunteers with type 2 diabetes were divided into three groups of sixty each and given a placebo, 100 mcg of chromium picolinate, or 500 mcg of chromium picolinate twice daily for four months. Researchers reported that improvements in the glucose/insulin ratio were very significant in those given 500 mcg of the mineral with less or no improvement in those given 100 mcg after two and four months. The mineral improves insulin binding, insulin receptor number, insulin internalization, beta-cell sensitivity, and insulin receptor enzymes, with an overall increase in insulin sensitivity.[8]

In an Israeli study involving type 2 diabetics, almost half of the volunteers were able to reduce dosages of their anti-diabetic medication after chromium supplements were given. Diabetics whose glucose levels are not well controlled with traditional medications may benefit from 300–1,000 mcg daily of chromium picolinate added to their dietary regimen.[9]

In a double-blind study, twenty-nine male and female volunteers, who were at a high risk for developing type 2 diabetes, were given either 1,000 mcg per day of chromium picolinate or a placebo for eight months, reported researchers from the University of Vermont College of Medicine. The mineral significantly improved the action of insulin in those who had a family history of type 2 diabetes. This suggested a direct effect on chromium picolinate on muscle insulin action.[10]

The beneficial effects of barley on blood glucose and water consumption in diabetics might be attributed to its high chromium content, according to a study at King's College, in London. Barley is often used in Iraq to treat diabetes because of its ability to modulate glycemic response to the ingestion of carbohydrates, as well as to inhibit weight loss and excessive water consumption. Barley contains about 5.7 mcg of chromium per gram. In the study, diabetic rats were fed a diet containing barley, starch, or sucrose. Only the barley-supplemented diet resulted in improved diabetic parameters.[11]

Jeffrey Gordon, M.D., a San Diego, California researcher, reported that taking chromium picolinate lowers total cholesterol, LDL cholesterol, and triglycerides, as well as improving the LDL-HDL ratio. He determined this by treating ten patients with high cholesterol using 200 mcg per day of chromium picolinate and 1–2 g per day of niacin, along with dietary suggestions. After four weeks of therapy, total cholesterol levels decreased 29 percent, LDL cholesterol decreased 27 percent, and triglyceride levels dropped 43 percent. HDL cholesterol in the blood remained unchanged, but there was a substantial improvement in the LDL-HDL ratio. He did not evaluate the effect of niacin.[12] These results indicate that the mineral may be useful for the cardiovascular complications that often accompany diabetes.

Chromium may be a secondary factor in the further progression of cataract changes in the lenses of diabetics, according to researchers in France. These observations came after evaluating the chromium concentrations in sixty-one human lenses and thirty-eight blood samples. An analysis of chromium in a human lens shows a significant difference between elderly and diabetic populations: the mean chromium concentrations in diabetic cataracts were 0.137 compared to 0.345 in the normal population.[13]

Taking Chromium

The best food sources of chromium include meat, cheese, whole grains, brewer's yeast, liver, wheat germ, spinach, apples, potatoes, and carrots.[14] However, most chromium is removed from grains when they are refined in today's processed foods, according to Robert Garrison, Jr., M.A., R.Ph., and Elizabeth Somer, M.A., R.D. "Low chromium levels in a highly refined diet combined with an increased intake of sugars and other processed carbohydrates that require chromium for metabolism might predispose some individuals to a chromium deficiency and aggravate adult-onset diabetes."[15]

The estimated safe dietary level of chromium is between 50 mcg and

200 mcg per day; however, most diets contain less than 60 percent of the suggested minimum intake of 50 mcg daily, according to Richard A. Anderson, Ph.D. Doses of up to 1,000 mcg per day have been used in supplements in laboratory work without toxicity.[16] Those with type 2 diabetes, impaired glucose tolerance, or hyperlipidemia (high levels of fats in the blood) should consider taking 400–600 mcg per day of chromium.[17]

Chromium losses in the urine may be caused by daily stresses such as chronic exercise, high sugar diets, lactation, and physical trauma. Elderly diabetics probably lack chromium because it is excreted in increasing amounts with aging.[18] Note that it takes about four hours for the mineral to become effective.

Magnesium

Magnesium is a co-factor in more than 300 enzymatic reactions, yet three-quarters of the U.S. population may have a dietary magnesium deficiency, according to Burton M. Altura, Ph.D., of the State University of New York Health Sciences Center, Brooklyn College of Medicine, in New York. Even more problematic is the fact that it is possible to have a normal blood level of the mineral and still have a total body deficit, because it is difficult to assess a deficiency in magnesium.[19] This is important because a magnesium deficiency is related to arrhythmias, heart attacks, hardening of the arteries, high blood pressure, diabetes, migraine headaches, toxemia of pregnancy, and kidney stones, among others.

Among diabetics, deficiency in magnesium ranges from 25 to 39 percent.[20] A magnesium deficiency can be due to lack of the mineral in the diet, malabsorption of the mineral, or expelling of magnesium by the kidneys due to drugs or genetic factors.[21] A deficiency of the mineral in type 2 diabetics may be related to environmental or genetic factors and may result in low oxygen uptake and decreased work capacity.[22]

Magnesium is essential for glucose balance, it helps in glucose transport, and regulates energy production in the liver. The mineral also is needed for the release of insulin and the maintenance of the pancreatic beta cells associated with insulin production and release. Magnesium deficiency contributes to the atrophy of beta cells. Magnesium increases the affinity and number of insulin receptors, sites on cell walls that react to insulin, which allows the cell to open and let glucose in. As mentioned, blood and tissue levels of magnesium are lower in diabetics, while the most frequent cause of low magnesium levels, other than acute ketoaci-dosis (sometimes called diabetic coma), is diabetes itself. The cause of a magnesium deficiency is complicated, but it includes increased urina-tion with glucose in the urine, an opposite association between plasma magnesium and blood glucose, an undersecretion of insulin and adren-aline, modification of vitamin D metabolism, and a lack of vitamin B_6. Magnesium supplements restore low blood and tissue levels, produce a protective effect against cardiovascular disease, and might aid in the pre-vention of vascular complications associated with diabetes, as well as in the development of the disease.[23]

Clinical Studies on Magnesium

A magnesium deficiency is prominent in patients with diabetes mellitus, according to Robert K. Rude, M.D. This can result in an increased risk for cardiac arrhythmia, hypertension, heart attack, and altered glucose metabolism. Actually, this association between low magnesium levels and diabetes has been known since 1946. For those patients with a magnesium deficiency, oral doses of 300 mg per day can be given, but the doses may have to be increased to 600 mg per day to achieve the desired therapeu-tic effect. To avoid diarrhea, a complication in susceptible individuals, the mineral can be taken in divided doses. For those with impaired kidney function, magnesium therapy should be reviewed by their doctor.[24]

Low blood levels of magnesium are found in about 25 percent of dia-betic patients, according to Lorraine Tosiello, M.D., of Overlook Hospi-tal, in New Jersey. Also, low levels of the mineral have been chronicled in childhood insulin-dependent diabetics and in adults with type 1 and type 2 diabetes. Low levels of magnesium are associated with insulin resistance in non-diabetic elderly patients. Dr. Tosiello noted that a mag-nesium deficiency is related to gastrointestinal loss of the mineral, excess excretion by the kidneys, nutritional deficiencies, endocrine disorders (internal secretions), redistribution problems, and other causes.[25]

Growing evidence and observational studies suggest that magnesium intake, from either diet or supplements, may favorably affect a cluster of chronic metabolic disorders, including insulin resistance, type 2 diabetes, cardiovascular disease, and high blood pressure, according to Yiqing Song, M.D., and colleagues at Brigham and Women's Hospital and Har-vard Medical School, in Boston, Massachusetts.[26] "The beneficial effects of magnesium intake have been explained by several mechanisms, including improvement of glucose and insulin homeostasis (balance), lipid (fat) metabolism, and vascular or myocardial contractility, antiarrhythmic effects, anticoagulant or antiplatelet effects, and increased endothelium-dependent vasodilation," the researchers stated. "Systemic inflammation, as measured by plasma C-reactive protein concentrations, is widely believed to be one of the common mechanisms underlying the development of these metabolic-related disorders. Magnesium intake may protect against diabetes and cardiovascular disease in part through reducing low-grade inflammation."

In evaluating 6,781 deaths in Taiwan from diabetes mellitus from 1990 to 1994, compared with 6,781 deaths from other causes, Chun-Y Yang, Ph.D., and colleagues said that there was a significant protective effect of magnesium in drinking water against the risk of dying from diabetes.[27] (It has long been known that people who live in areas with "hard" water, which is rich in minerals, are often protected from heart disease.)

Researchers have reported that low blood levels of magnesium may be a strong *predictor* of type 2 diabetes in white individuals. While studying blood levels of the mineral in 12,398 non-diabetic, middle-aged African-American and white volunteers over a six-year period, there was no association between magnesium levels and the development of diabetes in African Americans, but there was one in the white population. At the conclusion of the study, there were 807 new cases of type 2 diabetes in the white population, with the largest increase in risk for type 2 diabetes (94 percent) associated with those who had the lowest levels of magnesium in the blood.[28] Magnesium deficiency can adversely affect insulin metabolism, according to researchers from Johns Hopkins University, in Baltimore, Maryland.

In evaluating twenty-six fasting non-pregnant females, twenty normal pregnant females, and thirteen diet-controlled gestational diabetic women, Mordechai Berdicef, M.D., stated that, compared with non-pregnant controls, total and ionized magnesium were considerably lower in both normal pregnant and gestational diabetic women. Also, gestational diabetic women had significantly lower intracellular magnesium values. Ionized calcium rates were similar in all groups, which resulted in significant elevation of ionized calcium/magnesium ratios in both pregnant groups. These results confirm magnesium depletion as a factor in gestational diabetes. The research team concluded that magnesium depletion, or calcium excess, may predispose one to vascular complications in pregnancy.[29]

Researchers at Uppsala University Children's Hospital, in Sweden, reported that diabetic children have a chronic magnesium deficiency and insufficient liver synthesis of certain proteins in the blood. Their conclusions came after evaluating thirty-four children who were followed for five years from the onset of their diabetes. During that time, magnesium levels in their blood decreased to significantly lower levels than those in matched controls after two and five years. However, zinc levels in the blood were higher in the diabetic children than in the controls.[30]

Health problems associated with low levels of intracellular magnesium include high blood pressure and aging, which are also associated with insulin resistance, according to a team of researchers from the University of Naples, in Italy. Low levels of magnesium are especially noted in patients with diabetes, which show up as impaired insulin response in type 2 diabetes.[31] Magnesium supplements can improve beta-cell response and insulin action in insulin-dependent diabetics. Further, a magnesium deficiency may account for the atherosclerotic tendency in diabetics; that is, the development of hardening of the arteries. In patients given 4 g per day of magnesium for three weeks, it was reported that these non-insulin-dependent diabetics showed improved insulin secretion along with insulin sensitivity.

In a study involving seven type 2 diabetics with high blood pressure and low blood levels of magnesium, the participants were given 260 mg twice daily for six weeks. The volunteers without diabetes or high blood pressure received a placebo. The magnesium supplement increased blood levels of the mineral in the diabetic patients and led to a subsequent fall in blood pressure from an average of 157/96 mm Hg to 128/77 mm Hg. High blood pressure was controlled in the diabetics without medication, except for the magnesium. Platelets became less sticky and thromboxane was decreased. Jerry Nadler, M.D., notes that magnesium can be used by type 2 hypertensive diabetics with normal kidney function, but those with abnormal kidney function should confer with their physician about using the mineral.[32]

At the National Public Health Institute, in Helsinki, Finland, Johan Eriksson, M.D., Ph.D., gave fifty-six diabetics 600 mg per day of magnesium for ninety days. In another 90-day study, 2,000 mg per day of vitamin C was given. He reported that there was a decrease in systolic and diastolic blood pressure in type 1 diabetics given the mineral, and vitamin C improved glycemic control among type 2 diabetics in both fasting blood glucose and hemoglobin A_{1C} levels. Vitamin C also reduced cholesterol and triglyceride levels in type 2 patients.[33]

Low magnesium levels with elevated calcium increase the stickiness of platelets and blood clots, which have been implicated in the development of diabetes, heart attack, and eclampsia (convulsions during pregnancy), according to Mildred S. Seelig, M.D. Low magnesium levels can increase the release of thromboxane, one of a number of substances that can cause blood clots.[34]

Researchers at the University of Texas Southwestern Medical Center, in Dallas, evaluated 1,089 pregnant women who were given phenytoin (Dilantin) for eclamptic convulsions, compared to 1,049 women who received magnesium sulfate. Preeclampsia is a potentially serious complication of pregnancy; its most serious form (eclampsia) may bring on seizures and coma, which endanger both mother and fetus. Early symptoms include excessive fluid retention, an abnormal rise in blood pressure, and protein in the urine. It is theorized that magnesium sulfate may not act as an anticonvulsant but rather serve as a vasodilator. The research team found that ten of the women given the drug had convulsions compared to none getting the mineral. The magnesium therapy consisted of an initial 10 g dose of 50 percent magnesium sulfate given intramuscularly, then a maintenance dose of 5 g every four hours. For the pregnant women with severe preeclampsia, an additional 4 g initial dose was administered intravenously. The researchers concluded that magnesium sulfate is superior to Dilantin in preventing eclampsia in pregnant women with high blood pressure.[35]

S.E. Browne, M.D., initially used magnesium sulfate intramuscularly and intravenously in his practice to treat patients with gangrene, leg ulcers, Raynaud's disease, chilblains, intermittent claudication, peripheral vascular disease, congestive heart failure, angina, myocardial infarction, and cerebrovascular disease. He reported that magnesium has a significant vasodilating effect (widening of blood vessels) and can result in considerable flushing after intravenous injections of 4–12 mmol (millimole) of magnesium. It has excellent therapeutic results in all forms of arterial disease, he reported. This rapid infusion maintains very high initial blood levels of the mineral and it produces significant results that cannot be obtained by oral or other means. Of eight patients with leg ulcers, five healed quickly after failing to respond to other therapies.[36]

Taking Magnesium

Top food sources of magnesium include nuts, whole grains, green leafy vegetables, meat, fish and seafood, poultry, dried fruit, chocolate, and cottonseed, peanut, and soybean flours.

Magnesium supplements are available in a variety of formulations in health food stores and other outlets. The mineral is often combined with calcium and other minerals in supplements. The so-called Recommended Dietary Allowance (RDA) for the mineral is around 350 mg per day for men and 280 mg per day for women, but as we have seen, larger amounts may be prescribed by health-care professionals for diabetes and other disorders. It is helpful to take calcium and magnesium together. Researchers usually recommend a 2:1 ratio of calcium to magnesium; however, in some instances, others have recommended a 1:1 ratio.

Selenium

When you take selenium, it is absorbed in the intestines, mostly in the duodenum, where it is bound to a protein and transported in the blood to the tissues. It is then incorporated into tissue protein as selenocysteine and selenomethionine. Most of the mineral is excreted in the kidneys, although smaller amounts exit via feces and sweat. Deficiencies of selenium are sometimes hard to detect, because vitamin E, cysteine, and methionine may act as partial substitutes for selenium. Nutrients such as fat and protein may affect the body's need for selenium.[37] The metabolic roles of selenium and vitamin E overlap, so that each nutrient may replace the other to a limited extent in preventing certain types of disorders. But there are also unique functions for each nutrient, so each must be supplied in the diet to ensure good nutrition.

The liver is susceptible to damage by toxic substances released during fat metabolism unless it is supplied with selenium, vitamin E, and/or methionine and cysteine to prevent the build up of peroxides. Selenium is a constituent of an important antioxidant enzyme—glutathione peroxidase—that destroys free radicals. As reported by the National Research Council, selenium is involved in such human medical problems as cancer, cataracts, diseases of the liver, and cardiovascular or muscular diseases, along with the aging process.

Clinical Studies on Selenium

Selenium is known to help several insulin-like actions in humans, such as stimulating glucose uptake and metabolic processes such as glycosis (enzymatic breakdown of a carbohydrate such as glucose), gluconeogenesis (formation of glucose from fats and proteins), and fatty acid synthesis.[38] In studying 150 type 1 diabetics, between the ages of 11 and 60, it was found that the selenium content in diabetic patients was significantly lower than in the controls. In general, selenium, but not zinc and copper, concentrations in the blood are below normal in diabetic patients.[39] Other studies have also found a link between low blood levels of the mineral and diabetes.[40]

A research team in Vienna, Austria, evaluated twenty type 1 diabetics and twenty healthy controls and found that selenium levels were low in the red blood cells of the diabetics and that glutathione peroxidase activity in red blood cells was also low. The researchers said that reduced selenium levels in the red blood cells of diabetics could contribute to unnecessary bleeding.[41]

Selenium and the enzyme glutathione peroxidase protect cell membranes from damage by oxidation and thus are an important antioxidant source, according to researchers at Karolinska Hospital, in Stockholm, Sweden. Dietary intake between 50 mcg and 200 mcg per day is recommended, but deficiency symptoms are noted in less than 10 mcg per day. A deficiency in the mineral has been reported for cardiomyopathy (disorder of the heart muscle). Low levels of selenium in Finnish soils have been associated with an increased risk of ischemic heart disease and low levels of the mineral have been noted in smokers.[42]

Some researchers have suggested that deficiencies of selenium and vitamin E might contribute to heart disease, since these nutrients help to maintain adequate levels of coenzyme Q_{10} (coQ_{10}) in the heart muscle. If coQ_{10} is lacking, the production of energy in the heart and other muscles may diminish so that these tissues can no longer carry their workloads. Death rates in the United States from heart disease have consistently been highest in the states with low selenium in the soils—Washington, Oregon, Michigan, Florida, Ohio, Indiana, the New England states, and others.

Researchers at Erasmus University Medical School, in the Nether-lands, found that patients with heart attack had long-term low selenium levels (as indicated by the amount of the mineral found in their clipped toenails), which probably accounted for an increased risk for a coronary episode. The toenails often indicate how much selenium is stored in the body. As toenail selenium concentrations decreased, risk of myocardial infarction increased. The researchers concluded that low selenium levels were present before the heart attack and that this might have played a role in its development.[43]

Bodo Kuklinski, M.D., found that in a one-year, double-blind, con-trolled trial with heart attack sufferers, no patient died following antiox-idative treatment, but 20 percent of the controls expired. The treatment involved selenite (selenium), coQ_{10}, selenocysteine, beta-carotene, vita-mins B_6, C and E, and zinc. Researchers found that kidney excretion of albumin was lowered during administration of vitamin E, alpha-lipoic acid, and selenite in diabetic late syndrome patients. The term *late syn-drome* refers to complications in long-term diabetic patients with retinopathy (diseases of the retina), nephropathy (kidney disease), and neuropathy (disorder of the nerves). Peripheral diabetic neuropathy improved in 60 percent of the patients.[44]

The selenium content of the lens of the eye increases from birth to death, but it has been found that lenses with cataracts may contain less than one-sixth of the normal amounts of the mineral. Lack of selenium to activate the enzyme glutathione peroxidase may block the destruction of peroxides in the lens of the eye such that these toxic substances may accumulate in sufficient amounts to damage the lens. As reported in the *Journal of Nutritional Medicine,* Joseph Bittner, M.D., stated in 1977 that he had reversed macular degeneration in two patients using intravenous injections of selenium and zinc. Improvements also were noted when the two minerals were taken orally. Vitamin E and taurine, an amino acid, also were included in the therapy.[45]

Researchers at Hospital of Anbelholm, in Sweden, revealed the case of a 35-year-old male who had subcapsular cataract, atopic eczema, asthma, and other complications. He was treated daily with selenium (600 mcg), vitamin E (1,200 mg), vitamin B_6 (80 mg), vitamin B_2 (15 mg), and vita-min C (2 g). At the beginning of the therapy, vision in the right eye meas-ured 2/10 and the left eye was 3/10. Five months later, vision in the right eye was 4/10 and 8/10 in the left eye. After two months of treatment, signs of atopic dermatitis had vanished and there were no signs of asthma. The authors suggest that it is reasonable to try selenium and vitamin E treatment in other kinds of cataracts, such as diabetic cataracts. The use of selenium is safe, assuming the patient has normal kidney function.[46]

Taking Selenium

Selenium, which is available in breads, cereals, fish, poultry, and meat, stimulates glutathione peroxidase and thus is a powerful scavenger against damaging free radicals. Recommended daily amounts of selenium are 50 mcg to 200 mcg, but the average intake in the American diet is estimated about 60 mcg daily. Researchers often use larger amounts in supplements for specific health conditions. Taking selenium supplements totaling less than 800 mcg per day or eating Brazil nuts, the richest food source of the mineral, is a reasonable option for those facing a selenium deficiency.[47]

Vanadium

Vanadium has been studied for more than forty years, yet it is not classified as an essential nutrient for human beings. Pharmacologic doses of the mineral 10 to 100 times the normal intake can alter cholesterol and triglyceride metabolism, as well as the shape of red blood cells, and stimulate glucose oxidation and glycogen synthesis in the liver. Vanadium seems to assist in the metabolism of glucose by mimicking the action of insulin or altering the activity of the multifunctional enzyme glucose-6-phosphatase. Vanadium enhances the stimulatory effect of insulin on DNA synthesis in cultured cells.[48]

In the early 1900s, French physicians used vanadium as a cure-all for diabetes, anemia, chronic rheumatism, and tuberculosis. Vanadium treatment has been shown to reduce blood glucose levels and maintain normal glycemic states at least three months after withdrawal of treatment.[49] This mineral is a natural element that has worked for many diabetics. It is available in buffered form and it has insulin-like properties, which increase the uptake of glucose and protein by the muscles and liver.[50]

In *Anti-Fat Nutrients*, Dallas Clouatre, Ph.D., reported that problems with carbohydrate metabolism play a role in the tendency to put on excess weight. One of the main substances involved in fat storage is the hormone insulin, so it is reasonable to assume that foods and nutrients that make insulin more effective and can mimic insulin's actions in the body might aid in controlling appetite and weight gain. A great deal of scientific evidence is being directed at various nutrients that appear to perform these functions, including vanadium.[51] A 1985 article in *Science* suggested that vanadium controlled diabetes in laboratory animals. Other studies have confirmed these results and it is now known that the mineral plays a significant role in controlling blood sugar levels.

Clinical Studies on Vanadium

At Temple University Hospital, in Philadelphia, a research team gave 50 mg of vanadyl sulfate (vanadium), taken orally twice daily for four weeks, which resulted in a 20 percent reduction in fasting glucose concentrations and a decrease in glucose output in the liver in eight type 2 diabetics. However, researchers said that patients given the mineral for longer than one month should be evaluated for its metabolic effects.[52]

A research team at the University of Texas Health Science Center, in San Antonio, studied eleven type 2 diabetics, all fifty-nine years old, who had had diabetes for four years. Their hemoglobin A_{1C} (a measure of blood glucose) registered 8.4 percent; readings between 6 and 7 percent are considered satisfactory, so this reading was high. Each volunteer was given 150 mg per day of vanadyl sulfate for six weeks, with each 25 mg tablet of the mineral equal to 8 mg of elemental vanadium. Vanadium significantly improved glycemic control and fasting blood glucose level was reduced from 194 mg/dl (milligrams per deciliter) to 155 mg/dl; hemoglobin A_{1C} decreased to 7.8 percent. In addition, vanadyl sulfate reduced glucose production by about 20 percent, which correlated with a reduction in fasting plasma glucose. The mineral also lowered total cholesterol and LDL ("bad") cholesterol levels in the blood.[53]

Long-term treatment with vanadium brings a marked and sustained decrease in glucose, triglycerides, and cholesterol in the blood, according to researchers at the University of British Columbia, in Vancouver, Canada. Vanadium supplements have blood-pressure-lowering effects because of their ability to counter insulin resistance and weaken hyperinsulinemia (excess insulin in the blood).[54] Sodium vanadate (at 125 mg per day) can lower insulin requirements in type 1 diabetics and lower their cholesterol, according to J.J. Cunningham of the University of Massachusetts, in Amherst. Chromium, vitamin B_3 (niacin), vitamin C, vitamin E, and zinc can also benefit type 1 diabetics.[55] Researchers at the Albert Einstein College of Medicine reported that vanadyl sulfate (100 mg per day) given to seven type 2 diabetics and six non-diabetics lowered fasting glucose and hemoglobin A_{1C} in the diabetics.[56]

In an article in *Nutrition Reviews*, Karen Roberts, M.S., and colleagues reviewed the various nutrients that are available for dealing with metabolic syndrome, which can lead to type 2 diabetes. Among their recommendations were vanadium, which can improve blood glucose control and improve insulin action (vanadium salt at 100 mg per day, with an upper limit of 1,000 mg per day); chromium, which improves blood glucose control and insulin action (200 mcg per day); and magnesium, which has been shown to reduce blood pressure, improve blood glucose control, and improve insulin action (480 mg per day).[57]

Taking Vanadium

Vanadium is found in skim milk, lobster, vegetable oils, vegetables, grains, cereals, mushrooms, parsley, dill, and black pepper. The elevated levels of the mineral in processed foods are apparently due to stainless-steel processing equipment.[58] The estimated intake of the mineral in the American diet is 10 mcg to 60 mcg per day. Daily requirements for vanadium have not been established, but the suggested intake is about 10 mcg per day, according to researchers at the University of British Columbia, in Canada.

Doses of 0.083–0.420 mmol per day have shown therapeutic potential in clinical studies with both type 1 and type 2 diabetes. Doses from 50 mg to 125 mg per day of vanadyl sulfate have been beneficial for type 2 diabetics. Organic forms of the mineral are safer, more absorbable, and able to deliver a therapeutic effect up to 50 percent greater than inorganic forms.[59]

A chelated form of selenium—bis-maltolato oxovanadium (BMOV)—appears to be more biologically active and absorbable than vanadyl sulfate, according to Jack Challem, author of *Syndrome X*.[60] "Consumers should know that some researchers believe that, since vanadium mimics insulin, it may turn off pancreatic cells that make insulin," he states. "This suggests that if you take large amounts of supplemental vanadium for a long period and then stop, your body may under-produce insulin for a short time until the body increases its insulin production again." Robert C. Atkins, M.D., concurred about BMOV, saying that it may be a breakthrough, since it can be used at lower doses than vanadyl sulfate and so has less theoretical potential for long-term toxicity. Some of his colleagues have used BMOV at doses below 1 mg and are reporting benefits for their diabetic patients. Dr. Atkins has used BMOV for long-term management of diabetics once their blood sugar has been lowered with vanadyl sulfate.[61]

Vanadium toxicity can be prevented by giving EDTA (ethylenediaminetetraacetic acid), vitamin C, chromium, protein, ferrous iron, chloride, and aluminum hydroxide, which apparently inhibits the mineral's absorption.[62]

Fasting blood glucose and blood glucose levels after meals decreased significantly in diabetics following lithium therapy. An exception was the fasting blood glucose in the type 2 diabetics who were treated with diet and no medications. The researchers concluded that lithium could improve glucose metabolism in most diabetics. Lithium is said to have a hypoglycemic effect when it is combined with treatments for reducing blood glucose levels. However, when given at a dose of 300 mg four times daily, lithium can cause restless leg syndrome, so lithium intake should be monitored by a physician.[64]

Zinc

Zinc is an important mineral in the synthesis and action of insulin. Hyperglycemia (an abnormally high concentration of glucose in the

LITHIUM FOR DIABETES

At the Second Affiliated Hospital-Human Medical University in China, a research team said that lithium carbonate is an effective supplementary medication for oral hypoglycemia agents and/or insulin in treating diabetics. The dosage of 100 mg per day produced no significant side effects. In Chinese literature, lithium was used clinically before insulin was commercially available.[63] In the study, thirty-three type 2 diabetics and five type 1 diabetics, ranging in age from twenty to seventy, were evaluated for the effect of lithium on low blood sugar. Depending on the severity of the disease, the volunteers were treated by diet only with oral hypoglycemic drugs or with insulin. After their blood glucose levels were stabilized, the people were given 100 mg per day of lithium carbonate.

blood) in type 1 and type 2 diabetics causes loss of zinc from the body. Researchers have found that low levels of zinc may result in oxidative stress that damages the cells irreversibly, thereby making some of the complications of diabetes even worse.[65] Zinc increases the assimilation of glucose due to an insulin-like effect.[66]

The most likely cause of zinc deficiency, such as in diabetics, is a diet low in bioavailable zinc. A deficiency in the mineral causes dermatitis, abnormal pregnancy, immature sexual glands, poor eyesight, abnormal sense of taste and smell, macular degeneration, senile dementia, and other health problems.

Clinical Studies on Zinc

Obese patients, who are at high risk in developing diabetes, often have abnormal zinc and copper levels, according to a study at Surgical Research Laboratories, in Tennessee. The research team measured copper and zinc levels in the blood, urine, liver, and skeletal tissues of thirty-seven obese patients. Blood, liver, and urinary copper levels were significantly above normal, but blood levels of zinc were low and urinary zinc was elevated, which meant it was not being retained by the body.[67] Moderate zinc deficiency occurs frequently in type 2 diabetics, according to researchers at Ohio State University, in Columbus.[68]

At Umea University, in Sweden, researchers studied 2,957 cases of diabetes compared to 7,165 controls, ranging in age from 3 to 14, to look at the relationship between zinc in drinking water and the risk of diabetes. They reported that a high concentration of the mineral in groundwater ("hard" water) was associated with a significantly decreased risk of diabetes. In other words, people got reasonable amounts of zinc in the diet, presumably from the water. There was an even stronger association between zinc and diabetes in rural areas where drinking water came from local wells.[69] The so-called hard water contains a variety of minerals compared with "soft" water.

In ten volunteers with advanced cirrhosis of the liver and impaired glucose tolerance or diabetes, long-term supplementation with 20 mg of zinc, three times daily for sixty days, improved the dispersion of glucose by more than 30 percent, according to researchers at the Universita di Bologna, in Italy. Insulin sensitivity, which was reduced before the treatment began, did not change. The involvement of glucose was almost halved in cirrhosis patients before treatment and increased after zinc therapy. The normalization of zinc levels improved their ability to handle glucose. The researchers added that poor zinc status may contribute to the impaired glucose tolerance and diabetes found in cirrhosis patients.[70]

In a study of 110 diabetics who had had fasting glycosylated hemoglobin of less than 7.5 percent for at least five years, the volunteers, 51–55 years old, were randomly assigned to four groups that were given either zinc gluconate (30 mg), chromium picolinate (400 mcg), zinc (30 mg) and chromium (400 mcg), or a placebo. At the beginning of the study, it was thought that more than 30 percent of the volunteers may have been zinc deficient. Following supplementation, there was a significant reduction of plasma thiobarbituric acid reactive substances (TBARS) in the chromium group, the zinc group, and in the zinc-chromium group. TBARS are a marker for lipid peroxidation and often indicate free-radical damage in both type 1 and type 2 diabetics.[71]

As reported in the *Journal of the American College of Nutrition*, researchers evaluated 3,575 volunteers between the ages of 25 and 64, including 1,769 people from rural India and 1,806 urban dwellers. The research team found that the prevalence of coronary artery disease, diabetes, and glucose intolerance was significantly higher among those consuming lower amounts of zinc. After eating, insulin and blood glucose levels declined as zinc intake increased in rural men and urban men and women.[72]

Taking Zinc

Meat, poultry, and fish provide about 50 percent of the zinc in the omnivore diet and red meat has twice as much zinc as white meat. Cereals and legumes provide about 30 percent of dietary zinc, but phytate and fiber in those foods may impede zinc absorption. Foods prepared from cow's milk provide only about 20 percent of dietary zinc. According to the U.S. Department of Agriculture, 50 percent of those who follow the Dietary Guidelines for Americans have zinc intakes that are less than 75 percent of the Recommended Dietary Allowance (RDA) of 15 mg per day.[73]

CHAPTER 11

Other Nutrients to Help Diabetics

Alpha-Lipoic Acid

Alpha-lipoic acid has a number of beneficial effects, both in prevention and treatment of diabetes. At its most fundamental biological level, alpha-lipoic acid (also known as thioctic acid) serves as a coenzyme in the Krebs cycle, which breaks down glucose in every cell and converts it to energy. However, without alpha-lipoic acid, this breakdown cannot occur. For the process to occur, insulin must shuttle glucose from the blood into the cells. In type 2 diabetes, the body overproduces insulin in response to diets that are high in refined carbohydrates. After years of such a diet, glucose-burning cells stop responding to the insulin, which leads to insulin resistance, and glucose is increasingly stored as triglycerides in fat cells.

Burt Berkson, M.D., has said that alpha-lipoic acid is an effective treatment for the prevention, treatment, and reversal of type 2 diabetes. First, the supplement is a powerful antioxidant that neutralizes hazardous free radicals, which cause many diabetic complications. Second, the substance improves the efficiency of insulin and lowers blood sugar (glucose) levels. Third, alpha-lipoic acid slows the aging process, which is accelerated by diabetes.[1]

The supplement may act in a number of ways that are especially protective in diabetes. For example, it prevents beta-cell destruction leading to type 1-diabetes and it enhances glucose uptake in type 2 diabetes. In addition, it prevents glycation reactions in some proteins. Its antioxidant effects may be useful in slowing the development of diabetic neuropathy and cataracts and in alleviating diabetes-induced reduction in intracellular vitamin C levels.[2] Few of these improvements will surface over the course of weeks or months. It is unrealistic to expect dramatic effects in weeks, since diabetic complications develop over years and decades.

Clinical Studies on Alpha-Lipoic Acid

Alpha-lipoic acid stimulates the glucose carriers to increase sugar uptake in the cells, but in the case of diabetes, cellular sugar intake is impaired. In one study, alpha-lipoic acid therapy at 100 mg intravenously (IV) or 500 mg IV for fourteen days increased the glucose utilization of diabetics by 20 percent to 50 percent. Another study, using 600 mg per day taken by mouth for 30 days in 10 polyneuropathy patients found that adenosine triphosphate (ATP) production in the muscles of diabetics was improved because the supplement improved the energy supply.[3]

In Germany, alpha-lipoic acid is an approved "drug" for the treatment of nerve disorders in diabetics, but recent research has also studied the benefit of the nutrient to lower blood sugar (glucose) levels in diabetics. In a study on the effect of alpha-lipoic acid on diabetic rats with elevated glucose levels, researchers reported that alpha-lipoic acid substantially lowered blood glucose levels after fasting and meals, thus reducing the principal symptom of diabetes and probably lowering the risk of diabetic complications. It was also found that blood glucose levels were about 23 percent lower after feeding and some were 45 percent lower after fasting, when compared to the rats on placebo. It seems that alpha-lipoic acid improved the transport of glucose in muscle cells, where most of the glucose is burned for energy.[4]

Alpha-lipoic acid enhances glucose uptake in muscle cells and prevents glucose-induced protein modifications, reported Thomas Konrad, M.D., of J.W. Goethe-University in Frankfurt, Germany. In the study, the intravenous glucose tolerance tests before and after oral treatment with 600 mg of the supplement twice daily showed fasting lactate and pyruvate levels were significantly increased in type 2 diabetics. Also, the supplement was associated with an increase in glucose effectiveness in both lean and obese type 2 diabetics.[5]

Using a specific fat cell, a research team evaluated the effect of alpha-lipoic acid, dihydrolipoic acid (which the body converts to alpha-lipoic acid), and N-acetylcysteine (NAC; another antioxidant), on the cellular transport of glucose, which is needed for energy for normal metabolic processes. The effect of these antioxidants on insulin concentrations was also measured. In the first experiment, the research team found that glucose transport was increased when the fat cells were exposed to alpha-lipoic acid and dihydrolipoic acid, but not with NAC. This suggests that the two forms of lipoic acid prevent insulin resistance or poor insulin function, the main symptom of type 2 diabetes. In the second experiment, all of the antioxidants reduced levels of insulin.[6]

Researchers in Germany looked at the role of alpha-lipoic acid in treating polyneuropathy, a nerve condition that affects between 25 and 50 percent of diabetics. They reported that hyperglycemia (elevated levels of sugar in the blood) is the most important factor in the development of polyneuropathy and that increased levels of oxygen free radicals contribute to the loss of neurologic function in diabetes.[7] Polyneuropathy affects peripheral nerves, such as cranial nerves in the brain and spinal nerves; hands and feet are also affected. Symptoms include leg pain, numbness, and muscle weakness. The condition is caused by toxic exposure, nutritional deficiency (especially of vitamins B_1, B_6, and pantothenic acid), and malabsorption.[8]

As a potent antioxidant, alpha-lipoic acid is able to regenerate the body's own antioxidants, such as vitamins C and E and glutathione. In a study in which thirty-four volunteers received 600 mg IV and then 600 mg per day by mouth, alpha-lipoic acid brought lasting improvement in the clinical symptoms of peripheral diabetic neuropathy. However, there was no improvement in nerve function in one study during fifteen weeks of treatment.[9]

In another study, researchers gave 600 mg per day of alpha-lipoic acid for three weeks to ten diabetics with polyneuropathy. Symptoms were evaluated with measurements of blood flow and clinical assessments of the symptoms. The researchers reported that clinical symptoms of polyneuropathy improved significantly following alpha-lipoic acid therapy. In addition, the supplement improved the movement of blood cells in capillaries, which is thought to influence nerve function.[10]

At Heinrich-Heine University, in Germany, 328 type 2 diabetics with symptoms of peripheral neuropathy were given an injection of either a placebo or alpha-lipoic acid, using doses of 1,200 mg, 600 mg, or 100 mg for three weeks. Dosages of 1,200 mg and 600 mg versus the placebo brought relief in foot symptoms right from the start. With regard to pain, burning, paresthesia (tingling), and numbness, all were lower in the 600 mg group after nineteen days. In another study, thirty-nine patients with type 2 diabetes and cardiac autonomic neuropathy were randomly given a daily oral dose of 800 mg of alpha-lipoic acid, while thirty-four volunteers were given a placebo for four months. Two of the four parameters of heart rate variability at rest were greatly improved in the alpha-lipoic acid group. No side effects of significance were reported.[11]

In a study involving diabetic laboratory rats, researchers tested alpha-lipoic acid, vitamin E, and vitamin C to see if they could reduce kidney damage. Alpha-lipoic acid was far more effective than the two vitamins in preventing kidney disease. In fact, diabetic rats given alpha-lipoic acid supplements did not experience the increases in markers of kidney disease when compared with untreated animals.[12]

In another human study, thirty-one volunteers were asked to take 600 mg per day of alpha-lipoic acid or 400 IU per day of vitamin E for two months, followed by the same amounts of both combined for an additional two months. The research team reported that alpha-lipoic acid significantly slowed free-radical oxidative damage to cholesterol, which might promote the development of coronary artery disease. Alpha-lipoic acid is both water-soluble and fat-soluble and works well with fat-soluble vitamin E in halting free-radical buildup.[13]

In a study involving diabetic rats, a research team suggested that alpha-lipoic acid, as a potent antioxidant, protects nerve cells by fighting free-radical damage. Diabetics often suffer from oxidative stress

BREWER'S YEAST

Supplementation with brewer's yeast, an excellent source of glucose tolerance factor (GTF), has been shown to improve glucose tolerance in type 2 diabetics, increase their sensitivity to insulin, and lower their level of blood fats, according to Melvyn Werbach, M.D. GTF occurs pre-formed in certain foods, especially brewer's yeast, and humans have a varying ability to synthesize it from inorganic chromium, vitamin B_3, and amino acids. There are many commercial GTF products on the market, but their actual GTF activity is variable and largely unproven. Unless you can find out how potent a GTF supplement is, Dr. Werbach recommends that you obtain GTF from brewer's yeast. As a supplement, he suggests 9 g per day of brewer's yeast during a trial period of eight weeks.[14]

because of large amounts of damaging free radicals and small amounts of protective antioxidants in the body. While blood flow to the nerves of the animals was 50 percent of normal, alpha-lipoic acid protected the nerves from damage by reducing oxidative stress. High doses of the supplement restored normal blood flow in diabetic rats after one month, but it did not affect blood flow in rats without diabetes.[15]

Taking Alpha-Lipoic Acid

Alpha-lipoic acid is found in spinach, broccoli, kidney beans, and liver. Alpha-lipoic acid has the potential to prevent diabetes, improve glucose control, and prevent chronic hyperglycemia-associated complications, such as neuropathy, according to Shari Lieberman, Ph.D. For cataracts, glaucoma, ischemia perfusion injury, and diabetic neuropathy, she recommends 300–600 mg of alpha-lipoic acid per day.[16]

Amino Acids

In order for a protein to be created, all of its constituent amino acids must be available. Amino acids synthesized in the body are called non-essential amino acids. If the body cannot synthesize an amino acid from materials normally available, it must be supplied by the diet or supplements—this is called an essential amino acid.[17] There are twenty-two amino acids, including nine essential and thirteen non-essential ones. The essential amino acids are histidine, isoleucine, leucine, lysine, methionine, phenylalanine, threonine, tryptophan, and valine. Arginine, cysteine, glycine, and tyrosine are among the non-essential amino acids. Taurine and carnitine are not considered essential or non-essential amino acids, but may be needed for some health problems.

Cysteine and methionine are the principal sources of sulfur in the diet, which is needed for the formation of coenzyme A and taurine. Lysine is involved in the synthesis of carnitine, which stimulates fatty acid synthesis within cells. Histidine is a powerful blood vessel dilator. Most of the phenylalanine not used in protein synthesis is converted to tyrosine. The latter is involved in the manufacture of the hormones norepinephrine and epinephrine by the adrenal glands and the hormones thyroxine and triiodothyronine by the thyroid gland.

Tryptophan is necessary for the production of serotonin, an important neurotransmitter of the brain that counteracts the effects of epinephrine and norepinephrine and improves the duration of sleep. Serotonin is also a powerful constrictor of blood vessels in tissues, including blood platelets, and cells of the intestinal mucosa. Some vitamin B_3 can be manufactured from tryptophan, but this is not enough to meet the body's need for niacin.

Clinical evidence has accumulated concerning the beneficial effects of amino acids. For example, glutamine and arginine may improve immune function. Glutamine, a non-essential amino acid, when included in a study of intensive-care patients, lowered six-month mortality. The researchers added that there is a lack of defined dose-response relation with regard to glutamine or arginine. "The absence of large, multicenter trials in nutritional support of these amino acids is astonishing in view of the beneficial effects so far reported," the authors stated. "The most likely explanation is the reluctance of pharmaceutical companies to put huge investments into international multicenter trials when the financial profits are going to be limited."[18]

A note on amino acid forms: "Just as hands and feet are mirror images of each other, amino acids occur as mirror image forms (optical isomers)," states Robert A. Ronzio, Ph.D. "The left-hand forms are designated as 'L' and the right-handed opposites are designated as 'D.' Only 'L' amino acids are supplied by food and synthesized in the body and only the 'L' forms occur in proteins. Therefore, unless indicated otherwise, an amino acid can be assumed to be the 'L' form when mentioned in nutrition literature. The only common amino acid that does not exist as optical isomers is glycine, the simplest of amino acids."[19]

Clinical Studies on Amino Acids

Although type 1 and type 2 diabetes are two distinct diseases, taurine is useful in stabilizing blood sugar in both, according to Robert C. Atkins, M.D. For those with type 2 diabetes, taurine improves cellular sensitivity to insulin. For patients with type 1 diabetes, 1.5 g per day of taurine keeps blood sugar lower over the long term and reduces abnormal platelet activity. Diabetics often have below normal levels of taurine, which might compound their susceptibility to retinopathy and heart damage.[20]

Although the mechanism by which it works is unknown, researchers at the University of Graz, in Austria, found that arginine improves insulin sensitivity in overweight patients, in type 2 diabetics, and in healthy people. The study involved seven healthy volunteers, nine obese patients, and nine type 2 diabetics. The research team said that arginine, given at 0.52 mg/kg/minute IV over three hours restored the impaired insulin-mediated vasodilatation (the dilation of blood vessels) that is seen in overweight people and those with type 2 diabetes.[21] A holistic physician should be asked if an equivalent amount of the amino acid can be given orally.

At the University of Sassari, in Italy, a research team evaluated thirty-nine type 1 diabetics and thirty-four controls for levels of taurine before and after 1.5 g per day of the amino acid was given for ninety days. It was reported that platelet taurine concentrations were lower in diabetic patients than in the controls. Oral administration of taurine decreased platelet aggregation and may reduce diabetic complications such as micro- and macro-angiopathies, which are associated with increases in platelet aggregation.[22] The study suggests that normal concentrations of taurine could be important in restoring normal clotting and subsequently preventing blood vessel damage in type 1 diabetics. The amino acid has antioxidant capability, which may protect cell membranes and other cellular components.

At the University of Rome in Italy, a research team headed by Filippo Rossi-Fanelli, M.D., evaluated twenty-five overweight type 2 diabetics. The volunteers were given either 750 mg per day of 5-hydroxytryptophan (5-HTP) or a placebo pill for two weeks. The amount of the amino acid tryptophan in the brain was significantly reduced in the diabetics when compared to the healthy controls. Those getting 5-HTP significantly decreased their daily energy intake by reducing carbohydrate and fat intake and also lowered their body weight.[23]

An increase in dietary protein associated with a decrease in carbohydrates could be useful in type 2 diabetes, according to an article in the *Journal of the American College of Nutrition.* When protein is eaten, it is broken down into amino acids. In the liver, most of the absorbed amino acids are deaminated (separated). The nitrogen is converted to urea and excreted in urine, while the remaining carbon elements can be converted to glucose. For example, 3.5 g of glucose can be produced from every gram of nitrogen produced from ingested protein. In other words, 28 g of glucose can be formed from the ingestion of 50 g of protein.[24]

Researchers have determined that protein results in a modest increase in circulating insulin in normal people but a large increase in type 2 diabetics, as well as increasing circulating glucagon concentrations. Glucagon is a hormone that raises glucose (sugar) in the blood. It has a significant anti-insulin effect and increases blood sugar levels by releasing glucose that is stored as glycogen in the liver and muscles.

Taking Amino Acids

The proportions in which the essential amino acids are required are as important as the amounts, according to Ruth M. Leverton. The body prefers that these amino acids be available from food in about the same proportions each time for use in maintenance, repair, and growth. Meat, fish, poultry, eggs, milk, cheese, and some legumes contain complete protein.[25] "Often the proteins in grains, nuts, fruit and vegetables are classed as partially complete or incomplete because the proportionate amount of one or more of the essential amino acids is low or because the concentrations of all of the amino acids are too low to be helpful in meeting the body's needs," Leverton stated. When animal sources are not readily available, as in some developing countries, foods can sometimes be combined to make a complete protein. For example, corn can be combined with wheat to increase the proportion of tryptophan.

Coenzyme Q$_{10}$

CoQ$_{10}$ (or ubiquinone) could represent one of the major medical advances in the treatment of heart disease, says heart specialist Stephen T. Sinatra, M.D. CoQ$_{10}$ is a naturally occurring substance in foods and is

PHOSPHATIDYLCHOLINE (PC)

Phosphatidylcholine should be considered an important supportive therapy for the treatment of lipid (fat) disorders in diabetics, according to an article in *La Clinica Therapeutica*. In the study, twenty-nine diabetics were divided into two groups. PC was given at a dose of 1,200 mg per day, in the form of three 200-mg capsules at two main meals. The PC therapy led to a rapid fall in blood cholesterol, which was evident after thirty days and was statistically significant at ninety days, resulting in a 15.1 percent reduction in cholesterol. There was an increase in HDL ("good") cholesterol and a significant decrease in LDL ("bad") cholesterol from sixty days onward.[26]

synthesized in all cells of the body. While the average dietary intake is approximately 5–10 mg per day, the dominant source in humans is biosynthesis. This is a complex process involving tyrosine, an amino acid, and at least seven vitamins and several minerals. "As an antioxidant," says Dr. Sinatra, "CoQ_{10} inhibits lipid peroxidation in both cell membranes and serum low-density lipoproteins and it also protects proteins and DNA from oxidative damage."[27]

The biomedical and clinical applications of coQ_{10} continue to generate tremendous interest throughout the world, says Dr. Sinatra. There have been at least 10 international symposia on the biomedical and clinical aspects of coQ_{10} since 1976, comprising over 450 papers presented by more than 250 physicians and scientists from 18 countries, who have investigated coQ_{10} supplementation in a wide range of medical disorders. The majority of these clinical studies have demonstrated coQ_{10}'s positive impact on heart disease and they have been remarkably consistent in their conclusions: treatment with coQ_{10} significantly improved a wide variety of cardiovascular diseases while producing no adverse effects or drug interactions.[28]

Clinical Studies on Coenzyme Q_{10}

Robert C. Atkins, M.D., reported that coQ_{10}, at a dose of 60 mg per day, can help to reduce high blood sugar within six months. Since hardening of the arteries is a frequently encountered complication of diabetes, coQ_{10} is doubly important.[29]

A 35-year-old woman with diabetes, aspiration pneumonia, respiratory failure, and other complications was treated with antibiotic therapy, but after one week her consciousness remained unclear. Later, she was given 160 mg per day of coQ_{10} for six months. In a one-year follow-up, the patient only needed diet restriction to control her diabetes.[30]

Dr. Sinatra has been using coQ_{10} for over a decade. He points to a study of 115 patients with hypertensive heart disease, in which coQ_{10} resulted in clinical improvements, lowering of elevated blood pressure, improved diastolic function, and a decrease in myocardial thickness in 53 percent of the patients. In a study involving seven patients with heart problems, all of them reported improvements in symptoms of fatigue and shortness of breath on an average of 200 mg per day of coQ_{10}. "I recommend that when patients fail to respond to standard levels of coQ_{10}—

90 to 150 mg per day—it is best to obtain a blood level," Dr. Sinatra said. "If a serum coQ_{10} level is not feasible, treat the patient clinically by doubling or even tripling the dose according to their clinical symptoms as cardiologists frequently do with diuretics and/or ACE inhibitors when treating congestive heart failure. The higher doses of coQ_{10} are required for patients with 'right-sided' cardiac symptoms, particularly rather serious myocardial coQ_{10} deficiencies have been found in cases with high right atrial pressures."[31]

Coenzyme Q_{10} (coQ_{10}) is present in the mitochondria, or "energy factories," of human cells, and it is a co-factor in several enzyme systems related to energy production, according to Per H. Langsjoen, of Scott and White Clinic, in Temple, Texas. Since myocardial cells have a high percentage of mitochondria and energy needs are great, it is believed that a deficiency of coQ_{10} would have a significant effect on heart function. In a study of nineteen patients with cardiomyopathy (a disorder of the heart muscle) who were treated with coQ_{10}, Langsjoen reported that there was a subsequent improvement in heart function and clinical status.[32]

A longer study was undertaken involving patients with chronic dilated cardiomyopathy, in which 126 patients were given 33.3 mg of coQ_{10} or a placebo three times daily. All of the patients, of whom 75 percent were 60–80 years of age, had symptoms of heart disease before the study began and all had been prescribed various medications. In 99 percent of the patients, heart failure was deemed the main complaint and 86 percent were experiencing pulmonary edema (fluid in the lungs). Other complaints were chest pain, arrhythmias, thromboembolism (blood clots), and heart blocks. As the study began, coQ_{10} levels in the heart patients were significantly below that of the fifty-four control patients. It was found that 71 percent of the patients improved on the coQ_{10} therapy within three months. After six months, 16 percent more had improved.[33]

Researchers in Denmark pointed out that a defective myocardial energy supply due to a poor utilization of oxygen may be a common final pathway in the progression of myocardial disease. However, coQ_{10} is a natural antioxidant to combat the problem. After taking myocardial tissue samples from 45 patients with a variety of cardiomyopathies, it was found that coQ_{10} was significantly lower in those with more advanced heart failure when compared to those with milder cases of the disease.

The researchers said that myocardial tissue coQ_{10} deficiency might be restored significantly with oral supplementation in selected cases.[34]

Doses of between 30 and 600 mg per day of coQ_{10} have been shown to benefit some patients with angina pectoris (chest pain), according to the *European Journal of Clinical Nutrition*. In addition, doses of between 60 and 200 mg per day provide some benefit in reducing blood pressure and other complications. The nutrient may also be useful when given one week before cardiovascular surgery.[35]

At the University of Firenze Medical School, in Florence, Italy, eighteen patients with essential hypertension (high blood pressure) were taken off all high blood pressure medications for two weeks and given either 100 mg per day of coQ_{10} or a placebo for ten weeks. After the ten-week period, no supplements were given for two weeks and then the two groups switched protocols for an additional ten weeks. It was reported that, after ten weeks of coQ_{10} therapy, systolic blood pressure (when the heart is beating) dropped about 10 points, while the diastolic pressure (when the heart rests between beats) dropped 7 points on average. The researchers concluded that coQ_{10} is beneficial as a hypertensive agent.[36]

In another study at the University of Firenze Medical School, researchers reported that coQ_{10} has shown potential in treating congestive heart failure, angina pectoris, high blood pressure, and arrhythmias. Their study involved five men and five women with a mean age of sixty-one. The patients with essential arterial hypertension were given 50 mg of coQ_{10} twice daily for ten weeks. At the end of the study, systolic blood pressure decreased from 161.5 mm Hg on average to 142.2 mm Hg; diastolic pressure decreased from 98.5 mm Hg to 83.1 mm Hg. Total blood cholesterol dropped from 227 to 203, while HDL cholesterol increased.[37]

At Hamamatsu University in Japan, twelve patients, average age of fifty-six, with stable angina pectoris, were given 50 mg of coQ_{10} three times daily for four weeks. The researchers found there was a reduction in anginal frequency and nitroglycerine use and an increase in exercise time. One patient had a loss of appetite, but continued the therapy.[38]

In an article in *American Journal of Cardiology*, Ram B. Singh, M.D., discussed a study in which two capsules of coQ_{10} were given twice daily to patients with myocardial infarction (heart attack). He found the supplement more effective than vitamins in controlling arrhythmias, angina, and left ventricular failure, as well as other cardiac events. He also found that the supplement can decrease hyperinsulinemia (too much insulin in the blood) and possibly lipoprotein-a, which is thought to be a risk factor for coronary disease.[39] Gerard K. Nash, D.O., said research showed that heart failure patients with coQ_{10} deficiency had a favorable eight-year survival rate when coQ_{10} supplements are given.[40]

Coenzyme Q_{10} treatment is indicated in high-risk cardiac surgery patients who have coQ_{10} deficiency, according to Karl Folkers, Ph.D., of the University of Texas, in Austin, a pioneer in coQ_{10} research. The study involved ten high-risk patients during heart surgery compared to ten people who did not have a high risk, who were given 100 mg per day of the supplement for fourteen days prior to and thirty days after surgery. The recovery course, 3–5 days, was uncomplicated in the coQ_{10} group. In an open trial conducted by S.A. Mortensen, M.D., coQ_{10} therapy at 100 mg per day resulted in almost two-thirds of the patients having clinical improvements. Double-blind studies have confirmed the efficacy of coQ_{10} as an adjunctive treatment in heart failure.[41]

Since heart disease is a major concern for diabetics, it would seem prudent for them to review the coQ_{10} research with their health-care provider.

Taking Coenzyme Q_{10}

Food sources include beef muscle, beef heart, and eggs.

Robert C. Atkins, M.D., prescribed coQ_{10} for anyone with a health problem related to the heart, blood pressure, metabolism, energy level, or cancer. A minimum dose of 90 mg per day is required for a therapeutic response. For cancer protection, he recommended 200–400 mg per day.[42]

CHAPTER 12

Herbs

H erbal medicine has been used worldwide for centuries for treating a wide variety of health conditions. A number of herbs and supplements have proven useful in dealing with diabetes.

- Onion (400 milligrams of a standardized extract) improves glucose utilization.

- Bitter melon improves glucose utilization, when used as a 5 ml tincture two to three times a day to a total as high as 50 ml per day.

- *Gymnema sylvestre* lowers blood pressure, when given as 0.75 teaspoon in a glass of hot water as a tea.

- Fenugreek (625 mg, 2–3 times daily) improves glucose utilization.

- Stevia, a sweetener, improves glucose utilization, when taken at 200 mg twice daily.

- St. John's wort (425 mg of standard extract twice daily) helps to control depression and possibly diabetic neuropathy.

- Ivy gourd enhances glucose metabolism, when taken as six tablets a day in divided doses.[1]

Combinations of herbs may also be useful for the complications associated with diabetes. In studying 370 women and 526 men in Morocco, 61 percent had diabetes, 23 percent were hypertensives, and 16 percent were hypertensive diabetics, yet two-thirds of the patients regularly used medicinal plants to control their disease. For diabetics, forty-one plants were used, the most popular being *Trigonella foenum-graecum* (fenugreek), *Artemisia vulgaris,* and *Citrullus colocynthis* (colocynth). For high blood pressure, the patients were using eighteen different herbs, including garlic, *Olea europea* (olive), *Arbutus unedo* (cane apples), *Urtica doica* (nettle), and *Petroselinum crispum* (parsley).[2]

Bitter Melon (*Momordica charantia*)

Indian researchers have reported on the ability of bitter melon to reduce blood sugar. In animal studies, the herb delayed the development of diabetic complications. In a later human trial, those with diabetes who consumed 2 ounces of bitter melon juice a day saw their blood sugar levels decline by 54 percent. Dried fruits and seeds from the plant also help to reduce blood sugar.[3]

Bitter melon has some ninety names around the world, including ampalaya, cundeamor, bitter gourd, balsam pear, and karela. Clinical studies with animals and humans provide sufficient evidence that ampalaya's leaf and fruit extract, its dried powdered leaf, as well as the whole fruit can significantly reduce blood sugar, according to William D. Torres, Ph.D., of the University of the Philippines, in Manila. A number of studies have described the many constituents in ampalaya, including vitamins A, B_1, B_2, B_3, and vitamin C, calcium, iron, phosphorus, amino acids, aromatic oils, alkaloids, lectins, polypeptides, and fatty acids.[4]

A tea or capsule made from bitter melon, taken after each meal, dramatically lowers blood sugar levels in diabetics. Guia Abad, M.D., president of the Association of Municipal Health Officers in the Philippines, said, "After a few days, or within a month, of drinking ampalaya tea to fortify their usual diet, regular exercise, and medication, many of our patients with diabetes have an easier time of lowering their blood sugar levels. While having their blood-sugar levels monitored by their doctor, many of these people have been able to gradually reduce their medications for diabetes." Many type 1 and type 2 diabetics have benefited from using ampalaya as a tea or capsule, or by eating the vegetable:

- S.L., a 69-year-old type 2 diabetic has had the disease for ten years. With ampalaya tea and an improved diet, her blood sugar has decreased from 200 mg/dl to 153 mg/dl.

- C.P., a 66-year-old Filipino, had to have his right foot amputated because of diabetes. At the time, his blood sugar registered 265 mg/dl. By using ampalaya tea, his reading has gone down to 122 mg/dl.

- A.T., a 73-year-old Filipino, has had type 2 diabetes for sixteen years. With ampalaya tea and an improved diet, his blood sugar reading went from over 200 mg/dl down to 110 mg/dl.

- P.M., a 35-year-old Austrian, discovered he had diabetes when his blood sugar reading soared to 300 mg/dl. With a better diet, exercise, medication, and ampalaya tea, his blood sugar reading is now 90 mg/dl on an empty stomach and 150 mg/dl after he has eaten.[5]

Capsaicin

While capsaicin cream (from chili peppers) has been recommended for treating arthritis, it is also useful in dealing with diabetic neuropathy, according to researchers at Case Western Reserve University School of Medicine, in Cleveland, Ohio. Purified capsaicin depletes Substance P, which contributes to pain and inflammation.[6]

Fenugreek

At the National Institute of Nutrition, in Jamai-Osmania, Hyderbad, India, ten type 1 diabetics were given 100 mg of fenugreek seed powder, divided into two equal dosages and placed in the diets. The patients, ranging in age from twelve to thirty-seven, were given this therapy for two 10-day periods. The fenugreek diet considerably reduced fasting blood sugar levels, improved glucose tolerance, and led to a 54 percent reduction in daily urinary glucose excretion. Total cholesterol, LDL ("bad") cholesterol, and triglyceride levels also decreased, while HDL ("good") cholesterol remained unchanged.[7]

Fig Leaves (*Ficus carica*)

Drinking a decoction of fig leaves lowered the required insulin dose by 12 percent in a group of six men and four women, twenty-two to thirty-eight years of age, who had suffered with type 1 diabetes for nine years. The fig leaf decoction was taken for one month, followed by consuming a non-sweet commercial tea for the second month in a crossover design. Following a meal, the amount of glucose in the blood was significantly lower during the fig leaf supplement period when compared with the tea.[8]

Garlic Oil

A research team at John Bastyr College of Naturopathic Medicine, in Seattle, Washington, reported that garlic oil could be effective as part of a program to control and prevent hardening of the arteries and coronary artery disease, since it lowers cholesterol, blood pressure, and platelet aggregation. Coronary artery disease is a potential complication of diabetes. In the study, twenty healthy volunteers were randomly divided into two groups and rotated for four-week periods through two different sequences of oral garlic oil or placebo (18 mg per day). The amount of platelet aggregation dropped and serum cholesterol levels and blood pressure also declined with the garlic oil therapy.[9]

Ginseng (*Panax ginseng*)

Ginseng has been used for treating diabetes, cancer risk, high blood pressure, and colds and flu. For example, in one Korean study involving twenty-six volunteers with high blood pressure, those receiving 4.5 grams per day of red ginseng for eight weeks experienced a decrease in 24-hour mean systolic (beating) blood pressure and a slight decline in diastolic (resting) blood pressure.[10]

Researchers at the University of Oulu in Finland treated thirty-six type 2 diabetics for eight weeks, giving them 100 mg or 200 mg per day of ginseng or a placebo. They reported that the ginseng elevated mood, improved mental and bodily processes, and reduced fasting blood sugar and body weight. The larger dosage improved glycosylated hemoglobin and other parameters of diabetes.[11]

A study reported in *Archives of Internal Medicine* involved ten non-diabetics and nine type 2 diabetics. The participants were randomly selected to receive 3 g of ginseng or placebo pills either 40 minutes before or together with a 25-gram glucose challenge. The results showed no difference in the non-diabetic volunteers in after-eating sugar levels between placebo and ginseng when given with the glucose challange, but when ginseng was taken 40 minutes before the glucose challenges, significant reductions were recorded.[12] In type 2 diabetics, the same was true, whether the ginseng was taken before or together with the glucose challenge. It was found that American ginseng (*P. quinquefolius*) reduced after-meal glucose levels in both treatment groups.

Standardized ginseng extracts should contain 4 percent ginsenosides. Those who use this form should take 100 mg twice daily. For those who use non-standardized raw ginseng powder, the recommended dose is 1–2 g per day for up to three months. While the World Health Organization has recorded two incidents in which ginseng interacted with phenelzine, a monoamine oxidase (MAO) inhibitor (drugs designed to treat depression, high blood pressure, and other conditions), there have been relatively few adverse effects using the herb.

Gurmar (*Gymnema sylvestre*)

Gymnema sylvestre is an Ayurvedic herb that may be useful for diabetics. It is thought that the herb may regenerate or revitalize pancreatic beta cells. There may be an increase in insulin levels or a decrease in insulin resistance, but these mechanisms are still hypothetical.

In a study involving twenty-two type 2 diabetics, who were given 400 mg per day of gurmar in addition to conventional oral hypoglycemia agents for 18–20 months, there was a reduction in glycosylated hemoglobin levels (a measure of blood sugar) from 12 to 8.5 percent. In another study, involving twenty-seven type 1 diabetics, whose condition was followed for up to thirty months, volunteers were given 400 mg per day of gurmar for 6–8 months. Their average insulin requirement dropped from 60 to 45 units per day (30 percent) and their serum lipids returned to near normal levels.[13]

Jackass Bitters (*Neurolaena lobata*)

When this plant's ability to control type 2 diabetes becomes better known, jackass bitters will become easier to find. Its use in treating diabetes surfaced in 1989, when a Florida physician sent a sample to Walter Mertz, M.D., then director of the U.S. Department of Agriculture Health Nutrition Research Center, in Beltsville, Maryland, wondering what the plant was. One of his patients with type 2 diabetes had found the herb on a trip to the island of Trinidad. She made her own concoction and sipped it twice daily for six months. Her blood sugar normalized. Subsequent animal studies have found that jackass bitters tincture significantly lowers blood sugar levels.[14]

Marshmallow (*Althaea officinalis*)

This root is very high in a soluble plant fiber known as pectin (35 percent on a dry-weight basis). Taking pectin is an effective way of keeping blood sugar levels down, according to James A. Duke, Ph.D., a leading expert on herbs.[15]

Milk Thistle (*Silybum marianum*)

Silymarin is the main active component in milk thistle. At Hospital Monfalcone, in Italy, Mari Velussi, M.D., and colleagues studied sixty cirrhotic diabetic patients, ranging in age from forty-five to seventy, who were getting insulin and who had high insulin levels. The patients received either 600 mg per day of silymarin or no silymarin for six months. After six months of therapy, the silymarin-treated diabetics had levels of fasting glucose, daily blood glucose, daily glycosuria (sugar in the urine), glycosylated hemoglobin, daily insulin need, fasting insulinemia, and basal and glucagon-stimulated C peptide measured. All of these parameters were lower than in the untreated patients and lower than when the study began.[16]

These results suggest that milk thistle can reduce lipoperoxidation of liver cells in diabetics with cirrhosis of the liver and increase production of insulin inside the body, thus decreasing the need for insulin injections. Lipid peroxides are toxic molecules that can harm the body. Silymarin apparently restores the plasma membrane of liver cells and increases the sensitivity of insulin receptors.

Red Wine

A moderate amount of red wine during meals may help to prevent cardiovascular disease in diabetics, according to the *European Journal of Clinical Investigation*. The study involved twenty type 2 diabetics, average age of fifty-five years and they had had diabetes for nine years. The patients were evaluated during fasting consumption of 300 ml of red wine or during a meal in which they were given red wine or abstained. The researchers reported that red wine consumption during a meal significantly preserved antioxidant defenses in the blood and reduced low-density lipoprotein (LDL) cholesterol oxidation and development of blood clots. The beneficial nutrient in red wine is thought to be resveratrol.[17]

Tulasi (*Ocimum sanctum*)

Eugenol, a major component of the essential oil in tulasi leaves, has been found to inhibit lipid peroxidation. It is suspected that eugenol protects the beta cells in the pancreas from free-radical damage, thus allowing increased insulin secretion. Twenty-seven type 2 diabetics received 1 g of tulasi powder, which was consumed in a fasting state each morning for thirty days. Following one month of therapy, there were lower levels of blood glucose (20.8 percent), glycated proteins (11.2 percent), and uronic acid (13.7 percent; an oxidation product of sugars). In addition, total cholesterol was reduced 11.3 percent, LDL cholesterol went down 14 percent, very-low-density lipoprotein cholesterol was reduced 16.3 percent, and triglycerides were reduced 16.4 percent. There was no change in HDL cholesterol.[18]

CHAPTER 13

Why You Need to Exercise

Exercise can provide a host of benefits for diabetics. Type 2 diabetics can get impressive improvements in health and reductions in health care costs just by making modest increases in physical activity. This optimistic message about physical activity and type 2 diabetes doesn't mean it's necessary for patients to do a lot of strenuous exercise to reap health benefits. Diabetic patients should be encouraged to walk regularly, because it is probably one of the best things they can do for their health.[1]

Western and developing countries face two serious health problems, namely, the rising prevalence of obesity and diabetes and the fact that people no longer feel the need to be physically active in their daily lives, according to Chiara Di Loreto.[2] "Many studies have shown that regular physical activity improves the quality of life, reduces the risk of mortality from all causes, and is particularly advantageous in subjects with impaired glucose tolerance or type 2 diabetes," Di Loreto stated.

Over half of the U.S. population is overweight or obese, and the prevalence is especially high among women. Obesity increases the risk of coronary heart disease, type 2 diabetes, high blood pressure, stroke, colon cancer, and postmenopausal breast cancer. Physical activity may provide a low-risk method of preventing weight gain and promoting maintenance of weight loss in overweight and obese women. And unlike dieting, weight loss from exercise increases cardiorespiratory fitness.[3]

Moderate-intensity exercise produces significant changes in body weight, total body fat, and intra-abdominal and subcutaneous abdominal body fat. Previously sedentary postmenopausal women who exercised about 200 minutes per week lost 4.2 percent of total body fat and

6.9 percent of intra-abdominal fat while maintaining their energy intake. In addition, 84 percent of the exercisers in the study improved their cardiorespiratory fitness, which reduces the rate of cardiovascular morbidity and mortality, independent of obesity. Overweight women (and men) should be encouraged to begin moderate-intensity exercise as a way of obesity reduction and chronic disease prevention.[4]

In diabetics, exercise can reduce insulin resistance. Obese children tend to have elevated insulin levels, which can normalize with exercise. Daily participation in a prescribed exercise program is highly beneficial to health for many reasons. It increases blood supply to all organs and tissues; improves muscle/tendon/ligament strength, mobility and flexibility; releases endorphins, the body's "feel good" hormones; enhances bone formation; and stimulates creativity.[5] Exercise can also help to prevent high cholesterol and bone loss, reduce anxiety and stress, and elevate mood.

Clinical Studies on Exercise and Diabetes

In a study conducted between 1970 and 1993 of 1,263 fifty-year-old male type 2 diabetics, the participants were given a thorough physical. During an average follow-up of twelve years, eighteen had died. After adjusting for variables, the researchers found that those in the low-fitness group had an adjusted risk for all-cause mortality of 2.1, compared with those who were fit. The diabetics who said they were physically inactive had an adjusted risk of death that was 7.7-fold higher than those who were physically active.[6]

Low-fat diets and a half hour of walking and other exercise daily can reduce the risk of developing diabetes by 58 percent among those at high risk, according to a national survey by the National Institutes of Health, in Bethesda, Maryland. All of the 3,234 volunteers in the study were overweight and had trouble controlling the amount of sugar in their blood, a major contributor to type 2 diabetes. Those who were counseled on lifestyle changes, such as diet and exercise, lost on average 15 pounds during the three-year study. "Diabetes is not inevitable," reported Robert E. Ratner of the MedStar Research Institute, in Washington, D.C., one of the participants in the study.[7] While the study doesn't prove that these interventions will permanently prevent diabetes, even delaying the onset of the disease could prevent many costly complications, such as blindness and kidney failure. In the study, one-third of the participants were given individual counseling about diet, exercise, and other lifestyle changes. Another third took the diabetes drug metformin, while the remaining third were given a placebo. In each year of the study, 11 percent of those getting the placebo developed diabetes, 7.8 percent getting the drug developed the disease, and only 4.8 percent in the counseling group developed diabetes.

Researchers at the University of Ottawa report that exercise training can reduce glycosylated hemoglobin (hemoglobin A_{1C}) sufficiently to decrease the risk of diabetic complications. Hemoglobin A_{1C} is the substance formed when glucose is attached to hemoglobin molecules. Their conclusions came after reviewing a meta-analysis of controlled clinical trials, which showed that exercise can reduce hemoglobin A_{1C} by about 0.66 percent, a small amount but one that could cut the risk of diabetic complications significantly.[8] "Two of the major goals of diabetes therapy are to reduce hyperglycemia (abnormal amounts of glucose in the blood) and body fat," the researchers said. "Chronic hyperglycemia is associated with significant long-term complications, particularly damage to the kidneys, eyes, nerves, heart, and blood vessels. Obesity, especially abdominal obesity, is associated with insulin resistance, hyperinsulinemia, hyperglycemia, dyslipidemia, and hypertension. These abnormalities tend to cluster and are often referred to as the metabolic syndrome."

At Ohio State University College of Medicine, in Columbus, a research team concluded that exercise is also beneficial to type 1 diabetics. They reported that exercise increases insulin sensitivity (the normal state in which the cells of the body are receptive to the action of insulin) and reduces blood glucose levels. They added that an appropriate diet and insulin monitoring enables type 1 diabetics to exercise safely and regularly. To prevent hypoglycemia, the researchers suggested that the insulin doses may have to be reduced 30 to 50 percent before exercise begins. Avoiding taking regular insulin at bedtime and reducing the evening insulin dose may help to prevent nocturnal hypoglycemia after exercising.[9]

At Nagoya University, in Japan, ten type 2 diabetics were managed by diet alone and fourteen other diabetics were placed on a diet and exercise program. The exercise group was required to walk at least 10,000 steps daily, which were monitored by a pedometer. The other group followed its usual daily routine. While the body weight of both groups went down significantly during the study, the exercisers lost the most weight. In addition, the glucose infusion rate and the metabolic clearance rate went up substantially in those who were exercising. The authors said that walking can be safely incorporated into a daily routine and it can be recommended as an adjunctive therapy in the treatment of obese type 2 diabetics.[10]

Epidemiological studies reveal that those who have a physically active lifestyle are less likely to develop type 2 diabetes or impaired glucose tolerance. The protective effect of exercise is strongest for those who are at the highest risk of developing type 2 diabetes. Older people who have vigorously exercised on a regular basis have a greater glucose tolerance and lower insulin response to glucose than sedentary elderly people of similar height and weight. Exercise results in loss of fat from the central regions of the body and this should significantly prevent or alleviate insulin resistance. Several months of weight training can significantly lower the insulin response to a glucose challenge without affecting glucose tolerance. Exercise should be done on a regular basis and exercising

THE IMPORTANCE OF RESISTANCE TRAINING

Type 2 diabetes increases with age partly due to a reduction in muscle mass associated with aging. However, muscle mass can be enhanced with resistance training. An optimal exercise program consists of a combination of aerobic endurance training and circuit-type resistance training.[11]

Two sessions a week of progressive resistance training, even without a companion weight loss diet, significantly improves insulin sensitivity, fasting glycemia, and decreases abdominal fat in older men with type 2 diabetes, according to Javier Ibanez, M.D., Ph.D. "Exercise training results in preferential loss of fat from the central regions and it seems that this loss of visceral adipose tissue is closely related to an improvement in insulin sensitivity," Dr. Ibanez stated. "Moreover, exercise alone in the absence of body composition change is able to enhance glucose homeostasis (balance)."[12] This study provides support for the safety and effectiveness of twice-weekly exercise bouts for older men with type 2 diabetes. After sixteen weeks of progressive resistance training, the researchers observed significant improvements in muscle strength, insulin sensitivity, and glucose tolerance, and a significant decrease in abdominal fat.

with a variety of different exercises and using different large muscle groups helps to prevent and treat insulin resistance.[13]

Researchers at the University of Miami School of Medicine, in Florida, evaluated ten male adolescents with type 1 diabetes and ten youngsters who were not diabetic, to see the effect of an aerobic, strength, and callisthenic circuit training program. Mean age of the diabetics was 17.2 years. For twelve weeks, the volunteers underwent a 45-minute exercise program, three times weekly, to work all the major muscle groups. The researchers reported that the diabetics improved their cardiorespiratory endurance, muscle strength, lipid profile, and glucose regulation with the exercise, and that such a program is safe for properly trained and monitored adolescent diabetics.[14]

Insulin resistance is associated with large amounts of abdominal body fat and may cause 25 percent of cardiovascular disease in men and 60 percent of that found in women. However, low-intensity exercise, including walking briskly for forty-five minutes on a treadmill or outdoors, can lower a diabetic's insulin resistance and need for insulin. As an example, the risk of type 2 diabetes was reduced by 25 percent and heart disease risk reduced by 50 percent in those who were moderately active.[15] Researchers have found that insulin resistance is not associated with the total amount of excess fat on a person, but rather on how much fat is found in the abdominal area. In fact, one out of every four men, age forty and over, has excess abdominal fat and insulin resistance. Researchers have further found that abdominal fat is associated with a 20 to 25 percent increase in apolipoprotein-b (apo-b) levels, which is a reliable predictor of ischemic heart disease. Elevated insulin levels raise triglycerides and reduce high-density lipoprotein (HDL) cholesterol, which increases the risk of hardening of the arteries. Raised levels of insulin and apo-b, which are found in insulin resistance syndrome, are said to bring an 11-fold increase in heart disease risk.

Exercise is necessary for the prevention and treatment of high blood pressure. As an example, a meta-analysis of thirteen controlled studies on exercise showed a mean reduction of 11.3 mm Hg in systolic blood pressure and 7.5 mm Hg in diastolic pressure.[16]

Tips and Precautions

Researchers have long known that exercise increases cardiac output, redistributes blood flow, and increases blood flow to the muscles. For most people, exercising at 65 to 75 percent of the VO_2 maximum is a suggested goal. VO_2 measures oxygen consumption. For a 40-year-old, a safe pulse rate ranges between 117 and 135 beats per minute. For a 60-year-old, the safe range is between 104 and 120 beats per minute.[17]

While exercise is an important therapeutic tool for diabetics, it also produces oxidative stress, which, theoretically, can increase the risk of blood vessel complications. Oxidative stress is associated with an increase in free radicals, since oxygen molecules are usually involved in the creation of these destructive elements. For example, hyperglycemia (too much glucose in the blood) can stimulate the production of oxidative free radicals in the blood of diabetics. Also, exercise results in a significant increase in oxygen uptake at the whole-body level and in skeletal muscle.[18]

However, exercise increases the activity of catalase, superoxide dismutase, and glutathione in skeletal muscle and the heart and liver. Catalase is an enzyme that aids in the decomposing of hydrogen peroxide into water, superoxide dismutase is an enzyme that helps to deactivate harmful free radicals, and glutathione is an antioxidant that protects against free radicals. It is suggested that a lot of exercise in a type 2 diabetic who is untrained would result in more sustained oxidative stress. A trained diabetic would sustain less oxidative stress, presumably due to the induction of certain antioxidant enzyme systems.

CHAPTER 14

Treating Diabetes in Women and Children

Diabetes and Women

Several lifestyle factors affect the incidence of type 2 diabetes, especially in women. Obesity and weight gain dramatically increase the risk, and physical inactivity further elevates the risk independently of obesity. Cigarette smoking is associated with a small increase, and moderate alcohol consumption is associated with a decrease in the risk of diabetes. Also, a low-fiber diet with a high glycemic index (which reflects the effect of diet on blood glucose levels) has been associated with an increased risk of diabetes, and specific dietary fatty acids may differentially affect insulin resistance and the risk of diabetes.

The glycemic index (GI) of a carbohydrate is a measure of how much that food raises blood glucose compared with a standard carbohydrate, usually glucose or white bread. Several studies have shown a positive association between a high-glycemic diet and the risk of type 2 diabetes. Consumption of these foods may increase the risk of type 2 diabetes. Substituting lower glycemic, high-fiber forms of carbohydrates such as whole grains for high-glycemic foods should be encouraged.[1]

Researchers followed 84,941 female nurses from 1980 to 1996. The volunteers were free of diagnosed cardiovascular disease, diabetes, and cancer as the study began. A low-risk group was defined according to various variables: a body mass index (BMI; weight in kilograms divided by the square of the height in meters) of less than 25; a diet that was high in cereal fiber and polyunsaturated fat and low in trans-fat and glycemic load; amount of moderate-to-vigorous physical activity for at least half an hour per day; no smoking; and the consumption of an average of at least half a drink of an alcoholic beverage daily. During 16 years of follow-up, they documented 3,300 new cases of type 2 diabetes. Being overweight or obese was the strongest predictor of diabetes, and sedentary lifestyle, poor diet, cigarette smoking, and abstinence from alcohol were also associated with an increased risk.[2]

A research team at Sansum Medical Research Foundation, in Santa Barbara, California, reported that using low-carbohydrate diets to minimize glucose changes and decrease insulin secretion might decrease the prevalence of diabetes in women who had previously been diagnosed with gestational diabetes, which develops during a woman's pregnancy. In the study, calories consisted of nutritional supplement bars, except for the evening meal, which consisted of one-third of caloric needs based on two carbohydrate levels (55 percent and 40 percent). The twelve-week trial involved twenty-three obese women, thirteen of whom had had gestational diabetes. The women with previous gestational diabetes had higher results on a glucose tolerance test and higher fasting insulin levels that were consistent with greater insulin resistance. The participants all had higher triglyceride levels while on a 55 percent carbohydrate diet than while on the 40 percent carbohydrate diet. The researchers pointed out that a weight loss regimen that consists of 40 percent carbohydrates results in lower triglyceride levels than those attained with a 55 percent carbohydrate diet in obese women. Further, the hypoglycemic diet with the higher fat content brought the more favorable amounts of fat to all of the obese women. Those who switched to a 55 percent carbohydrate diet from 40 percent showed an increase in serum triglycerides, whereas those who switched to 40 percent from 55 percent showed a decrease.[3]

Gestational Diabetes

Approximately 135,000 cases of gestational diabetes are diagnosed in the U.S. annually, according to Dana Dabelea, M.D., Ph.D., and colleagues at the University of Colorado Health Sciences Center, in Denver. This condition appears to be more prevalent among Native-American, Asian, African-American, and Hispanic populations than among non-Hispanic whites. Exposure to high levels of glucose in the blood of the mother during pregnancy is associated with birth defects and it affects childhood growth and glucose regulation. As many as 50 percent of women with gestational diabetes may develop type 2 diabetes within five years of delivery.[4]

Gestational diabetes reflects a metabolically altered fetal environment because of an increased maternal supply of carbohydrates that leads to high levels of insulin in the blood of the fetus. Stimulation of the insulin-sensitive tissue results in increased fetal growth, predominantly of the abdomen, and the delivery of large-for-gestational-age newborns. Children of mothers with diabetes in pregnancy may develop an increased disposition for obesity and glucose intolerance. Effective preventive intervention must start at the earliest possible age, as accelerated intrauterine growth is a major antenatal factor for later overweight. In addition, in offspring of mothers with gestational diabetes, shared familial dietary and physical activity habits may strongly influence the risk of childhood obesity. So, promoting healthy diet and lifestyle factors, combined with closely following the child's development, is critical to reducing the risk of obesity.[5]

Women with a diagnosis of gestational diabetes have a 35 to 50 percent chance of reoccurrence in future pregnancies, and a 40 to 60 percent increased risk of developing type 2 diabetes within ten years, according to researchers at Pennsylvania State University. Children of these women also have an elevated risk of developing obesity and diabetes in their lifetime. "One approach that may be effective for both treating and preventing gestational diabetes is engaging in regular exercise," the researchers said. "Exercise is recommended during pregnancy and it provides physiological benefits to women with gestational diabetes, such as lowering blood glucose and controlling excessive gestational weight gain. In addition, exercise may be less stressful and more acceptable to women than insulin injections."[6]

Offspring of diabetic mothers are at an increased risk of developing overweight and impaired glucose tolerance, even in childhood, but breastfeeding was shown to protect against later overweight and diabetes. The benefits of breastfeeding are related to the composition of mother's milk versus formula. The first week of life appears to be the critical window for nutritional programming of the offspring of diabetic mothers.[7]

In New York City alone, gestational diabetes has risen by almost 50 percent during the past ten years, according to a story in the *New York Times*. Barbara Hackley, a certified nurse-midwife at the Children's

Health Fund and Montefiore Medical Center, in the South Bronx, stated, "It's really disturbing to us that women come into their pregnancies obese and then leave them even more obese. I've seen weight gains during pregnancies of fifty to sixty pounds. We've had 11- and 12-pound babies that are very dangerous to deliver." Doctors have often disagreed on how ambitiously to regulate the conditions of mothers-to-be with gestational diabetes. They usually recommend diet changes, such as cutting down on carbohydrates, juices, and sugared soda, and exercising. These women often take insulin injections, and they are advised to monitor their blood sugar four times daily.[8]

Osteoporosis

Researchers at the University of Pittsburgh reported that type 1 diabetes in middle-aged women was associated with a 3 to 8 percent bone mineral density at the total hip, femoral neck, and whole body, and a 15 percent lower bone ultrasound, after adjustments for fat mass and other potential mediators. "Type 1 diabetic women with lower bone mineral density before menopause may be at an even greater risk for osteoporosis and osteopenia after the menopausal transition compared with nondiabetic women," reported Elsa S. Strotmeyer, Ph.D. "Type 1 diabetic women may experience an earlier decrease in bone mineral density due to aging, given their younger age at menopause. Since type 1 diabetic women are at a markedly increased risk for fractures, osteoporosis screening or fracture prevention efforts may be appropriate."[9]

Cardiovascular Disease

Cardiovascular disease is a leading cause of death in the Western world, but the risk of heart disease in women is only half that of men. On the other hand, type 2 diabetes is associated with a two- to four-fold greater risk of CVD and, unlike the general population, women with diabetes are at a higher risk of CVD than are men with diabetes.[10]

A higher intake of cholesterol and saturated fat, and a low ratio of polyunsaturated to saturated fat is related to increased cardiovascular disease (CVD) among women with type 2 diabetes. In fact, among diabetics, the replacement of saturated fats with monounsaturated fats may be more effective in lowering cholesterol risk than is replacing carbohydrates. It is important to reduce intakes of cholesterol and to reduce saturated fat with unhydrogenated unsaturated fat. Further, researchers found that replacing 5 percent of the energy from saturated fat with equivalent energy from carbohydrates or monounsaturated fat was associated with a 22 percent or 37 percent lower risk of CVD, respectively.[11]

Specific Therapies for Women

Vitamins and Minerals

Thiamine (Vitamin B_1)—In evaluating seventy-seven mothers and newborns at birth, 19 percent of the pregnancies were found to be deficient in thiamine (B_1), in spite of vitamin supplementation and treatment for gestational diabetes. The newborn's blood had significantly higher levels of vitamin B_1 than did the pregnant women. Cord blood from newborns born to mothers who were treated with insulin for gestational diabetes had significantly higher vitamin B_1 concentrations than other newborns. Low levels of B_1 are frequently found in pregnant women in spite of vitamin supplementation, suggesting that the fetus is getting first dibs on the vitamin.[12]

Chromium—A deficiency in chromium might be related to gestational diabetes in pregnant women, according to a study at the Israel Institute of Technology, in Haifa. The results were determined after analyzing hair samples from normal and pregnant women.[13]

Calcium—Researchers reported in *Diabetes Care* that intakes of calcium and vitamin D from supplements, rather than from diet, were significantly associated with a lower risk of type 2 diabetes. This may be the first prospective study to suggest that the two nutrients may reduce the risk of type 2 diabetes in women. Women who consumed 800 IU per day or more of vitamin D had a 32 percent lower risk of developing diabetes when compared to women who consumed 200 IU per day. And women who consumed around 1,200 mg per day of calcium had a 21 percent lower risk of developing diabetes than women who were getting less than 600 mg per day.[14] If these results are confirmed, it will have important public health implications, since these two interventions can be implemented easily and inexpensively to prevent type 2 diabetes.

Researchers at Brigham and Women's Hospital, in Boston, Massachusetts, have concluded that a high calcium intake and dairy products are associated with a lower prevalence of metabolic syndrome in middle-aged and older women.[15] Metabolic syndrome is a precursor to the development of diabetes. Other epidemiologic studies have also suggested that low calcium intake may be a risk factor for primary high blood pressure.

Calcium supplementation lowers diastolic blood pressure (when the heart is resting between beats) in women with pregnancy-induced high blood pressure, but not in those with normal blood pressure, according to a research team at Auburn University, in Alabama. The study involved twenty pregnant women with high blood pressure and thirty pregnant women without the problem, ranging in age from eighteen to twenty-eight. During the twenty-week study, the women received 1,000 mg per day of calcium.[16]

Multivitamin and Mineral Supplementation—At the Sansum Medical Research Foundation, in Santa Barbara, California, Lois Jovanovic-Peterson, M.D., found that pregnant women with diabetes need extra vitamins and minerals because of increased nutrient losses in the urine due to frequent urination. For example, deficiencies are often found in magnesium, potassium, chromium, and vitamin B_6. Vitamin and mineral supplements may help to prevent pregnancy-related glucose intolerance, especially when the above-mentioned nutrients are taken.[17]

Healthy Fats

Excess body fat due to an imbalance between energy intake and physical activity is a major risk factor for type 2 diabetes, according to researchers at the Harvard School of Public Health. Their study suggests that total and saturated fat intakes as well as monounsaturated fatty acid intake are not associated with risk of type 2 diabetes in women. However, trans-fatty acids increase the risk, and polyunsaturated fatty acids reduce the risk of developing the disease. Substituting non-hydrogenated polyunsaturated fatty acids for trans-fatty acids would likely reduce the risk of type 2 diabetes substantially. Their study, based on a fourteen-year follow-up to the Nurses' Health Study, estimated that replacing 5 percent of energy from saturated fats with polyunsaturated fatty acids was associated with a 35 percent lower risk of developing diabetes. Replacing 2 percent of energy from trans-fatty acids with polyunsaturated fatty acids was associated with a 40 percent lower risk of developing the disease.[18]

In a study of 85 diabetic volunteers compared to 1,071 controls, the offspring of mothers who took cod liver oil during their pregnancy had a 30 percent lower risk of diabetes. Mothers given multivitamin supplements during their pregnancy and infants given cod liver oil, as well as vitamin D supplements, during the first year of life were not significantly associated with diabetes. It is believed that either vitamin D or the omega-3 fatty acids EPA (eicosapentaenoic acid) and DHA (docosahexaenoic acid) found in cod liver oil, or a combination of the two, have a protective effect against type 1 diabetes.[19]

Physical Exercise

In the Nurses' Health Study, researchers evaluated 5,125 female nurses with diabetes during a 14-year follow-up. During that time, 323 cases of cardiovascular disease were recorded, including 225 with coronary heart disease and 98 with strokes. Levels of exercise were inversely associated with coronary heart disease and ischemic stroke. Also, a faster walking pace was independently associated with a lower risk for cardiovascular disease.[20]

Diabetes and Children

Diabetes mellitus has always been classified as either juvenile-onset (type 1) or adult-onset (type 2), due to distinct differences in the usual age of presentation of the two conditions, explains David S. Ludwig, M.D., Ph.D., and Cara B. Ebbeling, Ph.D., of Children's Hospital in Boston, Massachusetts. However, with the increasing prevalence of type 2 diabetes in children, these terms are now inaccurate. "Recent estimates suggest that type 2 diabetes mellitus may now account for as many as half of all new cases of diabetes in certain pediatric populations," the authors reported in the *Journal of the American Medical Association*. "This apparent epidemic, attributable to the increased rates of obesity in children, carries enormous long-term public health implications."[21]

Currently, there are no nationwide epidemiological data focusing on type 2 diabetes in children, but prevalence has been estimated at between 2 and 50 per 1,000 in various populations. These rates have increased as much as tenfold in the last two decades. In two studies from the 1990s of people aged 10–19 years of age, type 2 diabetes accounted for 33 to 46 percent of all diabetes in those age groups. In addition to obesity, risk factors for type 2 diabetes in children include ethnicity, age, sex, sedentary lifestyle, family history, and perinatal influences. Type 2 diabetes is more common in American Indian, African-American, and Hispanic children. Risk appears to increase with either low or high birth weight, perhaps because under-nutrition or over-nutrition in utero (in the womb) may cause permanent metabolic and hormonal changes that promote obesity, insulin resistance, and beta-cell dysfunction later in life. (Beta cells make and release insulin in the pancreas, which controls the level of glucose or sugar in the blood.)

As a result of this epidemic, we face the prospect of coronary heart disease becoming a disease of young adulthood. This calls for a public health campaign to identify novel treatments for obesity and insulin resistance, public schools to promote physical activity and fitness, the commercial food industry to market healthful foods to children, and parents to model and support healthful lifestyle choices.[22]

Obesity

The incidence of type 1 and type 2 diabetes in children appears to be increasing in the United States, largely attributable (at least in type 2 diabetes) to the emerging epidemic of childhood obesity, according to Joyce M. Lee, M.D., and colleagues at the University of Michigan, in Ann Arbor.[23] In one small study, the prevalence of diabetes among adolescents aged 12 to 19 was 4.1 per 1,000. However, the Michigan researchers reported that the estimated prevalence of diabetes among U.S. children under the age of 18 was 3.2 per 1,000. "We found that obese children were over two-fold more likely to have diabetes than children of normal weight, offering evidence that obesity may be a significant contributing factor to the development of childhood diabetes," Dr. Lee stated. "If the association between obesity and diabetes in children is indeed causative, then public health strategies to prevent and treat obesity in children may help to reduce the future burden of diabetes in the U.S."

Low-fat diets do not result in more weight loss than higher-fat diets, according to David S. Ludwig, M.D., Ph.D., and Cara B. Ebbeling, Ph.D., of Children's Hospital in Boston, Massachusetts. Low-carbohydrate diets led to short-term but not long-term weight loss, and their safety in children has not been evaluated. "An alternative approach focuses on the glycemic index, rather than the restriction of any macronutrients," they added. "Highlights of over 100 studies indicate that children eat less after meals with a low-glycemic index than after those with a high-glycemic index."[24] Adolescents and adults lost more weight on diets that had a low-glycemic index than on control diets in randomized, controlled trials lasting up to one year. Also, laboratory animals fed a low-glycemic index diet had 40 to 50 percent less body fat than animals given a high-glycemic index diet.

Since magnesium is an important co-factor for enzymes involved in carbohydrate metabolism, it is not surprising that magnesium supplementation or increased intake of magnesium-rich foods may be an important tool in prevention of type 2 diabetes in obese children, according to researchers at the University of Virginia, in Charlottesville. The study, reported in *Diabetes Care*, is thought to be the first evidence that a magnesium deficiency is associated with insulin resistance in children. In insulin resistance, the pancreas produces insulin, but the body is unsure of what to do with it. The study indicates that the link between magnesium deficiency and risk for type 2 diabetes begins as early as childhood.[25]

Autoimmune Disease and Antioxidants

In a study involving 165 children, average age of three years, who had a parent or sibling with type 1 diabetes, 18 were found to have beta-cell autoimmunity. In autoimmune diseases, the immune system mistakenly destroys body tissue that it considers to be foreign. Type 1 diabetes is an example, in that the immune system produces antibodies that attack insulin-producing beta cells of the pancreas.[26] Two of the eighteen children had been given vitamin supplements during their first year of life. By comparison, 47 of the remaining 147 children who did not have beta-

CHILDHOOD STRESS AND DIABETES RISK

A research team in Sweden studied sixty-seven type 1 diabetics between the ages of newborn and fourteen years, and sixty-one healthy matched controls. They found that stress early in life increased the risk of type 1 diabetes, due to an autoimmune response. Negative events during the first two years of life were more prevalent in the diabetics than in the controls.[27]

cell autoimmunity had been given vitamin supplements during their first year of life. After controlling for other variables, the protective benefit of vitamin supplements remained. This prompted Jill Harris, Ph.D., of the University of Colorado Health Sciences Center, in Denver, to state that vitamin supplementation helps to prevent beta-cell autoimmunity rather than eliminate it. She believes that it is probably the antioxidants, specifically vitamin E, that help protect the beta cells from free-radical damage.

Celiac Disease

In evaluating forty-seven patients with type 1 diabetes, it was found that three had positive tests consistent with celiac disease. Celiac disease appears to be more common in patients with type 1 diabetes than those in the general population.[28] At Children's Hospital, in Valencia, Spain, a research team reported that all diabetic children should be routinely screened for celiac disease. This disorder, also called non-tropical sprue and gluten-induced enteropathy, is a severe allergy to the proteins in certain grains, specifically wheat, rye, oats, and barley. In the study, 141 type 1 diabetics were screened for serum immunoglobulin A (IgA) antigliadin antibodies. Twelve volunteers with positive IgA antigliadin antibodies in their blood on two or more consecutive measurements underwent a small intestinal biopsy, and four of them were diagnosed with celiac disease. Children who have diabetes and celiac disease have an onset of type 1 diabetes at a younger age than non-celiac patients, the researchers said. The prevalence of celiac disease in these type 1 diabetics is 2.85 percent greater than in the general population, which is one in 2,500 live births.[29]

Celiac disease causes a wide range of gastrointestinal symptoms. The classic syndrome of celiac disease consists of steatorrhea (excess fat in stools), diarrhea, and weight loss in adults and failure to thrive in children, with evidence of overt nutritional deficiencies due to small-bowel malabsorption. With a gluten-free diet, patients can often achieve substantial and rapid improvement of symptoms.[30] Gluten-free flours are quinoa, amaranth, corn, rice, and potato; millet and spelt can often be tolerated as well. Screening for celiac disease is rather simple using various antibody tests. Treating celiac disease with an appropriate diet can lead to tangible clinical benefits.[31]

Periodontal Disease

Periodontal (gum) disease is a complication of diabetes, one of the pathologic conditions often found in adults with diabetes, reported Evanthia Lalla, D.D.S., and colleagues at the Columbia University Medical Center, in New York. "Multiple studies have demonstrated that the prevalence, severity, and progression of periodontal disease are significantly increased in patients with diabetes," Dr. Lalla stated. Since periodontal diseases are largely preventable and progression can best be arrested when identified in early stages, screening for periodontal changes and implementing prevention and treatment programs should be considered as standard care for young patients with diabetes. This becomes even more important in the light of the emerging view that control of periodontal infections in adults with diabetes can further have a positive effect on the level of metabolic control in these individuals.[32]

Breastfeeding

A study was conducted of 720 Pima Indians, ranging in age from 10 to 39, of whom 325 were exclusively bottle-fed. They had significantly higher age-adjusted and sex-adjusted mean relative weights than 144 who were exclusively breastfed or 251 who were partially breastfed. However, those who were breastfed had significantly lower rates of type 2 diabetes when compared to those who were bottle-fed in all age groups. Those breastfed exclusively for the first two months experienced a significantly lower rate of type 2 diabetes.[33]

Cod Liver Oil

In Norway, cod liver oil is an important source of dietary vitamin D and

COFFEE, TEA, AND DIABETES?

In a study of 600 newly diagnosed diabetic children and 536 controls, researchers at the University of Helsinki, in Finland, evaluated the relationship of coffee and tea consumption in the children and their parents and the risk of diabetes. The research team found that the risk of type 1 diabetes was increased in children who drank at least two cups of coffee a day or those who consumed one or two cups of tea daily. Coffee consumption by the mother during pregnancy was not a factor.[34]

the omega-3 fatty acids eicosapentaenoic acid (EPA) and docosa-hexaenoic acid (DHA), which have biological properties of potential relevance for the prevention of type 1 diabetes, according to Norwegian researchers. A few studies have focused on the immunomodulatory effects of vitamin D in the prevention of type 1 diabetes. After vitamin D was found to prevent autoimmune diabetes in non-diabetic mice, two studies revealed an association between the use of vitamin D supplements in the first year of life and a lower risk of type 1 diabetes. In Norway, dietary vitamin D supplementation is recommended from infancy, preferably in the form of cod liver oil. Omega-3 fatty acids are incorporated into cell membranes and have anti-inflammatory properties that may help prevent of type 1 diabetes.[35]

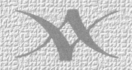

PART THREE

Treating the Complications of Diabetes

CHAPTER 15

High Blood Pressure

Almost 50 million Americans (25 percent of the adult population) have high blood pressure (140/90 mm Hg or more) or take anti-hypertensive medications. Hypertension (high blood pressure) increases with age and is more prevalent among African-Americans than in whites.[1] High blood pressure is a major risk factor for coronary heart disease. In one instance, the prevalence of hypertension in adults over eighteen years of age was 24 percent. In 1994, for example, 32.1 percent of all deaths were attributed to heart disease and 6.8 percent to stroke.[2]

To understand high blood pressure as a diabetes complication, let's first look at the basics of the heart. The heart is the center of the circulatory system, which supplies tissues and organs with blood, thus delivering vital nutrients and removing the products of metabolism. The heart's pumping action brings a flow of blood through a series of tubes (arteries) that have an ability to expand or contract. The arteries, which carry blood from the heart to the tissues, divert into vessels of progressively smaller diameter as they distance themselves from the heart, finally dividing into millions of tiny aristoles. Pulsatile high-pressure flow is converted to the continuous low-pressure flow that is needed for the exchange of material between capillaries (the smallest blood vessels in the body) and the cells. Finally, blood is returned to the heart through the veins.

A person's heartbeat changes the pressure inside the arteries. The maximum pressure, reached during the heart's contraction (systole), is called systolic or beating blood pressure. The minimum pressure, which occurs when the heart relaxes during beats (diastole), is diastolic blood pressure. Both systolic (the first number in a blood pressure readout) and diastolic (the second number) pressures are measured in millimeters of mercury (mm Hg).[3] Normal blood pressure is approximately120/80 mm Hg.

High blood pressure can be caused by a number of factors, including smoking, obesity, chronic stress, lack of exercise, excessive alcohol, and dietary fats and salt. It may also arise from other conditions, such as kidney disease, atherosclerosis, high cholesterol, and diabetes. When no cause is identified, hypertension is called "essential" or primary.

Diabetes and Hypertension

High blood pressure is reported with greater frequency in type 1 and type 2 diabetics than in the general population, according to Seymour L. Alterman, M.D., and Donald A. Kullman, M.D. Uncontrolled diabetes contributes to the accelerated buildup of fatty deposits in the arteries (atherosclerosis), and it plays a prominent role in the development of high blood pressure. It also has been suggested that hypertension may be related to insulin resistance found in diabetes and obesity. With insulin resistance, many type 2 diabetics produce enough insulin, but their bodies do not respond well to the hormone.[4]

A relationship between insulin and high blood pressure has been shown by epidemiologic studies since the mid-1980s. The relationship is most prominent in obese, hypertensive patients, as well as in lean hypertensives. Insulin is a vasodilator (expands blood vessels) and it also stimulates the sympathetic nervous system and promotes the absorption of sodium in the kidneys.[5]

In a study at the Saitama Medical School, in Japan, 470 men with a blood pressure exceeding 150 and/or 90 mm Hg had a significantly higher frequency of diabetes associated with excess cholesterol in the blood and mild obesity. When evaluating the men for too much insulin in the blood after a 75-gram glucose load, those with hyperinsulinemia (high levels of insulin in the blood) showed a higher blood pressure. Those with too much insulin had a greater incidence of glucose intolerance, abnormal amounts of triglycerides in the blood, low HDL ("good") cholesterol, elevated total cholesterol levels, and obesity. These individuals may be at a greater risk for cardiovascular episodes.[6]

How Foods and Nutrients Affect Blood Pressure

At the Kaiser Permanente Center for Health Research. in Portland, Oregon, William M. Vollmer, Ph.D., and colleagues reported that a diet rich in fruits and vegetables and low-fat dairy foods, along with reduced saturated and total fat, can significantly reduce blood pressure. The study evaluated 459 adults with systolic pressures of less than 160 mm Hg and diastolic pressures of 80–95 mm Hg. For three weeks, they were fed a control diet low in fruits, vegetables, and dairy products, with a fat content similar to the average American diet. The volunteers then ate a control diet for eight weeks that was rich in fruits and vegetables, or a combination diet rich in fruits, vegetables, and low-fat dairy products, along with reduced saturated and total fat. The research team reported that the combination diet reduced systolic and diastolic blood pressure by 5.5 and 3 mm Hg, respectively, when compared to the control diet. In 133 volunteers with high blood pressure who ate the combination diet, systolic and diastolic pressures were reduced by 11.4 and 5.5 mm Hg, respectively, more than the control diet.[7]

Studies have demonstrated that consumption of fruits, vegetables, wine, and tea may protect against stroke, which is a potential consequence of high blood pressure. Flavonoids (flavonols, flavones, and isoflavones) have been shown to be inversely associated with mortality from coronary heart disease and stroke. Therefore, increasing flavonoid intake may reduce the risk of high blood pressure.[8] Flavonoids, which were formerly collectively called vitamin F, are found in citrus fruits, berries, wine, green and black tea, onions, grapes, kale, cherries, red cabbage, broccoli, beets, radishes, apples, tomatoes, leeks, endive, green beans, and other foods.[9]

In evaluating forty-six studies on the relationship between blood pressure and diet in children and adolescents, it was found that in thirty-seven trials higher sodium intake was related to higher blood pressure. In fifteen studies, potassium did not give a clear picture of a relationship with hypertension, nine studies were inconclusive with regard to calcium and high blood pressure, and in five observational trials with magnesium was useful in lowering blood pressure.[10]

Salt Intake

Researchers at the Harvard School of Public Health studied 208 volunteers with high blood pressure (47 years of age, 59 percent females), who were on the Dietary Approaches to Stop Hypertension (DASH) diet, compared with 204 people (49 years of age, 54 percent females) on a control diet. The research team found that reducing salt intake from high to intermediate levels reduced systolic blood pressure by 2.1 mm Hg during the control diet and by 1.3 mm Hg on the DASH diet. Reducing salt intake from the intermediate level to the low level brought additional reductions of 4.6 mm Hg during the control diet and 1.7 mm Hg during the DASH diet. When compared to the control diet with a high sodium intake, the DASH diet with a low salt level led to a mean systolic blood pressure reduction that was 7 mm Hg lower compared with control diet patients without high blood pressure, and 11.5 mm Hg lower in those with hypertension.[11]

The DASH diet proved that a diet emphasizing fruits, vegetables, and low-fat dairy products, and which included whole grains, poultry, fish, and nuts, and only small amounts of red meat, sweets, and sugar-containing beverages, with lower amounts of total and saturated fat and cholesterol, can lower blood pressure in those with and without hypertension.

Potassium

In a study involving eight patients over 68 years of age, each was given potassium supplements for five months. This reduced their systolic blood pressure by an average of 15 points. The mineral can be found in cantaloupe, potatoes, avocadoes, bananas, broccoli, milk, and citrus fruits. However, in patients with poor kidney function, excessive potassium may be of concern.[12] The U.S. Food and Drug Administration allows health claims for potassium supplements in reducing the risk of high blood pressure and stroke. It was found that more than 80 percent of Americans do not get the recommended dietary allowance (RDA) for the mineral, which is 400 mg per day. An 8-ounce glass of orange juice contains about 450 mg of potassium.[13]

Garlic

A research team at the University of South Australia evaluated eight trials using dried garlic powder in 415 volunteers to determine the herb's effect on blood pressure. The dose range was between 600 mg and 900 mg per day (equivalent to 1.8–2.7 g of fresh garlic daily). The median duration of the trials was twelve weeks. Of the seven studies that compared the effect of garlic with placebo, three showed a significant reduction in systolic blood pressure and four found lower diastolic blood pressure. The researchers suggested that garlic preparations may be beneficial for patients with mild hypertension.[14]

Coffee

At Johns Hopkins, in Baltimore, Maryland, a research team evaluated 11 studies on the effect of coffee consumption on blood pressure in 522 people. The median duration of the studies was 56 days and the median dose of coffee was 5 cups per day. It was reported that systolic and diastolic blood pressures increased 2.4 mm Hg and 1.2 mm Hg, respectively, with coffee consumption, compared to those who did not drink coffee. The researchers added that there was an independent, positive relationship between cups of coffee consumed and subsequent changes in systolic pressure. The effect of coffee on blood pressure was more pronounced in younger people.[15]

At Royal Perth Hospital, in Western Australia, researchers evaluated twenty-two normotensive and twenty-six hypertensive, non-smoking men and women (mean age of 72.1 years), following two weeks of a caffeine-free diet. Participants were then randomized to continue with a coffee-free diet as well as abstaining from caffeine-containing drinks or to drink instead 5 cups per day of coffee (equal to 300 mg of caffeine daily), in addition to a caffeine-free diet for an additional two weeks. In the group with high blood pressure, the rise in mean 24-hour systolic blood pressure was greater by 4.8 mm Hg, and the increase in mean 24-hour diastolic pressure was higher by 3 mm Hg in the coffee drinkers, when compared to abstainers. The researchers suggested that coffee intake restriction may be of benefit to older people with high blood pressure.[16]

Vitamin C

At the Boston Medical Center, in Massachusetts, twenty volunteers given a placebo were compared with nineteen participants who were given 2 grams per day of vitamin C, followed by thirty days of 500 mg daily of the vitamin. One month following supplementation, there was a reduction in systolic blood pressure from a mean of 155 mm Hg to 142 mm Hg. There was no effect among the placebo takers. After one month, vitamin C reduced diastolic blood pressure; however, this response was not significantly different from that obtained by placebo.[17]

Another study evaluated blood pressure changes over an eight-year period in more than 1,800 white, middle-aged men. It was found that, over time, changes in systolic blood pressure were inversely related to the intake of vitamin C and beta-carotene (provitamin A). In other words, those with the highest intakes of vitamin C and beta-carotene would be expected to have a less than 2 mm Hg rise in blood pressure over ten years. Diastolic pressure was similarly affected, although the association was weaker than with systolic pressure. The researchers believe that dietary antioxidants (vitamin C, vitamin E, and others) may help to protect against blood pressure changes often seen in aging Americans.[18]

Magnesium

At the Norrlands University Hospital, in Sweden, researchers conducted a randomized, crossover study with magnesium or placebo in thirty-nine patients, ranging in age from 26 to 69. Magnesium was given at 365 mg three times daily for eight weeks. The researchers reported that the mineral, when given to mild to moderate hypertensive patients treated with beta-blockers, could bring a significant decrease in resting and standing blood pressure.[19]

At the Center of Hope Medical Center, in Duarte, California, Jerry Nadler, M.D., gave 260 mg per day of magnesium, twice daily for six weeks, to seven type 2 diabetics with high blood pressure and low magnesium levels in their blood. The controls were seven patients without diabetes or high blood pressure. The mineral brought a fall in blood pressure from an average of 157/96 mm Hg to 128/77 mm Hg. The magnesium therapy controlled the blood pressure in these patients. In addition, platelets became less sticky and thromboxane was decreased. Those with abnormal kidney function need to be monitored if using magnesium therapy. The effect on type 1 diabetes was not reported.[20]

Calcium

In nine studies involving people with normal blood pressure for their age group, calcium supplements resulted in lower blood pressure, while ten other studies found that calcium did not help. In those with high blood pressure, twelve studies found an inverse association with calcium supplements and twelve did not. Reasons for these inconsistencies are not known, but the possibilities include single-nutrient supplementation; high calcium levels in the blood when the study began; small sample size; short follow-up periods; inconsistent screening of participants for other factors (salt intake, salt sensitivity, and calcium imbalance); inadequate doses of calcium; variable blood pressure readings; and calcium absorption variables. However, the researchers said that it is evident from epidemiologic literature that dietary calcium plays an important part in the maintenance of normal blood pressure and that an adequate intake of the mineral may help to reduce the risk of hypertension. They added that it is also necessary to evaluate the mineral's interaction with potassium, magnesium, and sodium.[21]

At the University of Mississippi, thirty normotensive and twenty hypertensive pregnant women, between the ages of 18 and 28, were randomly assigned to either a control or supplemental group getting 1,000 mg per day of calcium for twenty weeks. The researchers reported that there was a significant inverse relationship between dietary calcium intake and blood pressure.[22]

In another study at the University of Mississippi, researchers evaluated seventy-five adults, between the ages of 19 and 25, who either were in a control group, or received 1,000 mg per day of calcium, or were given 24 fluid ounce of milk (skimmed, 2 percent, or whole) daily while following their normal diets. All systolic blood pressures, regardless of the treatment group, declined during a six-week period. Diastolic pressures went down only in the two calcium-supplemented groups. When total calcium intakes through diet and supplements were studied, the treatment group intakes were above the Recommended Dietary Allowance (RDA) for this age group.[23]

Coenzyme Q_{10} (CoQ_{10})

Ten patients, mean age of sixty-one, with essential high blood pressure were treated at the University of Firenze Medical School, in Italy. Each was given 50 mg of coQ_{10} twice daily for ten weeks. Following treatment, systolic blood pressure decreased from 161 mm Hg on average to 142 mm Hg. Diastolic pressure went down from 98 mm Hg to 83 mm Hg. During this time, total serum cholesterol dropped from 227 to 203, and serum HDL ("good") cholesterol went up from 42 mg/dl to 45.9 mg/dl.[24]

In another study at the University of Firenze, eighteen volunteers with essential hypertension were taken off all blood pressure medications for two weeks and then given either 100 mg per day of coQ_{10} or a placebo for ten weeks. There was a washout period for two weeks in which no supplements were given, and then the groups were crossed over to the other treatment for an additional ten weeks. Following ten weeks of coQ$_{10}$ therapy, the systolic blood pressure went down about 10 points, while diastolic pressure dropped 7 points on average.[25]

Fish Oils

At the University of Iowa Hospitals and Clinics, in Iowa City, researchers found that a high dose of 15 grams per day, but not a low dose of 3 g per day, of omega-3 fatty acids (fish oils) brought a significant decline in systolic and diastolic blood pressure. This data was confirmed in a large population-based trial in Norway, in which patients with high blood pressure who did not habitually eat fish had a reduction in blood pressure with 6 g per day of eicosapenataenoic acid (EPA) but not with a similar amount of corn oil.[26]

At Memorial Hospital of Rhode Island, researchers conducted a randomized, double-blind study of sixteen patients, eight of whom were given 50 g of vegetable oil while the others received 50 g of marine oil. It was found that diastolic blood pressure went down significantly in the fish oil group; however, systolic blood pressure did not change. Triglycerides dropped 30 percent in the fish oil group.[27]

Fiber

In a four-year study at Harvard University, it was found that 30,000 men who ate more than 24 grams (or 1 ounce) of fiber daily were less likely to develop high blood pressure compared to those who ate less than 12 g per day of fiber. Fiber from fruit was the most protective. The men who ate more than 24 g per day of fiber reduced their risk of developing hypertension by 57 percent.[28]

Vitamin E

Preeclampsia, which affects about 7 percent of pregnancies, is a serious disorder in which high blood pressure, fluid retention, and protein in the urine develop during the second half of a woman's pregnancy. It is a common problem for diabetics. Preeclampsia can lead to eclampsia, which brings seizures and may lead to the death of the woman or her fetus. High amounts of vitamin E may relieve high blood pressure during pregnancy and lower the risk of preeclampsia. A research team found low levels of the vitamin and high levels of lipid peroxides in women with severe gestational hypertension or preeclampsia. Lipid peroxides are fats that are damaged by free radicals, which increase the risk of preeclampsia.[29]

Lifestyle Modifications for High Blood Pressure

At the National Heart, Lung, and Blood Institute, in Bethesda, Maryland, Claude Lenfant, M.D., reported that the following lifestyle modifications can benefit people with high blood pressure.[30]

- Lose weight, if you are overweight.

- Limit alcohol intake to no more than 1 ounce (30 ml) per day for men, which is equal to 24 ounces of beer, 10 ounces of wine, or 2 ounces of 100-proof whiskey, and 0.5 ounces of alcohol per day for women and lighter-weight people.

- Increase physical activity to 30 to 45 minutes most days of the week. Researchers at the University of Auckland, New Zealand, studied 181 volunteers who followed a sedentary lifestyle and who were on drug therapy for high blood pressure. They were asked to walk briskly for forty minutes, three times weekly, with or without reducing salt in their diet. It was found that there was significant reduction of up to 7 mm Hg in systolic blood pressure after three months for brisk walking alone and salt restriction alone, but not for the combined intervention. There are no changes reported in diastolic blood pressure. The researchers concluded that it is possible to lower blood pressure for short periods, when hypertensive patients increase physical activity or reduce salt intake.[31]

- Reduce sodium intake to no more than 2.4 grams of sodium or 6 grams of sodium chloride (table salt) per day.

- Maintain an adequate intake of dietary potassium from fruits and vegetables.

- Maintain an adequate amount of dietary calcium and magnesium.

- Stop smoking.

- Reduce dietary saturated fat and cholesterol.[32]

Researchers at the University of Helsinki, in Finland, reported that dietary sodium is positively associated with blood pressure, and a reduction in salt intake can reduce blood pressure in some patients. Potassium, calcium, and magnesium can be protective electrolytes in some individuals. They added that omega-3 polyunsaturated fatty acids (fish oils) may help to lower blood pressure.

Coffee, alcohol, and habitual licorice consumption may increase blood pressure. While caffeine may increase blood pressure acutely, there is a tendency for the body to tolerate caffeine, a tendency which develops rapidly. A daily intake of more than 100 g of licorice is usually required to raise blood pressure markedly.[33]

CHAPTER 16

The Complications of Cardiovascular Disease

About three-fourths of the deaths among diabetics are caused by cardiovascular complications, according to the Columbia University College of Physicians and Surgeons *Complete Home Medical Guide*. In fact, those with diabetes have a much higher rate of heart disease and circulatory problems than the general population. These problems range from an increased risk of heart attacks, strokes, and high blood pressure to impaired circulation in both large and small blood vessels. In addition, hardening of the arteries (arteriosclerosis) and a buildup of fatty deposits in the arteries (atherosclerosis), which affect many in the general population, appear at an earlier age and advance more rapidly in diabetics.[1]

High total cholesterol and high triglycerides are common among both men and women with diabetes. Women ordinarily have lower blood lipid levels and a lower incidence of heart disease than men, but when they have diabetes they often have much higher levels of blood fats. High blood pressure is also very common among diabetic patients.[2]

How Diabetes Affects the Cardiovascular System

It is unclear how diabetes promotes cardiovascular and circulatory abnormalities, but a number of researchers believe the answer lies in the abnormally high blood glucose levels in diabetics. High blood glucose affects a number of blood components, especially red blood cells and platelets (which affect clotting), and these abnormalities may play a role in the development of hardening of the arteries.

Insulin seems to increase lipid synthesis in the artery walls, which may promote the buildup of fatty deposits. Since many type 2 diabetics have

181

high levels of insulin, even though their bodies do not correctly utilize it, a number of researchers think that this may be a factor in the high degree of fatty deposits among these patients. For type 1 diabetes, insulin therapy inhibits the atherosclerotic process by normalizing blood sugar.[3]

Diabetes also damages capillaries, or the microcirculation, which nourish body cells. However, with diabetes there is a thickening of the "basement" membranes, the substances that separate the epithelial cells lining the various body surfaces and the underlying structures. When the capillary membranes become thickened, the vessels are sometimes unable to carry sufficient blood to the tissues they serve, which causes poor circulation. Limbs are particularly vulnerable to these problems, which may be why diabetics have a greater incidence of leg and foot problems, such as skin ulcers, cramps or pain, and, in some cases, gangrene.[4]

Glucose Control

Insulin collects in the blood when cells fail to respond to the hormone's signal to take up glucose, as in the case of type 2 diabetes, states James B. Meigs, M.D., of the Massachusetts General Hospital and Harvard Medical School, in Boston. This increases a diabetic's risk of developing heart disease, and it goes beyond the dangers attributed to high blood pressure and elevated cholesterol. It is theorized that the insulin buildup inhibits the ability to break down blood clots efficiently.[5] The research involved 2,962 healthy volunteers, with an average age of fifty-three, who fasted overnight and then were tested for their metabolism of glucose. It was found that 80 percent of the volunteers processed the simple sugar normally, while 15 percent were glucose intolerant, a condition that often precedes type 2 diabetes; the remaining 5 percent had diabetes but did not know it. "Our data strongly suggest that insulin resistance is linked to arterial clotting, but it's still unclear whether physicians could determine patients' risk of heart disease by measuring insulin or other substances that influence clotting," Dr. Meigs said.

A study headed by David M. Nathan, M.D., at the Harvard Medical School suggests that strict glucose control can have long-term benefits by helping diabetics to avoid heart disease. Between 1983 and 1993, the researchers tracked 1,441 type 1 diabetics. The team had chosen half of the volunteers to receive insulin and standard counseling for their disease, while the remaining ones followed a program of checking blood glucose more frequently and taking insulin injections as needed.[6] All of the participants were placed on a strict glucose program. After six more years, the research team utilized ultrasound to measure the thickness of each patient's carotid arteries, which supply the brain with blood. Thickness of the vessel wall is an indicator of the beginning stages of hardening of the arteries. Dr. Nathan reported that those who had been intensively monitored and treated for ten years had only 76 percent as much artery thickening as those originally on standard treatment. This reinforces previous studies that show that strict glucose control reduces eye, nerve, and kidney complications stemming from type 1 diabetes.

Chronic Inflammation

Signs of chronic, low-grade inflammation precede the development of type 2 diabetes, according to Paul M. Ridker, M.D., of Brigham and Women's Hospital, in Boston. Various studies have shown that inflammation is the underlying factor that links obesity, heart disease, and diabetes. However, other researchers suggest that inflammation may not cause the disease but merely signals early stages of the disorders.[7] The researchers analyzed data from a subset of women in an ongoing study of heart disease. During the first four years of the study, 188 women in the subset developed diabetes. Their medical records were compared to 362 participants of similar ages who were not diabetics. The research team found that blood samples taken from both groups at the beginning of the study showed that those who had had higher concentrations of two biochemical markers of inflammation were more likely to develop type 2 diabetes. Other risk factors for the disease, such as obesity and high blood pressure, were factored in. The quarter of the women whose blood had the highest concentrations of C-reactive protein (CRP) were 4.2 times as likely to develop diabetes after four years as were the quarter of the women with the lowest concentrations. CRP is a protein in blood serum involved in inflammation. The quarter of women with the highest amounts of interleukin-6 (IL-6) were 2.3 times as likely to have developed the disease. IL-6 is involved in the body's immune system.

The Role of Nutrition

Nutrition can play a role in the prevention of diabetes, cardiovascular disease, hardening of the arteries, and other disabling diseases. Nutrition is the keystone of preventive health care, and the knowledge of nutrition as prevention is the responsibility not only of the physician but also of the general public. The prevention of disease could result in enormous cost savings to both physicians and hospitals.[8]

Carbohydrates

In a six-year study involving more than 65,000 women, those who ate diets high in carbohydrates from white bread, potatoes, white rice, and pasta had 2.5 times the risk for type 2 diabetes than those who ate a diet rich in high-fiber foods, such as whole-wheat bread and whole-grain pasta, according to Walter Willett, M.D., at the Harvard School of Public Health. He suggested that white bread and potatoes should be moved to the sweets category on the U.S. Department of Agriculture's food pyramid, since metabolically they are basically the same.[9]

"What's important in the diet is not just the total amount of carbohydrates but the type of carbohydrate and the food pyramid is remiss in not pointing that out," Dr. Willett said. Low-fiber carbohydrates such as pasta behave like white sugar during digestion, while fiber helps to reduce the rate of carbohydrate absorption. A number of studies have shown that whole grains lower the risk of coronary heart disease and other disorders.

Refined Grains

Refining splits the whole grain into bran, germ, and endosperm, and it also removes all but the endosperm, which is the kernel's starchy center. Ground fine, the endosperm is converted into flour that makes light and airy white bread, while the bran and germ are segregated to use in bran muffins and mixed into heavier breads that most Americans avoid. Enriched white flour is nutritionally stripped—of the fifteen key nutrients in white flour, including vitamin E, only five of them equal or surpass levels found in whole-wheat flour. In addition, unground whole wheat is better than ground whole wheat.

As Ruth Adams and I reported in *Improving Your Health with Zinc*, numerous scientists have pointed out that the refining of our grains and sugar cane has contributed to all kinds of ill-health, especially heart disease. For example, in refining grains to make white flour, 40 percent of the chromium is removed, along with 86 percent of manganese, 76 percent of iron, 89 percent of cobalt, 68 percent of copper, 78 percent of zinc, and 48 percent of molybdenum. Only some of the iron is restored in the so-called enrichment program, along with some of the B_1, B_2, and B_3.[10] In studying blood glucose levels in sixteen patients with diabetes who had eaten breads made with varying ratios of whole grains and milled flours, it was found that the higher proportion of whole grains (unmilled grains) the lower the blood glucose.[11]

Vitamin E

In a study at University Hospital, Queen's Medical Centre, in Nottingham, England, researchers reported that fatty deposits in the arteries account for 70 percent of the deaths in patients with diabetes, and a two- to fourfold excess mortality in those with impaired glucose tolerance. Vitamin E is lipophilic (it likes fats), and when it is incorporated into LDL ("bad") cholesterol, it inhibits oxidation. Dosages between 100 IU and 800 IU per day have been shown to reduce hardening of the arteries. The vitamin also improves insulin sensitivity.[12] Vitamin E, vitamin C, and other antioxidants fight off unstable free radicals that damage tissues and contribute to heart disease and other disorders.

Magnesium

A magnesium deficiency is prevalent in diabetes, and this may result in increased risk for cardiac arrhythmias, high blood pressure, myocardial infarction (heart attack), and altered glucose metabolism, reports Robert K. Rude, M.D., of the University of California School of Medicine, at Los Angeles. The association between low magnesium levels and diabetes has been documented since 1946. Insulin may enhance magnesium transport into the cells, and therefore insulin resistance may result in intracellular magnesium deficit. Insulin resistance is also linked to high blood pressure and high levels of fats in the blood. Magnesium supplements, either intravenously or by mouth, may prevent complications in those at risk for magnesium deficiency, such as diabetics and those using diuretics (water pills). Initial oral doses of 300 mg per day may be given, but doses gradually increased up to 600 mg per day may be needed to achieve maximum therapeutic effect. Divided doses are recommended in order to prevent diarrhea. However, caution should be taken for those with impaired kidney function.[13]

Chromium

Thirty-five years of research suggests that chromium plays a consider-able role in the progression of glucose intolerance and the increased risk of developing diabetes and cardiovascular disease, even though this suggestion has been generally ignored, reports Walter Mertz, Ph.D. Thir-teen out of fifteen studies evaluating the mineral's effect on glucose tol-erance show benefit by maintaining glucose levels with lower insulin output. In one study, chromium supplements reduced elevated total cho-lesterol and LDL cholesterol levels and increased levels of HDL ("good") cholesterol. A chromium deficiency results in insulin resistance, which can improve when chromium supplements are recommended. Insulin resistance is a significant risk factor for cardiovascular disease and it may be more significant in the cause of cardiovascular disease than LDL cholesterol. Since there is not a good way of diagnosing a chromium deficiency, many physicians ignore the potential benefits of chromium supplementation.[14]

Carl C. Pfeiffer, Ph.D., M.D., reported that chromium is essential in regulating blood sugar levels, yet much of it is removed during the refin-ing of grains. He wondered whether or not this is one reason that statis-tics on diabetes are soaring. Chromium and zinc are essential for the health of the eyes, and the removal of these minerals from grains may play a role in the increasing rates of glaucoma, cataract, and other prob-lems. He added that zinc is essential for the proper activity of the pan-creas, which is disordered in diabetics. Yet, few doctors prescribe zinc. Manganese is also related to blood sugar regulation.

Red Wine

In a study reported in the *European Journal of Clinical Investigation*, twenty type 2 diabetics—average age of fifty-five years and who had had dia-betes for an average of 9.2 years—were studied during fasting consump-tion of 300 ml of red wine, or during a meal with or without wine. The researchers found that red wine consumption during a meal significant-ly preserved plasma antioxidant defenses and reduced LDL cholesterol oxidation and thrombotic (clotting) activation. Therefore, a moderate amount of red wine during meals may help prevent cardiovascular dis-ease in diabetics.[15]

Sugar Consumption

When sugar cane is refined into white sugar, 93 percent of the chromium is removed, along with 89 percent of manganese, 98 percent of cobalt, 83 percent of copper, 98 percent of zinc, and 98 percent of magnesium.[16] In *Is Low Blood Sugar Making You a Nutritional Cripple?*, Ruth Adams and I reported that, as long ago as 1933, British researcher Dr. J.H.P. Paton wrote in *Lancet* that the great increase in the intake of refined sugar may be the cause of the great increase in coronary heart disease and heart attack. He added that there are a number of diseases—obesity, hardening of the arteries, and diabetes—that have long been associated clinically with the excessive carbohydrate intake, which is largely, if not entirely, due to the prodigious increase in the use of sugar.[17]

In an article in the *American Journal of Clinical Nutrition* (April 1974), Richard A. Ahrens, Ph.D., said that smoking, obesity, sedentary lifestyle, and stress have been implicated as possible causes of heart attacks, but that "the most striking dietary change (in the past 100 years or so) has been a sevenfold increase in the consumption of sucrose (sugar)." He went on to say that "it is relevant to observe that the pandemic of arteriosclerotic heart disease continues to increase on a worldwide scale in rough proportion to the increase in sucrose consumption, but not in proportion with saturated fat consumption."

You should consider eliminating from your meals all foods that contain the quickly absorbed carbohydrates (sugar and refined starches mostly), and instead eat considerable amounts of protein and moderate amounts of fat. You should eat often during the day so that you do not become hungry and fatigued. Snacks must be high-protein foods such as chicken, cheese, and nuts. Since they contain considerable carbohydrates, the following foods should be eaten in moderation: baked beans, pasta, rolls, bread, corn, split peas, sweet and white potatoes, lentils, rice noodles, and all cereals. Because of their sugar content, fruits should be eaten in limited quantities.

Physical Exercise

In studying 31,432 person-years from 5,125 female nurses with diabetes in the Nurses' Health Study, over a 14-year follow-up period there were 323 new cases of cardiovascular disease, of which 225 were coronary heart disease and 98 were strokes. It was found that physical activity was inversely associated with coronary heart disease and ischemic stroke. A faster walking pace was independently associated with a lower risk of cardiovascular disease.[18]

CHAPTER 17

High Cholesterol

holesterol is an important constituent of body cells and it is involved in the formation of hormones and bile salts, as well as in the transport of fats in the bloodstream to tissues throughout the body. Mark D. Altschule, M.D., points out that cholesterol is the material from which cortisone and other adrenal gland hormones are derived. During exercise, cholesterol can serve as a source of energy. The fatty substance is oxidized to carbon dioxide and water like any other source of energy (sugar, fat, and so on), and it is changed by the body into bile constituents (gallstones are almost pure cholesterol). Digestion would be difficult without bile salts to emulsify fats in the digestive tract so they can be absorbed into the body. Cholesterol is present in every body cell and it may help to regulate the transport of nutrient and waste products in and out of the body.[1]

Most of the cholesterol in the blood is made by the liver from foods, especially saturated fats. However, some cholesterol is absorbed directly into the bloodstream from cholesterol-rich foods, such as eggs and dairy products.[2]

Cholesterol and triglycerides (the most abundant fats in the body) are transported through the body in the form of lipoproteins. These particles are made up of cholesterol and lipoproteins and an outer wrapping of phospholipids and apoproteins (carrier proteins). The most abundant cholesterol in the blood is high-density lipoproteins (HDL cholesterol), which seems to protect against arterial disease. It is referred to as "good" cholesterol. If most cholesterol in the blood is low-density lipoprotein (LDL or "bad") cholesterol or very-low-density lipoprotein (VLDL) cholesterol, the risk of developing disease is increased. The level of cholesterol in the blood is influenced by dietary factors, genetics, and diseases such as diabetes. High blood cholesterol increases the risk of developing atherosclerosis, coronary heart disease, and stroke.[3]

While we are constantly bombarded in the media with details of how cholesterol is killing us, the eminent heart surgeon Michael E. DeBakey, M.D., states that only about 30 percent of his heart patients have any form of abnormality in their cholesterol. The majority of heart patients have perfectly normal cholesterol levels and have been eating almost anything they want without dietary restrictions. While Dr. DeBakey has not ruled out the importance of diet, he has said that it is not the specific cause of heart disease. "We don't know the cause and we need to take a much saner attitude towards diet in relation to the disease, since it is obvious that diet, as far as 65 to 70 percent of the patients are concerned, has not been related or associated with the disease in our experience."[4]

Joseph L. Goldstein, M.D., and Michael S. Brown, M.D., of the University of Texas Southwestern Medical School, in Dallas, state that the cause of high cholesterol levels is abnormal cholesterol *synthesis*, that is, how it is made. The key seems to be the enzyme that controls the rate of cholesterol synthesis. The genetic defect underlying inherited high cholesterol is in the gene that makes fat proteins that usually exert feedback control over the enzyme.

How to Measure Cholesterol

Cholesterol in the blood is measured as milligrams per deciliter (mg/dl); a deciliter is equivalent to 100 ml or 3.3 ounces of blood.

Cholesterol

200 mg/dl or below—Desirable

200 to 239 mg/dl—Borderline high

240 mg/dl or above—High; see physician for recommendations

Low-Density Lipoprotein (LDL) Cholesterol

100 mg/dl or less—No treatment needed

100 mg/dl to 130 mg/dl—Diet, exercise, lifestyle changes

130 mg/dl and over—Diet, exercise, lifestyle changes, medication

High-Density Lipoprotein (HDL) Cholesterol

40 mg/dl or more—No treatment needed

60 mg/dl—Ideal for protecting against heart disease

Triglycerides

150 mg/dl—No treatment needed

400 mg/dl and over—High; see physician for recommendations

Diet and Cholesterol

Ordinary diets are likely to supply 600–900 milligrams of cholesterol daily, according to the U.S. Department of Agriculture (USDA); a "low-cholesterol" diet usually provides about 300 mg of cholesterol each day. The USDA states that studies have not shown convincingly that a reduction of dietary cholesterol reduces the frequency of hardening of the arteries; however, people with atherosclerosis usually have higher blood cholesterol levels than those without the disease.

Blood levels of cholesterol are elevated in diabetes during periods of weight gain or low thyroid activity and with other conditions of depressed metabolism. Cholesterol is elevated by several dietary factors, including eating calories in excess of energy needs, by high intakes of fat (especially certain saturated fatty acids and dietary cholesterol), by high protein intakes (such as animal proteins and those high in the sulfur-containing amino acids methionine and cystine), and by choline and rapidly absorbed sugars.[5]

High cholesterol levels in the blood can be lowered by relatively high intakes of linoleic acid and perhaps by other polyunsaturated fatty acids, by high intakes of nicotinic acid (vitamin B_3), by dietary starches in place of sugars, and by strict vegetarian-type diets. Surprisingly, meat is not necessarily high in cholesterol, according to William C. Sherman, Ph.D. A standard serving (100 grams or 3.5 ounces) of beef, pork, or lamb has only about 70 mg of cholesterol. Veal is a little higher at about 90 mg per serving. Liver is relatively high in cholesterol, around 300 mg per serving, and kidney has 345 mg in an average serving. Also, stepped-up energy metabolism, such as regular exercise or taking thyroid hormone and other agents to speed up metabolism, may also reduce cholesterol.[6]

Nutritional Approaches to Reducing Cholesterol

There are numerous ways of lowering cholesterol naturally without resorting to drugs. There are hundreds of articles in medical journals that show how this can be done, and here are just a few of them.

Lecithin

To lower cholesterol levels, Roger Williams, Ph.D., of the University of Texas, in Austin, suggests consuming more lecithin. Lecithin has soap-like characteristics and is a powerful emulsifying agent; its presence in the blood tends to dissolve cholesterol deposits. When there is substantially more lecithin in the blood than cholesterol—a ratio of 1.2 to 1 is said to be favorable—the actual amount of cholesterol can be high without the blood plasma getting milky or showing a tendency to produce fatty deposits. Lecithin reduces cholesterol absorption by 34.4 percent at a dose of 300 mg.[7]

THE MALIGNED EGG

Eggs are certainly maligned by the health establishment, yet if they only had vitamin C, they would be the perfect food. They do not contain vitamin C because the hen manufactures what she needs. Meanwhile, a large egg contains 250–275 mg of cholesterol.[8] The egg has been referred to as "Nature's masterpiece." It is a perfect container for many important nutrients, especially the high-quality protein. Eggs also provide significant amounts of vitamin A, iron, and riboflavin (vitamin B_2) and they are one of the few foods that contain natural vitamin D. Eggs contribute smaller amounts of many other nutrients, such as calcium, phosphorus, and thiamine (vitamin B_1).

If you were to avoid all the cholesterol you could in your diet, your body would still manufacture cholesterol at a fairly steady rate and in a relatively profuse amount. It has been shown repeatedly that the less cholesterol a person eats, the more the body produces. The normal person's body will rid itself of just about the same amount of cholesterol as that eaten, according to the National Commission on Egg Nutrition in Illinois. For those who don't metabolize the cholesterol in eggs properly, this could cause hardening of the arteries and lead to heart attack and stroke, major health problems for diabetics. It has been estimated that between 5 and 13 percent of the population has inherited a condition in which they do not metabolize cholesterol properly and must take measures to lower it in the blood.

Niacin (Vitamin B₃)

In one study, twenty-eight men with normal cholesterol levels but with low plasma concentrations of HDL cholesterol were randomly selected to receive increasing doses of niacin, up to 3,000 mg per day or no vitamin for twelve weeks. Then, the men took the opposite treatment; fifteen completed the study. The vitamin treatment brought a 14 percent decrease in total cholesterol, a 40 percent decrease in triglycerides, an 18 percent decrease in LDL cholesterol, and a 30 percent increase in HDL cholesterol. Since the large dose of niacin can cause flushing, physicians should supervise the dosages.[9]

In a double-blind trial at Duke University Medical Center, in North Carolina, researchers studied 399 male and female volunteers, ranging in age from 21 to 75. During the test, 173 were randomly selected to receive Niaspan (a timed-release niacin), at doses increasing from 1,000 mg to 2,000 mg at bedtime, or gemfibrozil (a lipid-lowering drug) at 600 mg twice daily. The research team reported that Niaspan at 1,500 mg and 2,000 mg versus the drug raised HDL cholesterol levels 21 and 26 percent, respectively. The 2,000 mg dose was given once daily and was well tolerated.[10]

Another study examined twenty-three men and women, between the ages of forty-one and eighty, who had hardening of the arteries. They were given either 600 mg of gemfibrozil orally twice daily or timed-release nicotinic acid (a form of vitamin B₃), starting at 100–250 mg three times daily. This amount was eventually increased to 1,500–3,000 mg per day for three months. For those who tolerated the therapy, HDL cholesterol increased by 15 percent while taking the drug, by 35 percent while taking vitamin B₃, and by 45 percent while taking a combination of the two substances.[11]

Bran

At Texas A&M University, researchers evaluated seventy-nine men and women whose mean age was 48.2 years; all had high cholesterol levels. They were given 20 g of cellulose, 3 g of barley oil extract, or 30 g of barley bran flour daily. Barley bran flour significantly lowered total serum cholesterol, as did the barley oil, following 30 days of treatment. LDL cholesterol went down 6.5 percent with the addition of barley bran flour and 9.2 percent with the barley oil; LDL did not decrease significantly in the cellulose group. HDL cholesterol dropped appreciably in the cellulose and barley bran flour group, but not with the barley oil.[12]

A research team at the University of California—Davis Medical Center and Sutter Heart Institute, in Sacramento, California, gave participants 84 g per day of rice bran, oat bran, or rice starch placebo added to their usual low-fat diet. Serum cholesterol went down significantly in the rice bran and oat bran groups by 8.3 and 13 percent, respectively; there was no change in the placebo group. The researchers attributed the change to a lowering of LDL cholesterol by 13.7 percent in the rice bran group and 17.1 percent in the oat bran group. There was no significant change in triglycerides or HDL cholesterol readings.[13]

Plant Fiber

In a study involving 197 volunteers, James W. Anderson, M.D., and colleagues gave them 5.1 g of psyllium (a high-fiber plant substance), compared with 51 people who took a cellulose placebo, twice daily for twenty-six weeks. The participants had high blood levels of cholesterol and followed the American Heart Association Step 1 diet for eight weeks. The researchers found that serum total cholesterol and LDL cholesterol were 4.7 and 6.7 percent lower, respectively, in the psyllium group than in the placebo group after 24–26 weeks.[14]

At the University of Alberta, in Edmonton, Canada, a research team studied ten men with high cholesterol levels who consumed 27 g of ground rhubarb stalk fiber daily for four weeks. This brought an 8 percent lowering of total serum cholesterol and a 9 percent lowering of LDL cholesterol; HDL cholesterol remained unchanged. One month after the fiber was stopped, total and LDL cholesterol returned to the same levels as at the beginning of the study.[15]

In two controlled studies involving some 250 volunteers, Cholestin, which is derived from red yeast rice, lowered blood levels of LDL cholesterol by 20 to 30 percent. The recommended dose at 2.4 g per day contains 4.6 mg of lovastatin, a constituent in the rice.[16]

Nuts

In a study involving four men and six women with moderately high cholesterol levels, they substituted 20 percent of their daily caloric intake with pistachio nuts for three weeks. It was found that there was a reduction in total cholesterol, an increase in HDL cholesterol, a decrease in total cholesterol/HDL ratio, and a decrease in LDL/HDL ratio. There was a slight reduction in triglycerides and LDL cholesterol. Blood pressure and weight were unchanged.[17]

Australian researchers evaluated sixteen men, average age of forty-one, who consumed a diet containing 36 percent of calories from fat for nine weeks. In the first three weeks, the diet was supplemented with raw peanuts at 50 g per day, coconut cubes at 40 g per day, and a coconut confectionary bar at 50 g per day. During the following three weeks, the diet was supplemented with monounsaturated fatty acid–rich raw almonds at 84 g per day, equivalent to 46 g of fat. In the final three weeks, the diet was supplemented with polyunsaturated fatty acid–rich walnuts at 68 g per day, equal to 46 g of fat. There was a 7 and 10 percent reduction in total and LDL cholesterol after supplementation with almonds and a 5 and 9 percent reduction after eating walnuts.[18]

Garlic

A search of Medline (the database of the National Library of Medicine) covering 1966 to 1991 reviewed twenty-eight studies on the use of garlic and blood cholesterol levels. It found that patients treated with garlic consistently showed a greater reduction in total cholesterol compared to those given a placebo. A meta-analysis estimated that cholesterol levels dropped 23 mg/dl; the average drop in total cholesterol in the blood was about 9 percent.[19]

Omega-3 Oils

At the Hospital of Valdinievole, in Pescia, Italy, sixteen patients with high blood levels of fats were given 1 gram (g) of omega-3 fatty acids daily for ninety days. This brought a decrease in blood triglyceride and cholesterol levels and an increase in HDL cholesterol. There were minimal side effects.[20]

Chromium

Researchers at Oklahoma State University studied forty-two elderly volunteers, sixty years of age or older, who were given 150 mcg per day of chromium or a placebo. This brought a reduction in LDL cholesterol; HDL cholesterol, triglycerides, and glucose were unchanged.[21]

Acidophilus

At the V.A. Medical Center in Lexington, Kentucky, James W. Anderson, M.D., and colleagues gave twenty-nine volunteers 200 ml per day of the "friendly" intestinal bacteria *Lactobacillus acidophilus* for three weeks. In a second, double-blind study, patients consumed fermented milk (yogurt) containing *L. acidophilus* or a placebo for four weeks.[22] The fermented milk brought a 2.4 percent reduction in serum cholesterol levels, while the *L. acidophilus* reduced serum cholesterol by 3.2 percent. Combined analysis of both trials showed a 2.9 percent reduction in serum cholesterol concentrations. Dr. Anderson pointed out that a 1 percent drop in blood cholesterol levels is associated with a 2 to 3 percent reduction in risk of coronary artery disease. Regular consumption of yogurt containing *L. acidophilus* may reduce coronary heart disease by 6 to 10 percent.

Grains and Pulses

A study involving thirty type 2 diabetics used a cereal-pulse mix given for 1–2 months, which was beneficial in controlling hyperglycemia and hyperlipidemia. The pulse mix per 100 g contained wheat grits (52 g), soybean (20 g), red gram dhal (6.5 g), lentil (6.5 g), black gram dhal (3.25 g), guar seed (3.25 g), fenugreek (1.6 g), turmeric (0.3 g), asafetida (a gum resin of various Asian plants related to the carrot family) (0.15 g), and toasted cumin seeds (0.15 g). The mix lowered total cholesterol, LDL cholesterol, triglycerides, and HDL cholesterol.[23]

A 98-day study at Illinois State University evaluated twenty-nine sedentary men with high cholesterol levels, who ranged in age from thirty-eight to seventy. The volunteers were given a low-fat, controlled diet plus 20 g of corn bran supplement or a low-fat, controlled diet with 20 g of wheat bran supplement. The low-fat diet significantly lowered all the lipid parameters except for HDL cholesterol. The corn fiber supplement brought an additional lowering of total serum cholesterol, triglycerides, and VLDL cholesterol concentrations. The corn and wheat fiber did not significantly alter LDL cholesterol and HDL cholesterol concentrations; however, the researchers agreed that supplementing a low-fat diet with corn bran is an effective way of reducing serum lipid concentrations in men with elevated cholesterol.[24]

General Recommendations

In 2001, the National Cholesterol Education Program, which is coordinated by the National Heart, Lung, and Blood Institute, in Washington, D.C., published guidelines suggesting that the number of Americans who should be using diet to lower their cholesterol levels should be increased to 65 million and the number of people who should be prescribed cholesterol-lowering drugs should go up to about 36 million. It was recommended that diabetics monitor their cholesterol levels in order to avoid a heart attack.[25]

The recommendations were hardly new, since we have known for some time that people should keep total cholesterol at 200 mg/dl or below, eat a diet low in saturated fats and cholesterol, increase physical activity, and lose weight if overweight. What was new was that many of the members of the panel that issued the guidelines have close ties with the drug companies that produce the leading cholesterol-lowering drugs. With these conflicts of interest, one wonders how these panel members and their colleagues can keep a straight face while urging Americans to take more cholesterol-lowering drugs, which often have debilitating side effects, rather than the numerous natural solutions.

A low level of HDL cholesterol is an independent risk factor for future cardiovascular events, according to M. Mominique Ashen, Ph.D., and Roger S. Blumenthal, M.D., of the Johns Hopkins Hospital in Baltimore, Maryland. A comprehensive approach to achieving optimal HDL cholesterol levels—40 mg/dl or more in men and 50 mg/dl or more in women—should include lifestyle modifications followed by the consideration of pharmacotherapy in high-risk patients.[26] As to specific recommendations, the authors recommend the following program:

- Regular exercise—a gradual increase to thirty minutes of brisk aerobic activity five days a week

- Weight loss of 1 pound per week, with a target body-mass index (BMI) of less than 25

- The substitution of polyunsaturated fats—such as oils (olive, canola, soy, and flaxseed); nuts (almonds, peanuts, walnuts, and pecans); cold-water fish (salmon and mackerel); and shellfish—for saturated fats and simple carbohydrates

- Smokers should be urged to quit

- Moderate alcohol intake is reasonable for those who so choose and for whom there are no contraindications

- Medication to raise HDL levels should be considered once the target LDL cholesterol level has been achieved in persons who have established atherosclerotic disease (hardening of the arteries) or major risk factors, such as diabetes, and in whom HDL cholesterol levels remain low. Niacin (vitamin B$_3$) is an effective alternative.[27]

CHAPTER 18

High Triglycerides

H igh blood levels of cholesterol and triglycerides are found in diabetics. Even women, who often have lower blood fat levels and a lower incidence of heart disease than men, often have very high levels of blood fats when they are diabetic. High blood pressure, which increases the risk of strokes and heart attacks, is also common among diabetics. High blood glucose affects various blood components and may have a role in arteriosclerosis. Insulin is thought to increase the production of fats in the artery walls and promote the buildup of fatty deposits. Since type 2 diabetics have high levels of insulin—although they do not effectively utilize it—it is thought that this might be a factor in the high degree of fatty deposits in these patients.[1]

Triglycerides are a pure fat composed of molecules of glycerol (a trihydroxy alcohol, the same as glycerin), with three fatty acids attached (monoglycerides have one fatty acid and diglycerides have two). Natural fats found in meats, grains, and nuts are made up mostly of triglycerides, with only trace amounts of the mono- and diglyceride forms and some free fatty acids. Processed fats, such as hydrogenated hardened shortenings, may contain up to 20 percent monoglycerides and diglycerides.[2]

In evaluating 740 coronary patients at the University of Maryland School of Medicine, in Baltimore between 1977 and 1978, 350 with coronary artery disease were recontacted beginning in 1988. It was found that high-density lipoprotein (HDL or "good") cholesterol was significantly lower and the triglycerides were higher in patients than in controls. Independent predictors of cardiovascular disease included diabetes, an HDL level less than 35 milligrams per deciliter (mg/dl), and triglycerides higher than 100 mg/dl. It was found that reduced survival rates from coronary artery disease were reported in those with triglyceride levels higher than 100 mg/dl compared with triglycerides below that level. Therefore, the cutoff points established in the National Cholesterol Education Program for elevated triglycerides (over 200 mg/dl) may need to be refined.[3]

Natural Ways to Lower Triglycerides

There are a number of natural ways to lower triglyceride levels—here is a review of some of them.

Fenugreek

At the National Institute of Nutrition, in Hyderabad, India, defatted fenugreek seed powder (100 mg, divided into two equal doses) was added to the diet of ten type 1 diabetics, ranging in age from twelve to thirty-seven. The therapy was given for two 10-day periods (five patients each) to see what effect there would be on blood glucose and serum lipid profiles. The researchers reported that the fenugreek diet significantly reduced fasting blood sugar and improved glucose tolerance and there was a 54 percent reduction in daily urinary glucose excretion. Total cholesterol, low-density lipoprotein (LDL or "bad") cholesterol, very-low-density lipoprotein (VLDL) cholesterol, and triglycerides were significantly reduced, while HDL cholesterol remained unchanged.[4]

Magnesium

At the Medical Hospital and Research Center, in Moradabad, India, researchers studied 400 patients between the ages of twenty-five and sixty-three, most of whom were men. In the controlled study, 206 volunteers were given a magnesium-rich diet, while 194 others received their usual diet for six weeks. After six weeks, there was a significant drop in total serum cholesterol, LDL cholesterol, and triglycerides in those getting the magnesium-rich diet. HDL cholesterol went down slightly in the control group, but increased 2.5 mg/dl in the magnesium diet group.[5]

Niacin (Vitamin B₃)

Swedish researchers treated eight patients with primary high triglyceride levels with 4 g per day of niacin (vitamin B_3) for six weeks. This reduced apolipoprotein-b by about one-third and triglyceride levels by almost half. The vitamin, in the form of nicotinic acid, either reduces VLDL cholesterol synthesis in the liver or increases the clearance of VLDLs. HDL cholesterol levels increased.[6] Apolipoproteins are ingredients in the blood that transport fat and cholesterol through the lymphatic system and bloodstream. There are nine different apolipoproteins. Apolipoprotein-a is associated with HDL cholesterol, while apolipoprotein-b is associated with LDL cholesterol. Other researchers have reported that, in studying 1,045 patients who had recently had a heart attack, those with high levels of apolipoprotein-b were eight times more likely to have a second heart attack than those with low levels. Those with elevated levels of apolipoprotein-b had low amounts of apolipoprotein-a, which pushes cholesterol to the liver.[7]

Omega-3 Oils

Elevated blood levels of triglycerides are associated with other cardiovascular risk factors, especially reduced levels of HDL cholesterol. However, omega-3 fatty acids from fish oil can effectively reduce blood levels of triglycerides at low doses of 1 g per day.[8] Researchers studied 234 men, between the ages of thirty-six and fifty-six, who were randomly selected to supplement with 3.8 g per day of EPA (eicosapentaenoic acid), 3.6 g per day of DHA (docosahexaenoic acid), or 4 g per day of corn oil for seven weeks. It was found that triglycerides decreased 26 percent in the DHA group and 21 percent in the EPA group compared with the corn oil group. Both DHA and EPA reduced serum triglycerides, but had different effects on lipoprotein and fatty acid metabolism. The data suggest that omega-3 fatty acids should be taken into consideration when evaluating triglyceride levels.[9]

Thirty-six postmenopausal women, 43–60 years of age, were given eight capsules daily of either placebo oil or omega-3 fatty acids (which contained 2.4 g per day of EPA and 1.6 g per day of DHA) for twenty-eight days. This brought a 26 percent lower serum triglyceride level and a 28 percent lower overall ratio of serum triglyceride to HDL cholesterol. The researchers suggested that this therapy could reduce the risk of coronary heart disease in post-menopausal women.[10]

Norwegian researchers gave sixty-four healthy male volunteers, ages thirty-five to forty-five, either 14 g per day of fish oil concentrate (55 percent omega-3 fatty acids) or 14 g per day of olive oil for six weeks. Plasma fibrinogen (a significant, independent cardiovascular risk factor) was reduced 13 percent and blood levels of triglycerides went down 22 percent with the fish oil supplement. Three weeks after the supplementation ended, both variables were back to where they had been at the beginning of the trial.[11]

At University Hospital, in Leiden, the Netherlands, researchers gave nine volunteers with high triglycerides 1 g per day of fish oil (containing 55.7 percent omega-3 fatty acids) and 1 unit of vitamin E oil for six weeks, followed by 5 g per day of fish oil for an additional six weeks. The 5-gram dose of fish oil brought a significant increase in omega-3 fatty acid content in VLDL cholesterol and LDL cholesterol and decreases in serum triglycerides, VLDL triglycerides, and VLDL cholesterol concentrations of 54, 56 and 40 percent, respectively. As is often the case with fish oil therapy, the LDL cholesterol went up by 23 percent.[12]

As reported in *Atherosclerosis*, sixteen type 2 diabetics with elevated triglyceride levels, between the ages of forty and seventy-five, took 3 capsules daily of fish oil (containing 2.5 g per day of omega-3 fatty acids) or a placebo (containing 3 g per day of olive oil) for two months. Then, for the last four months they took a dose of 1.7 g per day of omega-3 fatty acids or 2 g per day of olive oil. There was no improvement in LDL cholesterol, but there was a positive effect in lowering triglycerides.[13]

CHAPTER 19

Eye Problems

Diabetics are prone to eye problems, which can lead to blindness. To understand how eye problems develop, we first need to know something about the eye's structure. The eye is a ball covered with a tough outer membrane that is crystal clear. The curved area at the front of the eye is the cornea, which focuses light while protecting the eye. After light passes through the cornea, it travels through the anterior chamber (which is filled with a protective fluid called the aqueous humor), through the pupil (which is a hole in the iris, the covered part of the eye), and then through the lens for more focusing.

Finally, light passes through another fluid-filled chamber in the center of the eye (the vitreous), then it strikes the retina, the back of the eye. Similar to the film in a camera, the retina records the images focused on it, but unlike film, the retina also converts these images into electrical signals, which the brain receives and decodes. A part of the retina called the macula is specialized for seeing fine print or other detail. The retina is nourished by small blood vessels or capillaries.[1]

Types of Eye Problems for Diabetics

The most serious eye problems for diabetics are glaucoma, cataracts, and retinopathy. Macular degeneration is also a harmful eye condition that may occur.

Glaucoma

Diabetics are 40 percent more likely than others to develop glaucoma. The longer one has had diabetes, the more likely one is to develop glaucoma, in which pressure builds up in the eye. Generally, drainage of the aqueous humor slows down and fluid builds up in the anterior chamber. Pressure pinches the blood vessels taking blood to the retina and optic nerve and vision gradually diminishes as the retina and nerves are damaged.

Cataracts

When cataracts develop, the eye's clear lens clouds and blocks light from entering. If any light does pass through, it may be distorted. While everyone is subject to cataracts, diabetics are 60 percent more likely to develop this eye condition, according to the American Diabetes Association. Diabetics are likely to develop cataracts at a younger age and to have them progress faster. For mild cases of cataracts, diabetics may need to wear sunglasses or have glare-control lenses put in their glasses.

Retinopathy

The term *diabetic retinopathy* refers to all disorders of the retina caused by diabetes. Non-proliferative retinopathy is the common, milder form and it is also known as background retinopathy. While this form has no effect on vision and needs no treatment, it is important that diabetics have their eyes checked at least once a year to ensure that it is not progressing. In non-proliferative retinopathy, capillaries in the back of the eyes balloon to form pouches. While the disorder does not usually cause a loss of vision at this stage, the capillary walls may lose their ability to control the passage of substances between the blood and the retina. However, the retina may become swollen and fatty deposits form. If the swelling affects the center of the retina, the problem is called macular edema and it may cause the loss of vision.

Retinopathy may eventually progress to proliferative retinopathy, which is a more serious disorder. This is when the blood vessels are so damaged that they close off. Although new blood vessels may start growing in the retina, they are weak and can leak blood. This blocks vision and results in vitreous hemorrhage. The new blood vessels may generate scar tissue, and if the scar tissue shrinks, it can distort the retina or pull it out of place, resulting in retinal detachment.

Unfortunately, the retina can be damaged before a diabetic notices any vision changes. That is why patients should have their eyes examined by an eye doctor regularly even though there may be no symptoms of eye damage.

A number of factors determine whether or not a diabetic will develop retinopathy. Type 1 diabetics suffer various complications, such as problems with blood glucose control and high blood pressure levels, that may affect the eyes. Almost everyone with type 1 diabetes will develop retinopathy, but fortunately proliferative retinopathy is far less common. Those with blood glucose levels near normal are less likely to have retinopathy. Retinopathy is more common in Mexican Americans with type 2 diabetes than others; women are more likely to lose their eyesight than men.

To avoid eye problems, keep your blood glucose levels under tight control. In the Diabetes Control and Complications Trial, those on standard diabetes treatment got retinopathy four times as often as people who kept their blood glucose levels close to normal. In diabetics who had retinopathy, the condition progressed in the tight-control group only half as often. High glucose levels may cause vision to become temporarily blurry. It is also important to bring high blood pressure under control and stop smoking. Finally, see an eye doctor regularly, since a special

WHEN TO SEE AN EYE DOCTOR

According to the American Diabetes Association, diabetics should see an eye doctor if:

- Your vision becomes blurry
- You have trouble readings signs or books
- You see double
- Your eyes hurt
- You feel pressure in your eye
- Your eye gets red and remains that way
- You see floating spots or flashing lights
- Straight lines do not look straight
- You can't see things at the side (peripheral vision) the way you used to

examination can locate early stages of retinopathy. During this exam, the doctor will dilate (expand) the pupils with drops and check the retina. Only optometrists and ophthalmologists can detect retinopathy, and only ophthalmologists can treat it.

Macular Degeneration

As explained earlier, the macula is the part of the retina with the sharpest sight. In many Americans, mostly older people, the surface of the macula degenerates enough to cause legal blindness. The problem may be due to poor blood flow to the retina or it can be an inherited condition. In its early stages, magnifying glasses may enable the diabetic to read.[2] While macular degeneration might rightfully be covered under diabetic retinopathy, I have decided to give it a special section since a great deal of research deals specifically with this condition.

How to Deal with Glaucoma

A research team in Italy suggested that polyunsaturated fatty acids are a beneficial supportive therapy for the prevention and treatment of glaucoma. These substances have a vasodilating effect, which facilitates blood flow, perhaps because of increased nitric oxide levels. Nitric oxide, a potentially toxic compound of oxygen and nitrogen, is produced by endothelial cells that line blood vessels, where it relaxes the vessels and helps to maintain blood pressure. The study involved twenty-five males and fifteen females, with a mean age of 48.9 years, and a mean increase in ocular (eye) pressure of 22.4 mm Hg. In the double-blind trial, the volunteers were divided into two groups. One group was given 240 mg of DHA (docosahexaenoic acid) along with 340 mg of EPA (eicosapentaenoic acid), twice daily for three months; the other group was given a look-alike pill. After three months of therapy, there were significant improvements in various parameters involving glaucoma.[3]

In a study involving forty-nine sets of eyes, of which thirty-nine people suffered from various types of glaucoma and nine were normotensive (having typical blood pressure levels), the volunteers received a single oral dose of vitamin C (0.5 g/kg body weight), which brought a significant fall in intraocular pressure. In patients with hemorrhagic glaucoma or secondary glaucoma, the tension-lowering effect of the vitamin was less significant.[4] In a study involving twenty-five volunteers, with an average age of sixty-three, with moderate pressure in their eyes, 0.5 g of vitamin C four times daily for six days brought a significant decrease in intraocular pressure of 1.10 mm Hg, but there was no significant change in the facility of outflow. In nineteen patients, a 10 percent solution of vitamin C was given topically in one eye, three times daily for three days, while the other eye served as a control. The research team found that pressure in the test eye was significantly lower than in the control eye.[5]

Alpha-lipoic acid, when given to glaucoma patients, normalized the metabolism of the amino acid tyrosine along with their co-factors of vitamin B_6, vitamin C, and iron. This therapy improved the pressure in the eyeballs of the patients. The researchers suggested alpha-lipoic acid, vitamin B_1, vitamin B_2, pantothenic acid, vitamin B_6, and vitamin C for glaucoma patients.[6]

Nine volunteers with glaucoma were exposed to normal daylight and then given either a placebo or 0.5 mg of melatonin at 6 P.M. This brought a 30 percent reduction of pressure in the eyeball, whereas the pressure in the control group went down only 13 percent.[7] Melatonin, a hormone of the pineal gland, is also a major antioxidant to route free radicals. This over-the-counter supplement is prescribed for insomnia, jet lag, and heart disease, among other things. A deficiency is known to increase blood levels of cholesterol and triglycerides.

How to Deal with Cataracts

The prevalence of cataract increases from about 5 percent at age 65 to about 50 percent in those older than 75, according to Allen Taylor, M.D., of Tufts University in Boston. The disability and cost for age-related cataract in the United States is between $5 and $6 billion a year. Delaying cataract formation by about ten years would reduce the incidence of visual disability from cataract by about 45 percent. Risk factors for cataract include light exposure, high energy radiation, exposure to high levels of oxygen, smoking, and reduced levels of antioxidants. For example, optimum levels of vitamin C appear to be 250 mg per day—this would bring close-to-saturating levels of vitamin C in the blood and provide protection against cataracts. Poor education and lower socioeconomic status also increase the risk of cataract, he added.[8] An increased risk of cataracts has been found with elevated levels of salt and fat intake in the diet.[9] Epidemiologic data suggest that better nutrition (especially with vitamins C and E and the carotenoids) and fruit and vegetable consumption are the least costly and most practical measures to delay cataract formation. Two studies have shown that the consumption of vitamin C supplements for more than ten years decreased the risk of cataracts.[10]

It has long been suspected that free-radical damage might influence the formation of cataracts. Thus began a study at the Harvard School of Public Health, in Boston, which concluded that dietary intake of carotenoids and long-term supplementation with vitamin C might delay the development of cataracts and prevent the condition from reaching a severe stage requiring extraction. The study involved dietary analysis of more than 50,800 nurses, aged 45–67, in eleven states.[11] The researchers found that women in the upper fifth for total vitamin A intake, excluding supplements, had a 39 percent lower risk of developing cataracts in relation to the women in the lowest fifth. Although dietary intakes of vitamin B_2, vitamin E, multivitamins, or vitamin C were not associated with cataract risk, the researchers did find that women who had taken vitamin C supplements for ten years or more had a 45 percent lower risk of developing cataracts than unsupplemented women. In a surprise development, carrots, a rich source of beta-carotene (provitamin A), did not necessarily protect against cataracts, suggesting that other carotenoids might be more beneficial. There are more than 500 carotenoids that are synthesized from plants, including beta-carotene, lutein, lycopene, and zeaxanthin.

A number of studies have shown a strong association between abnormal levels of lutein and macular degeneration. Studies have also revealed that low levels of this carotenoid also increase the risk of cataracts. In a study of 36,000 male physicians that lasted more than eight years, it was found that men who consumed the greatest quantities of the carotenes lutein and zeaxanthin were 19 percent less likely to develop cataracts when compared to those who consumed little or none of the nutrients. Broccoli and spinach, both rich in lutein, were also associated with a lower risk of the disorder.[12] Lutein and zeaxanthin may also help to maintain normal visual acuity while reducing the risk of cataracts and macular degeneration. Macular pigment (containing lutein and zeaxanthin) may act like polarizing glasses, filtering out stray light and improving visual acuity, or it may keep eye tissues healthy by screening out harmful light thereby acting as an antioxidant.[13] Also, the presence of high levels of carotenoids in the ciliary (lens) of the eye, a tissue not exposed to intense light, suggests that they may be involved in antioxidant protection of this tissue.

It has long been known that vitamin A is essential for normal eyesight and that the body converts some beta-carotene (provitamin A) to vitamin A. As we have seen, lutein and zeaxanthin also play major roles in eye health, specifically by reducing the risk of cataracts and macular degeneration.[14] In one study, researchers obtained 200 human eyes within 24 hours after being donated to an eye bank. The eyes were dissected to determine the levels of carotenoids in eye tissues. The researchers found that nearly all tissues in the eyes had measurable levels of lutein, zeaxanthin, and their by-products. Also present were small amounts of beta-carotene, alpha-carotene, lycopene, and other carotenoids.

In studying more than 110,000 men and women, researchers at Harvard University found that those who consumed the most foods rich in lutein and zeaxanthin were less likely to develop age-related cataracts than those who ate the least. Foods rich in these carotenoids include dark green, leafy vegetables (spinach, broccoli, kale, collard greens, mustard greens), winter squash, corn, and peppers. Consuming at least three servings per week of these vegetables seems to offer protection.[15]

Researchers have found that lutein supplements can increase the density of the macular pigment, which is one sign of healthy eyes. A research team asked five patients with cataracts and five patients with age-related macular degeneration to take lutein ester capsules (from natural compounds found in vegetables and fruits) three times a week for an average duration of twenty-six and thirteen months, respectively. Each capsule contained 15 mg of lutein esters and 3.3 mg of vitamin E. The research team reported that visual acuity in the cataract patients improved by an average of 40 to 50 percent, which approached normal; tolerance of glare also improved. Four patients with macular degeneration, who remained in the study, reported stabilized or improved vision. No side effects were recorded.[16]

Cataracts may be associated with inadequate levels of antioxidants in the eye. Several studies have suggested that alpha-lipoic acid, an antioxidant, may reduce the risk of diabetes-associated cataracts. In one study, researchers induced diabetes in laboratory rats, noting that diabetes interferes with the way lens cells in the eyes burn glucose. After feeding some of the animals with alpha-lipoic acid, the animals getting the supplement were more resistant to glucose-related changes to the lenses of the eye when compared to the animals not getting the supplement.[17] Also, people with the highest intakes of folic acid (a B vitamin) and vitamin C were less likely to develop cataracts, according to researchers at Tufts University, in Boston.[18]

Cortical cataracts may be partially reversed with vitamin E supplements, according to a study of twenty-five patients with nuclear cataracts (located near the center of the lens) and twenty-five patients with cortical cataracts (found toward the outside of the lens). All were scheduled to have the cataracts surgically removed. Before surgery, twelve volunteers in each group were given 100 mg per day of vitamin E or a placebo for one month. The researchers said that the vitamin E levels increased and free-radical damage decreased in the lenses of those getting the vitamins. Also, cortical lens opacity decreased by almost 40 percent among those getting the vitamin, suggesting a reversal of their condition. For those getting vitamin E, nuclear lens opacity (due to sunlight exposure) decreased by 14 percent. The study found that cortical cataracts, which can result in blindness, may be partially reversed with vitamin E.[19]

During the day, the lens of the eye is exposed to ultraviolet radiation from sunlight and this generates cell-damaging free radicals. One of the side effects of this exposure is cataract, which is often associated with diabetes. In a study published in *Ophthalmology*, a research team evaluated the dietary habits, vitamin supplement usage, and blood levels of vitamin E in 764 volunteers in what was called the Lens Opacities Case-Control Study. Eye lenses of the participants were photographed at the beginning of the study and follow-up eye exams were scheduled. It was found that those who took vitamin E supplements had a 57 percent lower risk of developing cataract, especially after five years of supplementation, when compared to volunteers who did not take the vitamin. Also, those with high blood levels of vitamin E had a 42 percent lower risk of developing cataracts. Those who took multivitamin supplements that contained vitamin E had a 31 percent lower risk of developing the disease.[20]

Cataract is an age-related problem and surgery to replace the lens of the eyes is the most frequently performed surgical procedure in the United States. Vitamin E and other antioxidants could reduce the number of these operations and reduce eye-related health care costs as well. It is biologically plausible that oxidative damage may lead to cataract formation and that the antioxidants could potentially diminish the risk, according to Joel A. Simon, M.D., of the San Francisco V.A. Medical Center. However, rather than measure blood levels of vitamin C, Dr. Simon feels that it might be more prudent to underscore the public health importance of fresh fruit and vegetable consumption. A vitamin C supplement (250–500 mg per day) may also be reasonable for the potential prevention of cataracts, cardiovascular, and other diseases.[21]

In a study of 2,900 people, ranging in age from forty-nine to ninety-seven, higher intakes of protein and vitamins A, B_3, B_1, and B_2 were associated with a reduced risk of nuclear cataract. Polyunsaturated fatty acid intake was associated with a reduced risk of cortical cataract.[22] Researchers evaluated 3,089 people, 43–86 years old, for cataract incidence during a five-year study. Compared with those who did not take multivitamins or supplements of vitamins C and E, the risk for any cataract was 60 percent lower among those who, during follow-up, reported the use of supplements containing vitamins C and E for more than ten years.[23]

A research team at the University of Stockholm in Sweden studied a 35-year-old male who had posterior sub-capsular cataract, severe atopic eczema, asthma, and an inflamed cornea. He was treated with selenium (600 mcg), vitamin E (1,200 mg), vitamin B_6 (80 mg), vitamin B_2 (15 mg), and vitamin C (2,000 mg) daily. When the treatment began, vision was 2/10 in the right eye and 3/10 in the left eye. Three months later, vision was 4/10 in the right eye and 7/10 in the left eye. Five months later, the vision in the right eye remained at 4/10, but had increased to 8/10 in the left eye. The researchers said that in less than two months of treatment, all signs of severe atopic dermatitis had vanished and there were no signs of asthma. They believe that it is prudent to try selenium and vitamin E in other kinds of cataracts, such as senile and diabetic cataract.[24]

How to Deal with Diabetic Retinopathy

In a study involving pycnogenol, a brand of French maritime pine bark extract, researchers gave twenty men and women with retinopathy 50 mg of the extract or a placebo three times daily for two months. In a separate phase of the study, twenty patients were given the same dosage of pycnogenol. Eye exams were given before and after supplementation. Following the study, researchers found that patients given the supplement showed improvements in visual acuity and no decrease in retinal function. All of the patients reported some degree of improvement, while the retinopathies in those given placebos progressively worsened during the study. The supplement, which is available over the counter, is thought to be effective by quenching free radicals and by strengthening blood vessel walls.[25]

A prospective study demonstrated that blood levels of magnesium are inversely related to the occurrence or progression of retinopathy. Magnesium intake may be of significant benefit in patients with impaired glucose tolerance or who have beginning stages of type 2 diabetes. People at risk for magnesium deficiency also include those on certain drugs (such as thiazide and loop diuretics), those with inadequate nutrition, or those who consume alcohol, according to researchers.[26] Increased magnesium excretion in the urine of diabetics may be due to poor glycemic control (glycosuria), high insulin levels in the blood, a possible kidney defect, or inadequate nutrition. However, magnesium supplements can improve insulin sensitivity. For example, when magnesium (500 mg per day) was given to patients over a 21-week period, insulin requirements were reduced without changing glycemic control. It has been found that patients with severe diabetic retinopathy have lower blood levels of magnesium compared with patients without the eye problem.

There is a relationship between diabetic retinopathy and plasma homocysteine levels, according to an article in *Diabetes Care*. Homocysteine is a generally benign amino acid, a product of the synthesis and breakdown of proteins. However, when homocysteine builds up in the bloodstream, it can increase the risk of various disorders, especially heart attack, stroke, and blood clots. In the study, sixty-nine patients with type 1 diabetes, with blood pressure readings of 140/90 (mild hypertension), were free of cardiovascular disease and thirty-four did not have retinopathy, but it was found that twenty had non-proliferative diabetic retinopathy and ten had proliferative diabetic retinopathy.[27] A number of studies have reported that homocysteine levels can be lowered with daily doses of folic acid (5 mg), vitamin B_6 (100 mg), vitamin B_{12} (1,000 mcg), betaine hydrochloride (500 mg), and lecithin (1,000 mg).[28]

How to Deal with Macular Degeneration

A low-fat diet (less than 25 percent of the calories from fat) can help to improve the vascular system and may lessen the contributions of vascular disease to the wet form of acute macular degeneration. In addition, keeping diabetes under control or reducing glucose intolerance can inhibit lens glycosylation. Excess sugar in the diet can promote osmotic swelling and increase oxidant stress. In fact, diabetes can increase cataract prevalence three- to fourfold in those sixty-five years of age and younger. Smoking and exposure to high-energy radiation can also harm the eyes. To protect the eyes, researchers suggests taking antioxidant defenses (such as copper, iron, manganese, zinc, selenium, and vitamin B_2), consuming free-radical scavengers such as vitamins E and C and beta-carotene, consuming antioxidants that help to absorb UV light (including beta-carotene, lutein, and zeaxanthin), reducing fat intake to less than 25 percent, and reducing the risk of type 2 diabetes by being less than 20 percent overweight, exercising, and lowering calorie intake. Benefits can be achieved with 200–400 IU of vitamin E, 100–250 mg of vitamin C, and 25 mg of beta-carotene daily. Dark green vegetables such as spinach, peppers, and broccoli are especially helpful.[29]

Antioxidants help to protect the human macula from destruction by oxygen free radicals, which are generated through normal oxygen metabolism. The free radicals can be increased by environmental stressors such as certain wavelengths of light and chemicals, according to David A. Newsome, M.D., of the Retinal Institute of Louisiana, in New Orleans. Taking antioxidants can increase blood levels of these nutrients and there is increasing evidence that antioxidants can slow vision loss in macular degeneration.[30]

Macular degeneration is one of the "wear and tear" diseases due to oxygen stress. The macula is an oxygen-rich environment in which the metabolic rate is high; this generates a significant amount of free radicals, which can damage tissue by their continuous search for missing electrons. (Free radicals are oxygen molecules with an unpaired electron. This imbalance makes them highly reactive and they are constantly striving to connect with other molecules. In so doing, they will attack any part of the body, thus contributing to heart disease, cataracts, aging, and other health problems.)

The eye, especially the macula, contains various naturally occurring antioxidants, such as vitamins C and E, beta-carotene, zinc, selenium, and copper, and antioxidant systems such as catalase, superoxide dismutase, glutathione peroxidase (which involves selenium, zinc, and copper), glutathione reductase (which includes vitamin B_2), metallothionein (which includes zinc), and retinal dehydrogenase (which also includes zinc). Unfortunately, older people are more susceptible to macular degeneration and tend to eat a diet that is not rich in antioxidants. Also, older people have reduced intestinal absorption of nutrients, which begins with a lowered output of stomach acid and this reduces the bioavailability of many of these nutrients. In a study from the National Cataract Study Group, it was found that there was an approximate 35 percent reduction in cataract formation in those with higher levels of antioxidants. Newsome and his colleagues have reported a reduction in vision loss among those with macular degeneration who ingested zinc.[31]

Using data from the third National Health and Nutrition Examination Survey (NHANES III), a research team reported a relationship between lutein and zeaxanthin levels and age-related macular degeneration (AMD) among 8,222 men and women. The researchers used photographs of the volunteers' eyes, as well as dietary and blood levels of the two carotenoids. Overall results found no relation of dietary or blood lutein or zeaxanthin levels in the early or late stages of AMD. However, those between the ages of forty and seventy-nine with the highest dietary levels of the two nutrients had a 90 percent lower risk of pigment abnormalities in the retina, which is an early indicator of the disease. Those 60–79 years old who consumed the highest amounts of lutein and zeaxanthin had a similar lower risk for late-stage AMD.[32] In another study, the researchers found that eyes containing the largest amount of lutein and zeaxanthin were 82 percent less likely to have AMD.[33]

Outside of supplements, plant pigments are the only source of these nutrients. The researchers added that a growing body of evidence suggests that the two carotenoids help to maintain the health of the retina and vision. Since carotenoids help to protect plants from dangerous free radicals, which are generated by exposure to oxygen and light, researchers theorize that these antioxidants can also protect human beings when they consume carotenoids found in fruits and vegetables. Researchers have determined that lutein and zeaxanthin form the yellow macular pigment found at the center of the retina. This pigment filters out deleterious blue wavelengths of light and may reduce the amount of free radicals. It has been known for some time that AMD, the leading cause of blindness in the elderly, is related to lower amounts of macular pigment. Increased dietary intake of lutein-containing foods or lutein supplements increases blood levels of the carotenoid, thereby increasing macular pigment density. However, the normal diet may not contain sufficient amounts of lutein; lutein ester supplements (a common form of lutein) can be used to optimize levels of the nutrient in the eye.[34] In one study, supplemental lutein increased lutein levels in both the blood and the eyes: during the twelve-week study, lutein levels went up five times in the blood and the macular pigment density increased by 19–22 percent.[35]

Researchers have determined that lutein and zeaxanthin protect eye cells from damaging free radicals—however, this protection was most noticeable when the carotenoids were combined with vitamins C and E and other antioxidants. The antioxidants protected the carotenoids from being damaged by free radicals.[36] In a study involving sixteen volunteers, 27–54 years old, it was found that high consumption of lutein from vegetables such as spinach and kale may reduce the risk of macular degeneration. The study group had been diagnosed with retinitis pigmentosa or other forms of retinal degeneration, which can contribute to blindness. The volunteers were given 40 mg per day of lutein for nine weeks followed by a maintenance dose of 20 mg per day for seventeen weeks. Ten other volunteers received 500 mg per day of docosahexaenoic acid (DHA), B vitamins, and digestive enzymes. Based on vision tests and comments by the volunteers, visual acuity and field of vision improved significantly among those taking lutein. Interestingly, improvement in visual acuity was some four times greater among those with blue

SMOKING AND THE RISK OF MACULAR DEGENERATION

In two studies involving 21,157 male physicians and 31,843 registered female nurses, it was found that cigarette smoking is an independent risk factor for age-related macular degeneration.[37] Smoking reduces blood concentrations of several micronutrients that act as antioxidants and may provide protection against macular degeneration.

eyes and dark eyes. Some of the volunteers also said that they could adapt better to light and darkness, had improved color perception, and experienced reduced glare from light.[38]

In a study of 3,600 patients, ranging in age from 55 to 80, from eleven medical centers, volunteers were given one of the following supplements or a placebo for an average of six years: (1) a multivitamin formula containing vitamin C (500 mg), vitamin E (400 IU), and beta-carotene (15 mg) daily; (2) zinc (80 mg) and copper (2 mg) daily; or (3) a combination of the first two protocols.[39] Those with the highest risk of advanced AMD experienced the greatest benefit with the combination of vitamins and zinc, which reduced the rate of visual acuity loss by 27 percent. The copper did not seem to affect the outcome.

Vitamin E is an antioxidant instrumental in increasing resistance to age-related macular degeneration. The progressive development of AMD is thought to be influenced by oxidative stress. In one study, a research team evaluated blood levels of nutrients in twenty-five men and women with AMD and compared them to a control group of fifteen volunteers without the disease. The participants were sixty years of age. It was found that the patients with AMD had significantly lower blood levels of vitamin E and zinc. It was also found that those with AMD had greater exposure to sunlight, which increases free-radical damage to the eyes.[40] Many studies support the use of vitamin E in preventing macular degeneration. One of these studies involved tabulating diets, blood levels of nutrients, and visual health of more than 2,500 people. After analyzing the ratio of vitamin E to blood fats, such as cholesterol, it was reported that those with the greatest concentrations of vitamin E were 82 percent less likely to develop macular degeneration. People with higher levels of blood fats may be able to protect themselves by increasing their vitamin E intake.[41]

CHAPTER 20

Foot Problems

Foot problems in diabetics usually happen when there is nerve damage in the feet and when blood flow is poor, according to the American Diabetes Association. About one in five diabetics who enter the hospital have foot problems. It is important that diabetics inspect their feet daily and ask for professional help if they get a foot injury. A health-care provider should check the feet of a diabetics at least once yearly.[1]

Diabetics are more likely to have a foot or leg amputation than others. That's because they often have artery disease that reduces blood flow to the feet. Diabetics are also prone to nerve damage, which reduces sensation. These problems make it easy to get ulcers and infections that may lead to amputation. The biggest threat to a diabetic's feet is smoking, since this affects the small blood vessels, causing decreased blood flow to the feet and making wounds heal more slowly. Amputation is often prevented by improving blood flow to feet and legs. There are two systems in the feet that seem to go wrong with diabetics: the circulatory system and the nervous system. Problems range from relatively minor ones, such as discomfort, to major ones, including the need for amputation of the leg.[2] Here we discuss some of the more common foot problems encountered with diabetes.

Skin Changes

Diabetes can cause feet to become very dry and the skin may peel or crack, because the nerves that control sweating in the feet are no longer working. To alleviate this problem, after bathing, dry the feet and seal in the moisture that remains with a thick coat of lubricant, such as petroleum jelly, unscented hand cream, or other emollient. Do not put oil or cream between the toes since moisture can cause an infection. Do not soak your feet.

Calluses

Calluses build up faster on the feet of diabetics. Using a pumice stone daily will keep calluses under control. It is best to use a pumice stone on wet skin and apply lotion afterward. If calluses are not trimmed, they can get very thick, break down, and result in foot ulcers (see below). Diabetics should not cut calluses or corns themselves, since this can lead to open sores and infection. This is best done by a professional. Also, do not remove calluses or corns with chemical agents, since they can burn the skin.

Foot Ulcers

Foot ulcers generally occur over the ball of the foot or at the bottom of the big toe. Ulcers can also form on the sides of the foot, often caused by poorly fitting shoes. Even if ulcers do not hurt, they should be examined by a health-care provider since neglected sores can result in infections and a possible loss of a limb. A health-care provider should x-ray the feet of a diabetic to ensure that the bones are not affected. They can also cut out any dead and infected tissue. Diabetics should keep off of their feet, since walking on an ulcer will make it larger and force an infection deeper into the foot. High blood sugar levels make it difficult to fight an infection. If the ulcer is not healing and circulation is poor, the doctor may suggest a vascular surgeon. After the foot ulcer heals, it is still necessary to treat the foot carefully since scar tissue under the healed wound can break down easily.

Diabetics should wear special shoes after the ulcer has healed to protect the area and prevent the ulcer from returning. Diabetics are more prone to get foot ulcers if they are over forty years old, have had a foot ulcer before, have had diabetes-related changes in their eyes, or have kidney disease, nerve damage, or poor blood circulation to the feet.

Neuropathy

There are three types of diabetic neuropathy, a disorder of the nerves. Motor neuropathy affects the muscles that change the function and shape of the foot. Autonomic neuropathy often inhibits the ability of the foot to sweat, so that the feet become very dry and the skin may crack. Sensory neuropathy prevents the foot from feeling sensations—this is the form that causes the most trouble. Doctors who see patients with diabetic neuropathy have various options for treatment. They can prescribe various drugs or they may opt for topical creams such as those containing capsaicin, which is derived from hot peppers; acupuncture is often recommended.[3]

While it can hurt, diabetic nerve damage (neuropathy) can paradoxically lessen the ability to feel pain, heat, and cold. Loss of feeling often means that a diabetic may not feel a foot injury. For example, they might have a tack or stone in their shoe and walk all day without feeling it. Therefore, they may not notice a foot injury until the skin breaks down and becomes infected. Nerve damage can also lead to deformities of the feet and toes, causing the toes to curl up. Those with deformed feet should not force them into regular shoes, but ask their health-care provider about special therapeutic shoes.

Evan V. Shute, M.D., related the story of a 70-year-old Halifax fisherman who had been severely diabetic for many years and was taking large doses of insulin daily. He was suffering from extensive ulceration of the left foot, with gangrenous changes including the toes. The man was urged to check into a hospital where his blood sugar could be monitored

ACUPUNCTURE FOR PERIPHERAL NEUROPATHY

Researchers at the University of Manchester, in England, evaluated forty-six patients with a mean age of 57.2 years. Thirty-four of the volunteers were type 1 diabetics, while ten were type 2 diabetics who had had the disease for an average of 13.2 years. Twenty-one of the patients were on a diet and oral hypoglycemic drugs and twenty-three were taking insulin. The volunteers, complaining of chronic painful peripheral neuropathy, were treated with acupuncture analgesia. The patients were given six courses of classical acupuncture for ten weeks, using traditional Chinese medicine acupuncture points. Of the forty-four patients who completed the study, 77 percent showed significant improvement in their primary and/or secondary symptoms. During follow-up over 18–52 weeks, 67 percent were able to stop or reduce their medications significantly, 21 percent said their symptoms had cleared completely, and only 24 percent of the patients required further acupuncture treatment.[4]

and his leg possibly amputated if it could not be saved.[5] The man refused to go to the hospital but, at his physician's suggestion, he agreed to take large oral doses of vitamin E. The man, whose daily habit was to sit in the kitchen with his leg supported on a kitchen chair, became fully ambulatory and the ulcerative area completely healed. The areas of blackish discoloration disappeared and his grossly swollen foot soon became a match for the other foot.

Dr. Shute also relates the case of a 59-year-old woman with ulceration on her right foot. A diabetic, she was taking no medication when she came to the small-town hospital in Pennsylvania. The doctors immediately gave her insulin and 800 IU per day of vitamin E. Then, they packed the ulcerated area with cotton saturated with vitamin E. Two months later, all wounds were healed.[6]

Poor Circulation

Poor circulation (blood flow) can make the feet less able to fight infection and to heal. That's because diabetes causes blood vessels of the foot and leg to narrow and harden. It is possible to control some of the things that cause poor blood flow, such as to stop smoking, since smoking makes arteries harden faster. Also, it is important to keep blood pressure and cholesterol under control. If feet are cold, there is a natural desire to warm them. However, if the feet cannot feel heat, they can be burned with hot water, hot water bottles, or heating pads. To keep feet warm, wear warm socks.

Exercise is also good for poor circulation since it stimulates blood flow to the legs and feet. Walk in sturdy, comfortable shoes, but do not walk with open sores on the feet. Some people feel pain in their calves when walking fast, up a hill, or on a hard surface—this is called intermittent claudication. Stopping to rest every so often should end the pain. Those who have this problem should also stop smoking.

In one study, a research team reported that, while their study did not focus on diabetes, poor blood supply in the veins is a condition that increases blood pressure and sluggish blood flow in the legs. Common signs of chronic venous insufficiency are varicose veins, a heavy feeling in the legs, and swelling. In the two identical phases of their trial, the researchers gave twenty volunteers either a placebo or 100 mg of pycnogenol three times daily for two months. Pycnogenol is a French maritime pine bark extract that has been shown to reduce platelet aggregation (the stickiness of blood platelets). In the first phase of the study, the sense of heaviness in the legs was reduced by 60 percent in those given the extract and leg swelling went down 74 percent. In the second phase, heaviness and swelling went down by 44 percent and 53 percent, respectively. The researchers attributed the improvement to the supplement's antioxidant or blood vessel–strengthening effect or both.[7]

In the *Journal of Nutritional Medicine*, S.E. Browne wrote that intravenous magnesium sulfate has been used in cardiovascular disease for the past sixty years. He initially used magnesium sulfate intramuscularly and then intravenously in his practice in 1958 for patients with gangrene, leg ulcers, Raynaud's disease, chilblains, and intermittent claudication. In soft-water areas (where magnesium is in short supply), patients with claudication were markedly improved with magnesium sulfate. In hard-water areas (rich in magnesium), fourteen patients with claudication showed marked improvement after intravenous magnesium; and out of eight patients with leg ulcers, five healed quickly after failing to respond to other measures. Further, seventeen patients with minor inflammation in a vein were free of pain, tenderness, and inflammation, with only residual hardness observed after two weeks of treatment, and an additional seven were fully recovered after 3–4 weeks of treatment. Four patients with deep vein thrombosis (blood clots) showed rapid improvement on intravenous magnesium (given in addition to anticoagulant therapy).[8]

Gangrene

Gangrene, which is a dangerous complication of diabetes, is the result of the death of tissue, usually because of a loss of blood supply. This can affect a small area of the skin, a finger, or a large portion of a limb, such as a leg. Pain can be felt in the dying tissue, but once the tissues are dead they become numb and can turn black. A bacterial infection can develop that causes gangrene to spread and give off an unpleasant odor. Often there is redness, swelling, and oozing pus around the affected area.[9]

There are two types of gangrene. With dry gangrene, there is usually no bacterial infection and the deprived area simply dies because its blood supply is blocked. This type, which does not spread to other tissues, can be caused by diabetes, hardening of the arteries, thrombosis, an embolism, or frostbite. Wet gangrene forms when dry gangrene or a wound becomes infected by bacteria.

To treat dry gangrene, circulation must be improved to the affected area before it is too late. Medications can be prescribed to prevent wet gangrene from developing. If wet gangrene develops, amputation of the affected area is usually unavoidable. Some of the adjacent living tissue may also have to be removed.

How to Care for Your Feet

- Keep your blood sugar under control.

- Wash feet daily and dry them carefully, especially between the toes.

- Check feet daily for sores, calluses, red spots, cuts, swelling, and blisters. To see the bottom of feet, use a mirror or ask someone for help.

- Do not put feet in hot water until you've tested to see how hot it is.

- If feet are cold, wear socks.

- Do not cut off blood flow to the feet by wearing garters or other tight garments.

- Do not use over-the-counter chemicals on corns, calluses, or warts, since they are usually too strong for diabetics and can burn the feet.

- Cut toenails straight across and file the edges. Do not rip off hangnails.

- Wear flat shoes that fit the feet.

- If there is no sensation in the feet, ask a health-care provider for advice on proper shoes.

- Consider wearing comfortable walking shoes daily.

- Check inside shoes before putting them on to see that they do not contain pebbles, nails, or other sharp objects. Also, check to see that the lining is not torn or rough.

- Socks should not have seams or other bumpy areas and put on socks gently to prevent ripping a toenail. Select padded athletic socks to protect the feet. Do not wear mended socks.

- Do not walk barefoot. It is possible to burn or cut a foot and not notice it. Keep slippers at your bedside to use when getting up during the night.

- Do not smoke.

- See a health-care provider at the first sign of infection or inflammation.[10]

CHAPTER 21

Kidney Disease

idney failure is a serious potential complication for long-standing diabetes. The kidneys are complex, highly efficient organs for filtering waste materials from the blood for disposal from the body. Each of the two kidneys contains more than one million nephrons, which are minute filtering systems. Damage to the small blood vessels in the nephrons can lead to progressive kidney failure, which is characterized by the excretion of protein and other nutrients in the urine.[1] Researchers, using a diabetic rat model, have found that there is an increased level of thiobarbituric acid reactive substances (TBARS) and activity of the enzyme superoxide dismutase and CM5-Px in the kidney during the progression of diabetes. TBARS are toxic molecules that can damage the kidneys. The susceptibility of the kidney to oxidative stress, found early in diabetes, may be an important factor in the development of diabetic nephropathy.[2]

Because diabetes enhances the kidney's vulnerability to infections, diabetics should be aware of any symptoms of kidney or urinary tract infections (flank pain, difficult or burning urination, urgent need to urinate, blood in the urine) and should consult their physician at once. Improved treatments for kidney failure, notably melodialysis using an artificial kidney and replacement of diseased kidneys with transplants, have enhanced the outlook for patients with advanced diabetic kidney disease (diabetic nephropathy). However, these measures do not cure the disease and studies have reported that kidneys transplanted in patients with poorly controlled diabetes will develop diabetic nephropathy in a few years. Bringing elevated blood glucose into the normal range can reduce kidney damage.[3]

Dealing With Kidney Problems

At Washington University School of Medicine, in St. Louis, Missouri, Saulo Klahr, M.D., found that the progression of kidney disease may be slowed by reducing high blood pressure, lowering cholesterol levels, reducing the amount of protein in the diet or reducing protein in the urine, and reducing the amount of immune cells in the kidney. Reducing animal protein intake decreases blood pressure and plasma flow within the glomerulus (a small grouping of capillaries in the kidney). Protein restriction is also thought to affect immune function.[4]

Since dietary protein intake can increase blood flow to the kidneys, decreasing the amount of protein in the diet can reduce the blood flow to the kidney, according to Ping H. Wang, M.D., of the University of California at Irvine. This seems to provide a protective effect on a variety of kidney diseases. While previous studies have not consistently shown the efficacy of dietary protein restriction in reducing the risk of kidney disease progression, this study clearly shows that by lowering the amount of protein intake, the risk of end-stage kidney disease (requiring dialy-

LITHOTRIPSY INCREASES THE RISK OF DIABETES

The use of shock waves to pulverize kidney stones into sand-like material significantly increases the risk for diabetes and high blood pressure later in life. A study by the Mayo Clinic, in Rochester, Minnesota, found that patients who underwent the pulverizing procedure (lithotripsy) developed diabetes at almost four times the rate of those whose kidney stones were treated by other methods. The lithotripsy patients also developed high blood pressure about 50 percent more often than a group treated by other methods.[5]

The diabetes risk is partially related to the number of shocks given. The risk for high blood pressure was related to treatment of stones in both kidneys but not to the total number of shocks, which can number in the hundreds of thousands. The shock wave therapy for kidney stones apparently increases the risk for diabetes by damaging the insulin-producing cells of the pancreas, through which the shock waves may pass. The shock waves may increase the risk for high blood pressure by scarring the kidneys and affecting their secretion of hormones, like rennin, that influence blood pressure. An estimated one million people in the United States have undergone lithotripsy treatment since the procedure was introduced in 1984. Shock waves can demolish up to 90 percent of kidney stones.

sis) can be reduced by 30 percent in most diabetic and non-diabetic patients. Since the significant side effect of restricting protein is malnutrition, patients should be closely followed by a physician and dietitian. A low-protein diet for people with kidney disease should consist of 0.6 g of protein per kilogram of body weight, which is safe for the majority of patients.[6]

Michael T. Pedrini, M.D., and colleagues at the University of California at Irvine also agree that restricting dietary protein effectively slows the progression of both diabetic and non-diabetic kidney diseases. They evaluated the effects of a low-protein diet on chronic kidney disease in 1,413 volunteers from five studies of non-diabetic kidney disease and 108 patients in five studies with type 1 diabetes. In the type 1 diabetics, a low-protein diet significantly slowed the increase in urinary albumin levels and the decline in other parameters. Albumin is a water-soluble protein found in blood plasma.[7]

Diabetics with kidney failure must endure dialysis (a machine that filters their blood) or have a kidney transplant if a donated kidney can be found. Without dialysis, harmful levels of toxins can build up in their bodies. Kidney dialysis patients are subject to painful muscular contractions in their legs. Researchers advised sixty dialysis patients to follow one of four daily supplement regimens for eight weeks: 400 mg of vitamin E; 250 mg of vitamin C; a combination of both vitamins; or a placebo.[8] The patients taking a combination of vitamins E and C reaped the greatest benefit—a 97 percent reduction in leg cramps. When taken alone, vitamin E and vitamin C resulted in 54 percent and 61 percent reductions in leg cramps, respectively, while the placebo brought only a 7 percent reduction in symptoms.

A Swiss study evaluated the vitamin status of six patients, 45–66 years old, and four other volunteers, 28–40 years of age, who, due to nephropathy caused by analgesics or diabetes, underwent Continuous Ambulatory Peritoneal Dialysis (CAPD). Compared to healthy controls, vitamins B_1, B_6, C, and folic acid in the blood were in the lower range of normal, while vitamin A and B_{12} amounts in the blood were elevated. After supplementing with vitamin B_1 (8 mg), B_2 (8 mg), B_6 (10 mg), nicotinamide (B_3; 50 mg), calcium pantothenate (pantothenic acid, 10.9 mg), biotin (30 mcg), folic acid (2 mg), and vitamin C (100 mg), given twice daily over seven weeks, the levels of B_6 and C were normalized and the levels of folic acid greatly increased. However, levels of B_1 and B_2 remained unchanged. Pantothenic acid, biotin, and folic acid are B vitamins. During the thirteen-week study, levels of vitamin A and B_{12}, which were not supplemented, tended to normalize. The results of the trial show that increasingly efficient methods of dialysis lead to a growing loss of nutrients, whereby even substances regarded as insoluble in water are eliminated. This can lead to depleted body stores and malfunctions, especially during long-term dialysis. Researchers recommend vitamin B_1 (30 mg), B_6 (10–50 mg), folic acid (0.5–1.0 mg), and vitamin C (100–200 mg) twice daily.[9]

Malnutrition is one of the main factors in the death and disability of dialysis patients, according to Richard Schmicker, M.D., in Berlin, Germany. Food restriction, adequate protein and energy intake, electrolyte (mineral) balance, and vitamin intake are important when beginning dialysis.[10] Because of deficiencies, dialysis patients may need to take daily supplements of vitamins C (100 mg), B_1 and B_2 (1.5–1.6 mg), and B_6 (10–20 mg). Folic acid may need to be supplemented at 1 mg per day. Vitamin A may not be needed, since it is often higher in dialysis patients.

In a study in Rome, Italy, it was reported that of the forty-eight chronic hemodialysis patients, coenzyme Q_{10} levels were abnormally low in 62 percent of the cases. Reduced levels of coenzyme Q_{10} may increase the risk of oxidative damage in patients undergoing hemodialysis.[11]

At Schneider Children's Hospital, in New Hyde Park, New York, researchers pointed out that the kidney plays a significant role in maintaining taurine balance, an amino acid that acts as an antioxidant in the body. Taurine can prevent the oxidizing of fats in capillaries and tissues in the kidney that are exposed to high glucose in diabetes and other conditions. In experimental tests, dietary taurine ameliorates kidney disease, including refractory nephritic syndrome and diabetic nephropathy.[12]

CHAPTER 22

Thyroid Gland Complications

An organ of the endocrine system, the thyroid gland is located in the neck, just below the voice box. It consists of two lobes, one on each side of the windpipe, joined by a narrow portion of tissue called the isthmus. Thyroid tissue is made up of two types of secretory cells, follicular cells and parafollicular cells (C cells). Follicular cells are made up of hollow, spherical follicles, which secrete the iodine-containing hormones thyroxine (T4) and triiodothyronine (T3). Inside the follicles is a semifluid, colloid substance that is essential for the production of T4 and T3.[1] Parafollicular cells are found singly or in groups in the spaces between the follicles. These cells secrete the hormone calcitonin. Between the follicles are a number of blood capillaries, which are small lymphatic vessels, and connective tissue.

T4 and T3 hormones play a significant role in controlling body metabolism. For example, calcitonin acts with parathyroid hormone (produced by the parathyroid gland) to regulate calcium balance in the body. By regulating metabolism, the two hormones release energy from nutrients or use energy to create other substances, such as proteins. In children, the two hormones are essential for normal physical growth and mental development. The secretion of T4 and T3 is controlled by a hormonal feedback system that involves the pituitary gland and hypothalamus in the brain. Insufficient thyroid hormone production is called hypothyroidism—symptoms may include tiredness, dry skin, hair loss, weight gain, constipation, and sensitivity to cold. Hyperthyroidism (the overproduction of thyroid hormones) causes fatigue, anxiety, palpitations, sweating, weight loss, diarrhea, and intolerance to heat.[2]

Diabetes and the Thyroid

It was the late Broda O. Barnes, M.D., in his landmark book *Hypothyroidism: The Unsuspected Illness*, who highlighted the many health problems due to low thyroid function. Concerning diabetes, he called it an "iceberg" disease, in that sugar in the blood is only the tip of the iceberg. Today, diabetics are not so much troubled by metabolic crises, but may suffer from the complications of diabetes—blindness, kidney and nervous disease, skin infections, and, above all, degenerative changes in the heart and blood vessels. Diabetics have twice the rate of coronary heart disease as non-diabetics, and as many as 77 percent of diabetic deaths are due to blood vessel disease of one type or another.[3]

"The complications of diabetes are much like the manifestations of hypothyroidism," Dr. Barnes stated. "Many diabetics do, in fact, have low thyroid function. I am not the first to observe that the complications of diabetes, particularly the atherosclerotic complications (hardening of the arteries), are not due to the disturbance in carbohydrate metabolism but to something else. And that something else could well be hypothyroidism. I believe that thyroid therapy for people with low thyroid function who have not yet developed diabetes may do much to prevent appearance of the disease."[4]

Dr. Barnes discussed the clinical experience of C.D. Eaton, M.D., a Detroit physician, who published a report in *The Journal of the Michigan Medical Society* in 1954. Based on his experience with hundreds of diabetics, Dr. Eaton said that the symptoms of hypothyroidism and diabetes are quite similar, except for the disturbance in carbohydrate metabolism that occurs in diabetes. The patients with both complications suffered from

SMOKING AND THYROID PROBLEMS

Smoking appears to have a goitrogenic (or goiter-producing) effect, apparently from the action of thiocyanate and other compounds found in cigarette smoke, according to researchers in Pisa, Italy. A goiter is a visible enlargement of the thyroid gland. This is especially important for people who live in iodine-deficient areas. Smokers have a high prevalence of Graves' disease (an autoimmune disease of the thyroid gland) as well as Graves' ophthalmology (increased water in the eyes as a result of hyperthyroidism).[5]

similar symptoms, such as weakness, itching, constipation, somnolence, muscular pains, elevated blood fat levels, susceptibility to infections, poor healing of wounds, premature hardening of the arteries, and gangrene.

While controlling the sugar level in diabetic patients, Dr. Eaton found that the other symptoms persisted. Using the basal metabolic rate, he found that, even though that test is not very sensitive and may miss many cases of low thyroid function, it established that hypothyroidism was more frequent in diabetics than in non-diabetics. When Dr. Eaton began giving thyroid therapy in small doses to his hypothyroid diabetic patients, he found that the thyroid had no direct influence on diabetes. But when sugar metabolism was controlled by insulin, diet, or other measures, it *remained controlled* when thyroid doses were added. Also, there were fewer problems with blood clots in the arteries, which he interpreted as being due to improved circulation and less stagnation of blood. In addition, as a result of increased circulation in the extremities, there was less gangrene, even in those with hardening of the arteries.

"All of the diabetic patients I have personally treated to date have run subnormal basal temperatures and have had symptoms of hypothyroidism, and with thyroid therapy they have had not only relief of the hypothyroidism symptoms but have shown no detectable progression in atherosclerosis," Dr. Barnes added.[6]

Basal Body Temperature Test to Check Your Thyroid Status

The basal body temperature test is a relatively easy way to self-monitor your thyroid activity. Here is the procedure to follow.

1. Before going to sleep, shake down a thermometer to below 95°F and place it near your bed.

2. Upon waking, place the thermometer in your armpit for ten minutes. Do not move about, but rest with your eyes closed.

3. After ten minutes, record the temperature and date.

4. Record your temperature on successive mornings at the exact same time. Menstruating women should perform the test on the second, third, and fourth days of menstruation.

The correct basal body temperature should be between 97.6°F and

98.2°F. It will register below the normal reading of 98.6°F since you are taking your temperature under the arm rather than orally or anally. Show the readings to your physician to determine if you have hypothyroidism.[7]

Dealing With Thyroid Problems

The size of a proper starting dose of thyroid therapy will vary with the age and size of the patient, according to Dr. Barnes. A child under three years of age will usually not need more than 0.25 grain daily. By age six, 0.5 grain may be used in the beginning; a teenager or adult may be safely started on 1 grain daily; for overweight people, 2 grains may be used, but larger doses are not needed initially. The starting dose should be used for about two months and perhaps increased after that. Those who have had a heart attack should not begin therapy for at least two months after the incident, then the starting dose should not be more than 0.5 grain per day. The basal body temperature can serve as an excellent guide not only to the need for thyroid therapy, but also to determine the proper thyroid dosage. However, thyroid replacement therapy should only be done under the supervision of an experienced physician or endocrinologist.

Proper levels of thyroid hormone are necessary for the body to maintain proper levels of blood sugar, explain Ronald Klatz, D.O., and Robert Goldman, M.D. Therefore, hypothyroidism may be implicated in diabetes, especially type 2 diabetes. Basically, the thyroid allows the body to convert glucose into energy, but in cases of hypothyroidism, glucose cannot be utilized, resulting in glucose waste and hypoglycemia. Hypoglycemia causes the excretion of adrenaline, which causes toxicity of the circulatory system. These circulatory problems are common in diabetics, but they can be reduced or avoided with thyroid supplements. The authors added that thyroid supplements have also been shown to reverse other symptoms of diabetes and, in some cases, have reversed type 2 diabetes.[8]

The medical treatment for hypothyroidism involves taking desiccated thyroid or synthetic thyroid hormone (T4), according to Michael Murray, N.D., and Joseph Pizzorno, N.D. While synthetic hormones are popular, many naturopathic physicians prefer desiccated natural thyroid, complete with all thyroid hormones, not just thyroxine. The thyroid extracts sold in health food stores are required to be free of thyroxine in order to prevent serious problems such as heart disturbances, insomnia, and anxiety. The health food store products may provide support for those with mild hypothyroidism.[9]

"It is important to nutritionally support the thyroid gland by avoiding goitrogens and insuring adequate intake of key nutrients required in the manufacture of thyroid hormone. For this reason, most health food store thyroid products also contain supportive nutrients such as iodine, zinc, and tyrosine," added Drs. Murray and Pizzorno. Goitrogenic agents, which produce goiter, include members of the cabbage family (cabbage, turnip, rutabaga, kale; cooking usually inactivates the goitrogenic agent), milk from cows that have eaten plants containing goitrogens, raw soybeans, thiocyanate-containing drugs for high blood pressure, and arsenic.

Researchers in Brazil evaluated twelve hyperthyroid patients and seven hypothyroid patients to determine their zinc levels. They found that hyperthyroid patients showed a marked zinc loss with maintenance of serum zinc due to probable tissue depletion of the mineral and lower zinc incorporation into their tissues after being given a zinc supplement. The findings were probably due to the catabolic state of hypothyroidism. Catabolism is the breaking down of complex chemical compounds into simpler ones, such as glycogen into carbon dioxide and water. For the hypothyroid volunteers, there was a definite zinc deficiency, with lower intestinal absorption of the mineral.[10]

Subclinical hypothyroidism (too low to be diagnosed by conventional tests) is found in more than 10 percent of women over sixty, thus increasing serum lipids and lowering the threshold for developing major depressive disorders, according to Kenneth A. Weeber, M.D., of the San Francisco Mount Zion Medical Center. Subclinical thyrotoxicosis (excessive amounts of thyroid hormone) is a state in which there is normal serum T4 but with a level of thyroid-stimulating hormone (TSH) that is undetectable in an individual who is not ill. Subclinical thyrotoxicosis is sometimes associated with reduced bone mineral density in postmenopausal women and a threefold relative risk for the development of atrial fibrillation (irregular heart beat).[11] Inadvertently excess hormone in the treatment of hypothyroidism can result in subclinical hypothyroidism. It has been estimated that, even in thyroid disease clinics, excessive doses may occur in about 20 percent of the patients.[12]

CHAPTER 23

Impotence

E rectile dysfunction (ED), or impotence, is defined as an inability to have and maintain an erection rigid enough for sexual intercourse. It is estimated that more than 10 million American men are bothered by impotence, and it is three times more common in men with diabetes in all age groups.[1] An estimated 100 million men are affected worldwide and the prevalence of ED is expected to double by 2025. The risk of ED is related to age, smoking, diabetes, heart disease, depression, high blood pressure, and other illnesses.[2]

Recent data is perhaps the first evidence of a strong association between ED and a subsequent development of cardiovascular disease, and this should prompt investigation and intervention for cardiovascular risk factors, since the risks for the two disorders are similar. Researchers at the University of South Carolina, in Columbia, studied 3,250 men, ranging in age from twenty-six to eighty-three, who did not have ED at their first office visit. The men were studied for six to forty-eight months, at which time impotence was recorded in 2.2 percent of them during follow-up. The researchers found that high levels of total cholesterol and low levels of high-density lipoprotein (HDL or "good") cholesterol are significant risk factors for developing erectile dysfunction.[3]

Strong epidemiological evidence links the subsequent risk of erectile dysfunction to the presence of well-recognized risk factors for coronary heart disease, such as increased body weight, high blood pressure, and high blood levels of cholesterol and triglycerides, according to Katherine Esposito, M.D., and colleagues at the Second University of Naples, in Italy.[4] The researchers postulated an association between erectile dysfunction and the metabolic syndrome (a precursor to diabetes), because four of the five components of the metabolic syndrome are risk factors for ED. The adoption of a healthful lifestyle is strongly recommended in order to reduce the prevalence of the metabolic syndrome and the burden of erectile dysfunction.

The Massachusetts Male Aging Study (MMAS) and other studies show that diabetes in men over forty years of age is associated with impotence. Erectile dysfunction has a broad negative impact on health-related quality of life in people with type 2 diabetes. In one study, the onset of ED was associated with a further worsening in physical functioning, general health perception, and social functioning. ED was also associated with a highly significant increase in depressive symptoms and a marked decrease in quality of sexual life.[5] Impotence in diabetics may be the result of nerve damage, clogged arteries, decreased testosterone levels, prescriptions for high blood pressure (beta-blockers and diuretics), depression, ulcers, or drugs to prevent vomiting. Also, it is made worse by psychological factors, an injury, blood vessel disease with decreased circulation, and nerve damage. Other factors are stress, fears about aging, and worry about sexual performance.

Although impotence can occur for a number of reasons, in men forty and older, it is often associated with circulatory problems related to hardening of the arteries, according to Kenneth Goldberg, M.D., of the Male Health Center, in Dallas, Texas. The same fatty deposits that often clog

SMOKING AND IMPOTENCE

One possible cause of diminished hormones that contributes to impotence is smoking, which leads to large amounts of carbon dioxide in the blood, reducing the hormone levels and contributing to erectile dysfunction, states Robert M. Giller, M.D. Smoking not only affects hormonal levels, but it can clog the penile arteries and cause impotence, even in younger men. One study reported that men as young as thirty-five suffered from impotence due to smoking; men who smoked a pack of cigarettes a day for twenty years were four times more likely than non-smokers to become impotent because of clogged arteries.[6] A study involving 4,400 Vietnam veterans reported that impotence occurred at a 50 percent higher rate among current smokers than in non-smokers or past smokers. The rate of impotence among non-smokers was 2.2 percent; 2 percent for former smokers; and 3.7 percent for current smokers.[7]

arteries of the heart can also build up in the tiny arteries in the penis. Therefore, too little blood is available to pump up the spongy cylinders that cause an erection. Also, drugs prescribed to treat high blood pressure and nerve damage caused by diabetes can also cause erectile dysfunction.[8] Men with diabetes typically suffer from impotence—first, because of poor circulation, and second, because of autonomic nerve damage, according to Ronald L. Hoffman, M.D. This complication of diabetes can reduce potency in men as early as in their thirties and forties.[9]

In the standard work-up for ED, a urologist will measure penile blood flow and perhaps perform an angiogram, in which a dye is injected to see how it travels through the bloodstream. Less invasive is the penile Doppler test, in which a ring with a sensor is placed around the penis to test for nocturnal erection.

Lifestyle Changes for Overcoming Impotence

A number of lifestyle modifications may prove useful in overcoming impotency.

- Stop smoking.

- If you suffer from diabetes, hardening of the arteries, elevated cholesterol, or high blood pressure, your impotence could be connected to these problems. Follow appropriate measures to keep them under control.

- Check any medications to see if they affect potency. Ask your doctor about the side effects of your medications.

- If you have had a heart attack or other major illness, discuss with your doctor its effects on your sex life. Also, if you have had prostate or abdominal surgery, it's possible you have had nerve or vascular damage that can be reversed—ask your doctor.

- If you sense that your impotence has a psychological basis (fear of performing), get counseling.[10]

- In a study of diabetic men treated in ambulatory, secondary, and tertiary diabetes clinics in Israel, it was found that physical activity (leisure and work-related) and drinking small amounts of alcohol may have a protective effect against ED, according to Ofra Kalter-Leibovici, M.D., and colleagues at Tel-Aviv University, in Israel.[11]

Natural Remedies for Impotence

Men having trouble maintaining an erection might want to try natural remedies before opting for a Viagra prescription. Nutrition plays a role in determining sexual impotence, according to Julian Whitaker, M.D. Vegetables, fruits, whole grains, and legumes are key food groups, along with proteins (fish, chicken, turkey, and lean cuts of hormone-free meat). Nutrients such as zinc, essential fatty acids, and vitamins A, B_6, and E are also necessary for healthy sexual function.[12] Since it is concentrated in semen, frequent ejaculation depletes zinc stores. Food sources of zinc include nuts, seeds, legumes, and liver.

Some patients have improved potency and fertility after their zinc and vitamin B_6 deficiencies have been corrected, according to Carl C. Pfeiffer, Ph.D., M.D. Cadmium, a harmful metal, antagonizes zinc and can, in extreme cases, stop the formation of sperm in the testes.[13] Semen contains considerable amounts of zinc and sulfur. Semen is 25 percent calcium, 14 percent zinc, 14 percent magnesium, 3 percent sulfur, and 0.015 percent copper. The vitamin content of semen consists of 13 mg of vitamin C and 53 percent inositol, which is related to the B-complex.

Earl Mindell, R.Ph., Ph.D., recommends *Ginkgo biloba* (60 mg, three times daily); a combination of saw palmetto, zinc, and pumpkin seed oil (2–4 capsules daily); and arginine (4–5 g) taken forty-five minutes before sex. For men over fifty, he recommends DHEA (dehydroepiandrosterone), a steroid hormone (one tablet, 25–50 mg per day). DHEA should not be taken by those under forty unless blood levels of the hormone are low; men over fifty can take 50 mg per day.[14]

A study in Hawaii evaluated twenty-five male volunteers, 40–70 years of age, with mild to moderate erectile dysfunction. They were evaluated during a four-week period when they were given a supplement containing various vitamins, minerals, and herbs. The supplement contained *Ginkgo biloba* (24 percent flavone glycosides, 6 percent terpene lactones); Korean ginseng (30 percent ginsenosides); American ginseng (5 percent ginsenosides); L-arginine (an amino acid); vitamins A, B-complex, C, E, folic acid, pantothenic acid, and biotin; and the minerals zinc and selenium. The volunteers were given the supplement twice daily, once in the morning after waking and once in the evening. Of the twenty-one men who completed the study, 88.9 percent improved their ability to maintain an erection during sexual intercourse, and 75 percent had improved satisfaction with their sex life. There were no side effects reported.[15]

Yohimbine

In 1982, a group of physicians at Queens University in Kingston, Ontario, Canada, studied the effect of yohimbine on organic impotence. The study involved twenty-three patients, 32–72 years old, of which almost half were diabetics. The other volunteers had high blood pressure and other circulatory problems and were taking antihypertensive drugs. The patients were given 6 mg of yohimbine hydrochloride three times daily for ten weeks. Since that is virtually the maximum dose, a few of the patients experienced nervousness, unspecified gastric complaints, and mild tremors. They were told to reduce the amount to 2 mg three times daily and then to increase the amount until they were back to 18 mg per day. All of the volunteers eventually were able to tolerate that amount without further complications. Six men were able to experience sustained erections and to resume normal satisfactory sexual relations. Four others reported partial satisfaction. Yohimbine hydrochloride, extracted from the bark of a West African tree, is a stronger version of yohimbe and is approved by the U.S. Food and Drug Administration to treat impotence.[16]

At Valparaiso University, in Indiana, researchers recruited eleven men with erectile dysfunction from a urology outpatient clinic. When yohimbine was given at a dose of up to 10 mg three times daily, there was no effect in sexually functional men, but there were mixed effects in the sexual function of men with ED. The herb may have exerted an enhancing effect on sexual desire and improved sexual performance. In this study and others, the improved erection response was about 20 percent or higher.[17]

A study in Brazil evaluated twenty-two men, with a mean age of fifty-eight, who complained of ED. The volunteers were treated for thirty days with a placebo and then thirty days with oral yohimbine hydrochloride (100 mg daily). Fourteen percent and 55 percent of the men reported complete or partial response to the treatment, respectively. Common side effects included anxiety, increase in cardiac frequency, increased urinary output, and headache, but none of the men dropped out of the study. However, the authors said that a single dose would not have any effect on impotence.[18]

Rhodiola rosea

Researchers, in China, Russia, and the Far East have long used *Rhodiola rosea* (golden root) to ward off fatigue and treat a variety of conditions, such as weak erections. A three-month clinical trial revealed significant improvement in sexual function and other conditions. In a Russian study using experimental animals with diabetes, the research team found that golden root and ginseng increased the blood levels of insulin and decreased the level of glucagons, a hormone that promotes an increase in the sugar content of the blood by accelerating the rate of glycogen breakdown in the liver. Typical dosages of the over-the-counter supplement are 1–2 capsules or follow directions on the label.[19]

Other Foods and Herbs for Erection Problems and Increasing Libido

- Fava bean (*Vicia faba*): A source of L-dopa, the fava bean allegedly was used to incite the Roman poet Cicero to passion. An 8- to 16-ounce serving of the beans might be enough to give an erection a boost.

- *Ginkgo biloba:* In several studies, physicians have obtained good results with a standard ginkgo extract (60–240 mg per day). In a nine-month study, 79 percent of the men with impotence due to atherosclerotic clogging of the penile arteries reported significant improvement and no side effects.

- Velvet bean (*Mucuna* spp.): These seeds contain more L-dopa than fava beans and are considered an aphrodisiac.

- Anise (*Pimpinella anisum*): Anise has a reputation for increasing the male libido.

- Cardamom (*Elettaria cardamomum*): Arab cultures hold this herb in high esteem for its aphrodisiac qualities. It is often mixed with coffee.

- Cinnamon (*Cinnamomum* spp.): In a test at the Smell and Taste Research Foundation in Chicago, Illinois, researchers reported that the smell of cinnamon buns increased the blood flow in male medical students.

- Ginger (*Zingiber officinale*): Saudi researchers suggest that ginger extracts significantly increase sperm motility and quality.

- Ginseng (*Panax* spp.): Chinese philosophers maintain that ginseng makes an old man young again.

- *Muira puama:* One study shows that this little-known herb may be effective in restoring libido and treating ED.

- Oat (*Avena sativa*): Stallions that are fed wild oats supposedly become friskier and libidinous, which generated the phrase "sowing wild oats."

- Querbracho (*Aspidosperma quebracho-blanco*): In South America, this herb is considered a male aphrodisiac; it is not recommended for those with high blood pressure.

- Wolfberry (*Lyciumm chinese*): In one study, men over fifty-nine ate about 50 g of wolfberries a day for ten days and reported significantly raised testosterone levels.

- Ashwagandha (*Withania somnifera*): Occasional use of this Ayurvedic herb, in a tea, is said to increase male libido.

- Country mallow (*Sida corifolia*): This stimulant herb has a folk reputation as an erection-enhancing aphrodisiac. It contains 850 parts per million of ephedrine.

- Guarana (*Paullinia cupana*): This Brazilian herb contains lots of caffeine and is regarded as an aphrodisiac.

- Saw Palmetto (*Serenoa repens*): This herb, native to the southeastern United States, has been used to treat prostate problems and was once considered useful for treating impotence and loss of libido.[20]

Since the purpose of this chapter is to discuss possible natural and nutritional approaches to impotence, I won't be dealing with penile implants, injection therapy, hormonal treatments, vacuum devices, topical drugs, bypass surgery, and so on. These are subjects to discuss with your urologist.

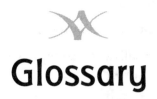

Glossary

ACE inhibitors. Drugs that can lower blood pressure and slow the progression of kidney disease.

Acetone. A chemical found in the blood when the body uses fat instead of glucose for energy. When acetone forms, it usually means that the cells do not have enough insulin or cannot use insulin in the blood to convert glucose (sugar) to energy. Acetone is eliminated in the urine and someone with lots of acetone in the body can have breath that smells fruity.

Acidosis. Too much acid in the body. For diabetics, this can lead to diabetic ketoacidosis.

Acute diabetic ketoacidosis (DKA). A serious condition found in type 1 diabetics due to insufficient insulin. Symptoms include high blood glucose levels (over 240 mg/dl), ketones in the urine, shortness of breath, nausea, and, in extreme cases, coma.

Adrenal glands. Two organs sitting atop the kidneys that release hormones such as adrenaline (epinephrine). This and other hormones, such as insulin, control the body's use of glucose (sugar).

Adult-onset diabetes mellitus. Former term for type 2 diabetes.

After-eating blood glucose. Blood that is taken one to two hours after eating to see the amount of glucose (sugar) in the blood.

Albumin. A water-soluble protein that is found in tissues and fluids.

Albuminuria. The presence of protein in the urine.

Alpha cell. A type of cell in the pancreas, in the area called the islets of Langerhans, that makes and releases a hormone called glucagon, which raises the level of glucose in the blood.

Amino acids. A group of twenty-two essential and non-essential nitrogen-containing compounds that form the basic structure of proteins.

Aminos. Compounds that contain nitrogen.

Amylase. A pancreatic or salivary enzyme necessary for breaking down starch so that it can be absorbed.

Amyotrophy. A type of diabetic neuropathy that brings muscle weakness and wasting.

Angina pectoris. Chest pain that may also involve the arm, jaw, and shoulder.

Angiopathy. A disease of the blood vessels (arteries, veins, and capillaries) that occurs when someone has diabetes for a long time. In macroangiopathy, fat and blood clots build up in large blood vessels, stick to the vessel walls, and block the flow of blood. In microangiopathy, the walls of the smaller blood vessels become so thick and weak that they bleed, leak protein, and slow the flow of blood through the body. Cells, such as those in the eye, do not get enough blood and may be damaged.

Antibodies. Proteins that the body makes to protect itself from foreign substances. For diabetics, the body sometimes makes antibodies to work against pork or beef insulins because they are not exactly the same as human insulin or because they have impurities. The antibodies can keep the insulin from working well and may cause a diabetic to have an allergic reaction.

Anticoagulants. Blood thinners that inhibit the formation of clots.

Antioxidant. A substance, such as vitamin E, that prevents free-radical or oxidative damage.

Apolipoprotein-a. A fairly new defined risk factor for hardening of the arteries, including coronary and cerebrovascular vessels. It is similar to low-density lipoprotein (LDL) cholesterol.

Apolipoprotein-b. A single protein found in low-density lipoprotein (LDL) cholesterol that allows LDL to attach itself to cells. LDL, the so-called bad cholesterol, is associated with cardiovascular disease by way of oxidation and free-radical damage. When LDL mixes with oxygen and becomes oxidized, it can clog arteries and lead to cardiovascular disease.

Arrhythmia. Irregular heartbeat.

Arteriole. The smallest blood vessel.

Artery. A blood vessel that carries oxygen-rich blood away from the heart.

Ascorbic acid. Vitamin C.

Atherosclerosis. Commonly called hardening of the arteries, this is a process in which cholesterol, triglycerides, and other fatty substances are deposited in artery walls, causing a blockage of an artery.

Autonomic neuropathy. Damage that is caused by elevated blood sugar levels.

Basal metabolic rate. The energy necessary for internal or cellular work, such as maintaining body temperature, when the body is resting.

Benign. Harmless.

Beta-carotene. Provitamin A. One of the carotenoids in plants that can be converted into vitamin A in the body.

Beta cell. A cell in the pancreas, located in the islets of Langerhans, that makes and releases insulin, a hormone that controls the level of glucose (sugar) in the blood.

Bilirubin. Breakdown product of the hemoglobin molecule in red blood cells.

Biotin. A B-complex vitamin.

Blood-brain barrier. A barrier that prohibits the passage of substances from the blood into the brain.

Blood glucose. The main sugar that the body makes from proteins, fats, and carbohydrates (mostly from carbohydrates). Glucose is the major source of energy for living cells and is carried to the cells via the bloodstream. Cells cannot use glucose without the help of insulin.

Blood glucose monitoring. A way of testing how much glucose is in the blood. A drop of blood, usually taken from the fingertip, is placed on the end of a testing strip, specially coated with a chemical that makes it change color according to how much glucose (sugar) is in the blood. Telling whether the level of glucose is low, high, or normal can be determined by comparing the strip's color to a reference color chart or by inserting the strip into a small meter. Blood testing is more accurate than urine testing in monitoring blood glucose levels, since it shows what the current level of glucose is rather than what the level was an hour or so previously.

Blood pressure. The force of the blood on the walls of the arteries. The higher, or systolic pressure, occurs each time the heart pushes blood into the vessels and the lower, or diastolic pressure, occurs when the heart rests between beats. In a blood pressure reading of 120/80, 120 is the systolic pressure and 80 is the diastolic reading. A reading of 120/80 is said to be normal. High blood pressure can lead to heart disease and strokes.

Blood urea nitrogen (BUN). A waste product of the kidneys, increased BUN levels in the blood may indicate early kidney disease.

Blood vessels. Tubes that carry blood to and from all parts of the body, including arteries, veins, and capillaries. The heart pumps blood through these vessels so that the blood can carry oxygen and nutrients the cells need or take away waste that the cells do not need.

Body mass index (BMI). A ratio of weight to height, which can accurately determine whether or not a person is obese. The BMI is determined by multiplying your weight in pounds by 703, multiplying your height in inches by itself, then dividing the first number by the second one. The CDC reports that a healthy range is between 18.5 and 24.9.

Brittle diabetes. A term used when a person's blood sugar level often swings quickly from high to low and from low to high; also called labile or unstable diabetes.

Bronze diabetes. A genetic disease of the liver in which the body takes in too much iron from food; also called hemochromatosis.

Calorie. A nutritional calorie is calculated as the amount of heat necessary to raise 1 kilogram of water 1°C.

Capillary. The smallest of the body's blood vessels.

Capsaicin. A topical ointment made from chili peppers that is used to relieve the pain of peripheral neuropathy.

Carbohydrates. Starches and sugars in foods.

Cardiomyopathy. Heart damage.

Cardiovascular disease. A variety of heart and blood vessel diseases that include heart attack, stroke, hardening of the arteries, and congestive heart failure.

Cataracts. Condition in the eyes that reduces lens transparency and results in a loss of visual acuity.

Celiac disease. A malabsorption disorder that brings on malnutrition, edema, abnormal stools, anemia, and peripheral neuropathy. These abnormalities in the intestinal tract require a gluten-free diet, which involves the avoidance of wheat, rye, oats, barley, and several other grains and grasses.

Cerebrovascular disease. Damage to the blood vessels in the brain, which can cause a stroke. Sometimes the blood vessels can burst, resulting in a hemorrhagic stroke. Diabetics are at high risk for this condition.

Charcot's foot. A deformity of the bones in the feet caused by diabetic nerve damage. It can cause foot ulcers.

Cholecalciferol. Vitamin D_3.

Cholesterol. A fat found in foods of animal origin and also produced inside the body. It is needed for the production of certain hormones as well as for obtaining vitamin D from the sun. Large amounts can cause a narrowing of the arteries in susceptible people.

Choline. A vitamin-like substance related to the B-complex vitamins.

Chronic. Long-standing or frequently recurring.

Cirrhosis. A severe liver disease characterized by the replacement of the liver cells with scar tissue.

Clinical trial. A scientifically controlled study using people, usually to test the effectiveness of a new treatment.

Cobalamin. Vitamin B_{12}.

Coenzyme. A necessary non-protein component of an enzyme, most often a vitamin or a mineral.

Congenital defects. Problems that are present at birth.

Congestive heart failure. Chronic disease that develops when the heart is not capable of supplying the oxygen demands of the body.

Contraindication. A condition that makes a treatment not helpful or possibly harmful.

Coronary artery disease. A condition that develops when the heart does not get an adequate supply of blood and oxygen due to hardening of the arteries.

Cortisol. A stress hormone that raises blood glucose levels.

Coxsackie B$_4$ virus. An agent that has been shown to damage the beta cells of the pancreas in laboratory tests. The virus may be one cause of type 1 diabetes.

C-peptide. A substance that the pancreas releases into the bloodstream in equal amounts to insulin. A test of C-peptide levels will show how much insulin the body is making.

C-reactive protein. An inflammatory marker in the blood that is strongly associated with heart disease.

Creatinine. A chemical in the blood that is passed in the urine. A test of the amount of creatinine in blood, or in blood and urine, shows if the kidneys are working right or if they are diseased.

D-alpha tocopherol. Natural vitamin E.

dl. Deciliter; 0.18 pint dry or 0.21 pint liquid.

Dl-alpha tocopherol. Synthetic vitamin E.

Delta cell. A cell in the pancreas, located in the islets of Langerhans. These cells make somatostatin, a hormone that is thought to control how the beta cells make and release insulin and how the alpha cells make and release glucagon.

Dextrose. Also called glucose, it is a simple sugar found in the blood and the body's main source of energy.

Diabetic amyotrophy. A disease of the nerves leading to the muscles, this condition affects only one side of the body and occurs most often in older men with mild diabetes. *See* neuropathy.

Diabetic coma. A severe emergency in which a person is not conscious because the blood glucose is too low or too high. If the level is too low, the person has hypoglycemia; if the level is too high, the person has hyperglycemia and may develop ketoacidosis.

Diabetic ketoacidosis (DKA). Out-of-control diabetes with high blood sugar, this condition needs emergency treatment. Blood sugar levels may get too high because of illness, taking too little insulin, or getting too little exercise. The body begins using stored fat for energy and ketone bodies (acids) build up in the blood. Signs of DKA include nausea and vomiting (which can lead to loss of water from the body), stomach pain, and deep and rapid breathing. Other signs include a flushed face, dry skin and mouth, fruity breath odor, a rapid or weak pulse, and low blood pressure. If the person is not given fluids and insulin immediately, ketoacidosis can lead to coma and even death.

Diabetic myelopathy. Damage to the spinal cord found in some diabetics.

Diabetic retinopathy. Disease of the small blood vessels of the eye.

Diabetogenic. Causing diabetes. Some drugs cause blood glucose levels to rise, leading to diabetes.

Diabetologist. A doctor who specializes in treating diabetes.

Dialysis. A procedure that substitutes for kidney function by filtering toxic chemicals from the blood and maintaining blood pressure and blood chemical balances.

Diastolic pressure. Blood pressure when the heart is resting between beats.

Disaccharide. Any sugar—lactose, maltose, sucrose—that yields to two monosaccharides when hydrolyzed.

Diuretic. A substance that increases the urine output.

DNA. Abbreviation for deoxyribonucleic acid, a chemical substance in plant and animal cells that tells the cells what to do and when to do it. DNA contains the genetic information about what each person inherits from his/her parents.

Double-blind crossover study. In a double-blind study, none of the participants or scientists knows which group of subjects is getting the medication or placebo. In a crossover study, each group is later switched to the medication or placebo they have not been getting. Between the switches may be a "washout" period in which neither group gets any medication for a week or several weeks.

Duodenum. Upper portion of the small intestine.

Dyslipidemia. High levels of cholesterol and triglycerides, which puts patients at risk for hardening of the arteries.

Dyspnea. Labored breathing.

Edema. A swelling or puffiness of some part of the body. Water or other body fluids collect in the cells and cause the swelling.

Eicosapentaenoic acid (EPA). A fatty acid found mostly in cold-water fish, such as salmon and sardines.

Endocrine glands. Glands that release hormones into the bloodstream. They affect how the body uses food (metabolism). One endocrine gland is the pancreas, which releases insulin so the body can use sugar for energy.

Endogenous. Grown or made inside the body. Insulin made by the pancreas is endogenous insulin. Insulin made from beef or pork pancreas or derived from bacteria is exogenous, since it is derived from outside the body and must be injected.

End-stage renal disease. A final phase of kidney disease, which requires dialysis or kidney transplant.

Enzyme. A special type of protein. Each enzyme usually has its own chemical job to do, such as helping to change starch into glucose (sugar).

Epidemiology. The study of a disease that deals with how many people have it, where they are, how many new cases develop, and how to control the disease.

Epinephrine. One of the secretions of the adrenal glands, it helps the liver release glucose and limits the release of insulin. It also makes the heart beat faster and can raise blood pressure. Also called adrenaline.

Epithelium. Cells that line most of the internal organs.

Essential fatty acids. Fatty acids, such as linoleic and linolenic acids, that the body cannot make and must be obtained from the diet.

Essential hypertension. High blood pressure for which a cause has not been found.

Etiology. The study of what causes a disease.

Euglycemia. A normal level of sugar in the blood.

Exogenous. Grown or made outside the body.

Extracellular. The space outside a cell.

Fasting blood glucose test. A method for finding out how much glucose (sugar) is in the blood. The test, using a blood sample taken in a laboratory or doctor's office, can show if a person has diabetes. The test is usually done in the morning before a person has eaten. The normal, non-diabetic range for blood glucose is 70–100 milligrams per deciliter (mg/dl), depending on the type of blood being tested. A level over 140 mg/dl usually means the person has diabetes, except for newborns and some pregnant women.

Fats. One of the three main classes of foods and a source of energy in the body. Fats help the body use some vitamins (A, D, E, and K) and keep the skin healthy. Saturated fats are solid at room temperature and come chiefly from animal sources. Examples are butter, lard, meat fat, solid shortening, palm oil, and coconut oil. These fats can raise cholesterol levels. Unsaturated fats, which include monounsaturated fats, are liquid at room temperature and come from plant oils, such as olive, canola, peanut, corn, cottonseed, sunflower, safflower, and soybean. These fats tend to lower cholesterol levels; however, too many unsaturated fats in relation to saturated fats can cause some health problems.

Fatty acids. A basic unit of fats. When insulin levels are too low or there is not enough glucose to use for energy, the body burns fatty acids for energy. The body then makes ketone bodies, which are waste products that cause acid levels in the blood to become too high. This can lead to ketoacidosis, a serious problem.

Fiber. A substance found in foods that come from plants. Fiber helps in the digestive process and is thought to lower cholesterol and help to control blood glucose. Soluble fiber, found in beans, fruits, and oat products, dissolves in water and is thought to help lower blood fats and blood sugar. Insoluble fiber, found in whole-grain products and vegetables, passes directly through the digestive system, helping to rid the body of waste products.

Flavonoid. A group of flavone-containing compounds found in nature. These include many of the plant pigments, such as anthocyanins, flavonols, bioflavonoids, anthoxanthins, epigenins, and flavones.

Folacin. Folic acid, a B vitamin.

Folic acid. A B vitamin.

Free radicals. Highly unstable molecules, characterized by an unpaired electron which can bind to and destroy cellular compounds.

Fructose. A type of sugar found in fruits, vegetables, and honey. It is considered a nutritive sweetener since it has calories. It is also called levulose or fruit sugar.

Fundus of the eye. The back or deep part of the eye, including the retina.

Galactose. A type of sugar found in milk products and sugar beets. It is also made in the body.

Gangrene. The death of body tissue, usually caused by a loss of blood flow, notably in the legs and feet.

Gastroparesis. A form of nerve damage that affects the stomach, in which food is not digested properly and does not move through the stomach in a normal way. This causes vomiting, nausea, or bloating and interferes with diabetes management. *See also* Autonomic Neuropathy.

Gestational diabetes mellitus. A type of diabetes that occurs in pregnancy. In the second half of the pregnancy, the woman may have glucose in the blood at a higher than normal level. When the pregnancy is terminated, blood glucose levels return to normal in about 95 percent of cases.

Gingivitis. An inflammation of the gums that, if left untreated, can lead to periodontal disease. Typical signs are bleeding gums and inflammation.

Gland. A group of cells that make substances so the other parts of the body can work. For example, the pancreas is a gland that releases insulin so other body cells can use glucose for energy.

Glaucoma. An eye disease caused by increased pressure in the eye. It can damage the optic nerve and cause impaired vision and blindness.

Glomerular filtration rate. A measure of the kidneys' ability to filter and remove waste products.

Glomeruli. Tiny blood vessels in the kidneys where the blood is filtered and waste products are removed.

Glucagon. A hormone that raises the level of glucose (sugar) in the blood. The alpha cells of the pancreas (in the islets of Langerhans) make glucagon when the body needs to put more sugar into the blood. An injectable form is often used to treat insulin shock. *See also* Alpha Cell.

Glucose. A simple sugar found in the blood. Also known as dextrose, it is the body's main source of energy.

Glucose tolerance test. A test to see if a person has diabetes. The test is given in a laboratory or doctor's office in the morning before the patient has eaten. A first sample of blood is taken, and then the person drinks a liquid containing sugar. After one hour, a second blood sample is drawn and, after another hour, a third sample is taken. The idea is to see how well the body deals with the glucose in the blood over time.

Gluten. A protein found in certain grains that give dough its elastic character.

Gluten intolerance. *See* Celiac Disease.

Glycemic index. Developed to quantify blood sugar responses caused by carbohydrates in different types of foods. Diets with a high glycemic index—sugar, bread, potatoes, rice, and so on—and low in fiber increase the risk of type 2 diabetes.

Glycemic response. The effect of different foods on blood glucose levels over time. Researchers have discovered that some kinds of foods may raise blood glucose levels more quickly than other foods containing the same amount of carbohydrates.

Glycogen. A substance made up of sugars, it is stored in the liver and muscles and releases glucose into the blood when needed by the cells. Glycogen is the chief source of stored fuel in the body.

Glycogenesis (glucogenesis). The process in which glycogen is formed from glucose.

Glycolysis. A breakdown of glucose into carbon dioxide and water.

Glycosuria. Having glucose in the urine.

Glycosylated hemoglobin (glycated hemoglobin). The attachment of glucose (sugar) to the hemoglobin protein in red blood cells. The amount of glucose attached to hemoglobin goes up when blood glucose levels are chronically high.

Glycosylated hemoglobin test. A blood test that measures a person's average blood glucose (sugar) level for the two- to three-month period before the test. *See also* Hemoglobin A_{1C}.

Gram. A unit of weight in the metric system, there are 28 grams in 1 ounce.

Gram-molecule. The amount of a substance with a mass in grams equal to its molecular weight. For example, a molecule of hydrogen weighs 2.016 g. A molecule of water weighs 18.015 g.

Hemochromatosis. Iron overload or bronze diabetes.

Hemodialysis. A method of cleaning the blood for those with kidney disease. *See also* Dialysis.

Hemoglobin A_{1C} (HbA_{1C}). The substance in red blood cells that carries oxygen to the cells and sometimes joins with glucose. Because the sugar stays attached for the life of the cell (about four months), a test to measure hemoglobin A_{1C} shows what the person's average blood glucose level was for that period of time.

Hepatic. Pertaining to the liver.

High blood pressure. When the blood flows through the vessels at a greater-than-normal force. High blood pressure strains the heart, harms the arteries, and increases the risk of heart attack, stroke, and kidney problems. Also called hypertension.

High-density lipoprotein (HDL) cholesterol. The beneficial or "good" cholesterol, these protein particles in the blood transport cholesterol from the blood to be broken down by the liver and help to reduce the risk of heart disease.

HLA antigens. Proteins on the outer part of the cell that help the body fight illness. These proteins vary from person to person. Scientists think that those persons with certain types of HLA antigens are more likely to develop type 1 diabetes.

Hormone. A chemical released by special cells to tell other cells what to do. For example, insulin is a hormone made by the beta cells in the pancreas. When released, insulin tells other cells to use glucose for energy.

Hypercholesterolemia. Large amounts of cholesterol in the blood.

Hyperglycemia. Too high a level of glucose in the blood, a sign that diabetes is out of control. It occurs when the body does not have enough insulin, or cannot use the insulin it does have, to turn glucose into energy. Signs of hyperglycemia are a great thirst, dry mouth, and a need to urinate often. For those with type 1 diabetes, this may lead to diabetic ketoacidosis.

Hyperinsulinism. Too high a level of insulin in the blood. This generally means that the body produces too much insulin. Researchers believe that this condition may play a role in the development of type 2 diabetes and hypertension. *See also* Syndrome X.

Hyperlipidemia/hyperlipemia. Too high a level of fats (lipids) in the blood.

Hyperkalemia. Large amounts of potassium in the blood.

Hypertension. High blood pressure.

Hypoglycemia. Too low a level of sugar in the blood. This occurs when a person with diabetes has injected too much insulin, eaten too little food, or exercised without extra food. The person may feel nervous, shaky, weak, or sweaty and have a headache, blurred vision, and hunger. Taking small amounts of sugar, sweet juice, food with sugar, cheese, or other foods will usually help the person feel better within ten to fifteen minutes. Also called low blood sugar. *See also* Insulin Shock.

Hypotension. Low blood pressure or a sudden drop in blood pressure. A person rising quickly from a sitting or reclining position may have a sudden fall in blood pressure, causing dizziness or fainting.

Iatrogenic. A condition caused by a physician or other health-care provider.

IDDM. Insulin-dependent diabetes, now called type 1 diabetes.

Idiopathic. A disease of unknown origin.

Ileum. Lower part of the small intestine between the jejunum and the cecum.

Impaired glucose tolerance (IGT). Blood glucose levels higher than normal but not high enough to be called diabetes. Those with IGT may or may not develop diabetes. Names for IGT no longer used include borderline, subclinical, chemical, or latent diabetes.

Impotence. Loss of a man's ability to have an erect penis and to emit semen. Some men may become impotent after having diabetes for a long time because the nerves or blood vessels to the penis have been damaged. If the problem is psychological, it may be treated with counseling.

Infarction. A quick drop in blood supply to an organ. A myocardial infarction is a heart attack.

Inositol. A vitamin-like substance associated with the B-complex vitamins.

Insulin. A hormone that helps the body use glucose (sugar) for energy. The beta cells of the pancreas (in the islets of Langerhans) make the insulin. When the body cannot make enough insulin, a diabetic must inject insulin from other sources: beef, pork, human insulin (recombinant DNA origin), or human insulin (pork-derived, semi-synthetic).

Insulin allergy. When a person's body has an allergic or bad reaction to taking insulin made from pork, beef, or bacteria, or because the insulin is not exactly the same as human insulin, or because it has impurities. A local allergy results when the skin becomes red and itchy around the site of injection. In a systemic allergy, a person's whole body can have a bad reaction—hives or red patches all over the body or changes in the heart rate and rate of breathing.

Insulin antagonist. Something that opposes the action of insulin. Insulin lowers the level of glucose in the blood, whereas glucagon raises it. Therefore, glucagon is an antagonist of insulin.

Insulin binding. This happens when insulin attaches itself to something else. When a cell needs energy, insulin can bind with the outer part of the cell. The cell then can bring glucose inside and use it for energy. With the help of insulin, the cell can do its work very well. However, sometimes the body acts against itself. In this case, insulin binds with the proteins that are supposed to protect the body from outside substances (antibodies). If the insulin is an injected form and not made by the body, the body sees the insulin as a foreign substance. When the injected insulin binds with the antibodies, it does not work as well as when it binds directly to the cell.

Insulin-dependent diabetes. Now called type 1 diabetes.

Insulin reaction. Hypoglycemia.

Insulin receptors. Areas on the outer part of the cell that allow it to bind with insulin in the blood. When the cell and insulin bind together, the cell can take sugar from the blood and use it for energy.

Insulin resistance. Many people with type 2 diabetes produce enough insulin, but their bodies do not respond to the action of insulin. This may happen if the person is overweight and has too many fat cells, which do not respond well to insulin. As people age, their body cells lose some of the ability to respond to insulin. Insulin resistance is linked to high blood pressure and high levels of fat in the blood. Insulin resistance may happen in those who take insulin injections. They may have to take high doses of insulin daily (200 units or more) to bring their blood sugar down to the normal range. This is also called insulin insensitivity.

Insulin sensitivity. This is said to be the normal state in which the cells of the body are receptive to the action of insulin.

Insulin shock. This occurs when the level of blood sugar drops quickly. The signs are shaking, sweating, dizziness, double vision, convulsions, and collapse. Insulin shock may occur when an insulin reaction is not treated quickly enough. *See also* Hypoglycemia and Insulin Reaction.

Intermittent claudication. Pain in the muscles of the leg that occurs off and on, usually while walking or exercising, and results in lameness (claudication). The pain results from a narrowing of the blood vessels feeding the muscle.

Intramuscular injection. Putting a fluid into a muscle with a needle or syringe.

Intravenous injection. Putting a fluid into a vein with a needle or syringe.

In vitro. A process carried out in laboratory glassware.

In vivo. A process carried out in a living organism.

Ischemia. A deficiency of blood due to an obstruction of a blood vessel.

Ischemic stroke. Caused by a lack of blood supply to the brain.

Islets of langerhans. Special group of cells in the pancreas that make and secrete hormones to help the body break down and use food. There are five types of cells in an islet: beta cells, which make insulin; alpha cells, which make glucagon; delta cells, which make somatostatin; and PP and D cells, about which little is known.

Jejunum. Middle part of the small intestine between the duodenum and the ileum.

Juvenile onset diabetes. Now referred to as type 1 diabetes.

Ketone bodies. Chemicals that the body makes when there is not enough insulin in the blood and it must break down fat for its energy. Ketone bodies can poison and even kill body cells. When the body does not have the help of insulin, the ketones build up in the blood and then spill over into the urine so that the body can get rid of them. The body can also rid itself of one type of ketone, called acetone, through the lungs. This gives the breath a fruity odor. Ketones that build up in the body for a long time lead to serious illness and coma. *See also* Diabetic Ketoacidosis.

Ketonuria. Having ketone bodies in the urine which is a sign of diabetic ketoacidosis (DKA).

Ketosis. A condition of having ketone bodies build up in the body tissues and fluids. Signs of ketosis are nausea, vomiting, and stomach pain. Ketosis can lead to ketoacidosis.

Kidney disease. Any one of several chronic conditions that are caused by damage to the cells of the kidney. Those who have had diabetes for an extended period may have kidney damage. Also called nephropathy.

Kidney threshold. The point at which the blood is holding too much of a substance, such as glucose, and the kidneys spill the excess sugar into the urine.

Kimmelstiel-Wilson syndrome. Lesions formed on the tubules of the kidneys, which are caused by blood-vessel degeneration related to poorly controlled diabetes.

Korsakoff's disease. Found in alcoholics and others with B-vitamin deficiencies, this syndrome is characterized by amnesia, confusion, and apathy.

Krebs cycle. The process that breaks down glucose in every cell and converts it to energy.

Kussmaul breathing. A rapid, deep, and labored breathing in those with ketoacidosis or who are in a diabetic coma. Also called air hunger.

Labile diabetes. A term that is used to indicate when a person's blood sugar level swings quickly from high to low and from low to high.

Lactic acidosis. The buildup of lactic acid in the body. The cells make lactic acid when they use sugar for energy. If too much lactic acid stays in the body, the balance tips and the person begins to feel ill. The signs of lactic acidosis are deep and rapid breathing, vomiting, and abdominal pain. This condition may be caused by diabetic ketoacidosis or liver or kidney disease.

Lactose. A sugar found in milk and milk products (cheese, butter). Also called milk sugar.

Lactose intolerance. Those who cannot metabolize lactose because they do not have the enzyme lactase.

Lancet. A fine, sharp-pointed blade or needle for pricking the skin.

Latent diabetes. Former term for impaired glucose tolerance.

Lente insulin. A type of insulin that is intermediate-acting: it begins working within four to six hours and stops after about twelve hours. It is a mixture of 30 percent Semilente and 70 percent Ultralente insulin.

Leukocytes. White blood cells.

Leukotrienes. Inflammatory substances that are produced when oxygen combines with polyunsaturated fatty acids.

Lipid. Another term for fat, such as cholesterol, triglycerides, and phospholipids. The body stores fat as energy for future use. When the body needs energy it can break down the lipids into fatty acids and burn them like glucose (sugar).

Lipid peroxidation. An interaction of fats and oxygen, which can lead to the destruction of cells.

Lipoatrophy/lipodystrophy. Lumps or small dents in the skin that form when a person keeps injecting the needle in the same spot. Avoid the problem by changing injection sites.

Lipogenesis. The formation of fats.

Lipoprotein. A complex of fat and protein found in blood and responsible for the transportation of fats in the bloodstream.

Lipotrophic. Substances that prevent the accumulation of fat in the liver.

Low-density lipoprotein (LDL) cholesterol. Also called "bad" cholesterol, these protein particles help cholesterol and triglycerides to build up in artery walls and can lead to heart disease.

Macrosomia. The development of abnormally large babies in some women with diabetes.

Macrovascular disease. Disease of the large blood vessels that can occur when a person has had diabetes for a long time. Fat and blood clots build up in the large blood vessels and stick to the vessel walls. Three kinds of macrovascular disease are coronary disease, cerebrovascular disease, and peripheral vascular disease.

Macula. Center of the retina.

Macular degeneration. A disorder of the eye in which central vision is impaired.

Macular edema. A swelling in the macula, an area near the center of the retina of the eye that is responsible for fine or reading vision. This is a common complaint associated with diabetic retinopathy.

Malondialdehyde. A marker for fatty acid oxidation.

Maturity-onset diabetes. Former term for type 2 diabetes.

Megaloblast. An immature red blood cell.

Meta-analysis. A compilation of various published studies.

Metabolic syndrome. This is a compilation of five conditions that are related to type 2 diabetes—glucose intolerance, obesity, high blood pressure, and high levels of cholesterol and triglycerides. Anyone with three of these five conditions may develop diabetes (formerly called Syndrome X).

Metabolism. The way cells chemically change food so that it can be used to keep the body alive. One part is called catabolism, when the body uses food for energy, and the other part is called anabolism, when the body uses food to build or mend cells. Insulin is necessary for the metabolism of food.

Mg/dl. Milligrams per deciliter. A measurement used to describe how much glucose is in a specific amount of blood. In self-monitoring of blood glucose (sugar), test results are given as the amount of glucose in milligrams per deciliter of blood. A fasting reading of 70–110 mg/dl is considered in the normal (non-diabetic) range.

Micelle. A microscopic amount of fats and bile salts.

Microaneurysm. A small swelling on the side of tiny blood vessels. They may break and bleed into nearby tissue. Diabetics sometimes get these swellings in the retina of the eye.

Microvascular disease. Disease of the smallest blood vessels that sometimes occurs when a person has had diabetes for a long time. The walls of the vessels become abnormally thick but weak and tend to bleed, leak protein, and slow the flow of blood through the body.

Millimole (mmol). One-thousandth of a gram-molecule.

Mononeuropathy. A form of diabetic neuropathy affecting a single nerve, often in the eye.

Monosaccharide. A simple sugar, such as fructose or glucose.

Monounsaturated fat. Found in olive oil, canola oil, and nuts, this is considered a heart-healthy fat.

Morbidity rate. The number of people who are sick or have a disease compared with the number who are well.

Mortality rate. The number of people who die of a certain disease compared to the total number of people. Mortality is often stated as deaths per 1,000, 10,000, or 100,000.

Myocardial infarction. Heart attack. It results from permanent damage to an area of heart muscle, which happens when the blood supply to the area is interrupted because of a narrowed or blocked blood vessel.

Myocardium. Heart muscle.

Myoglobin. Hemoglobin that is found in muscle.

Myoinositol. A substance in the cell that is thought to play a role in helping the nerves to work. Low levels of the substance may be involved in diabetic neuropathy.

Necrobiosis lipoidica diabeticorum. A skin condition usually on the lower part of the legs. The lesions can be small or extended over a large area. They are usually raised, yellow, and waxy in appearance and often have a purple border. Young women are most often affected. It occurs in people with and without diabetes.

Necrosis. Death of living tissue.

Neovascularization. When new, tiny blood vessels grow in a new place, such as from the retina.

Nephropathy. Disease of the kidneys caused by damage to the small blood vessels or to the units in the kidneys that clean the blood. People who have had diabetes for a long time may have kidney damage.

Neuritis. Inflammation of the nerves.

Neuropathy. Disease of the nervous system. Those with long-standing diabetes may have nerve damage. The three major forms are peripheral neuropathy, autonomic neuropathy, and mononeuropathy. The most common form is peripheral neuropathy, which mainly affects the feet and legs.

Neurotransmitters. Substances that transmit nerve impulses.

Niacin. Vitamin B_3. Also called niacinamide and nicotinic acid.

Nitric oxide. A potentially toxic compound of oxygen and nitrogen that is also a beneficial free radical. It relaxes blood vessels and may play a key role in penile erections and impotence.

Non-essential amino acids. Amino acids necessary for human health, but which can be synthesized by the body.

Non-insulin-dependent diabetes. Now called type 2 diabetes.

Non-ketonic coma. A type of coma caused by a lack of insulin. A non-ketonic crisis entails very high levels of sugar in the blood, absence of ketoacidosis, great loss of body fluid, and a sleepy, confused, or comatose state. This coma often results from some other problem, such as a severe infection or kidney failure.

Norepinephrine. A nerve transmitter derived from the amino acid tyrosine.

Nucleic acid. Molecular structures, such as DNA, that carry the cell's genetic code or are necessary for protein synthesis.

Obesity. When people have 20 percent or more extra body fat for their age, height, sex, and bone structure. Fat works against the action of insulin. Extra body fat is thought to be a risk factor for diabetes.

Oral hypoglycemic agents. Pills or capsule that lower the level of sugar in the blood.

Overt diabetes. Diabetes in those who show clear signs of the disease, such as great thirst and urgent need to urinate.

Oxalic acid. A dicarboxylic acid found in spinach, chard, rhubarb, and other foods. Spinach, a good source of iron, is a poor source of calcium, since the oxalic acid in the spinach converts the calcium to calcium oxalate and removes large amounts from the body.

Oxidation. A chemical reaction in which a substance combines with oxygen, such as oxygen free radicals, often to the detriment of health.

Pancreas. An organ behind the lower part of the stomach that is about the size of a human hand. It makes insulin so that the body can use glucose for energy. It also makes enzymes that help the body digest food. Spread over the pancreas are areas called the islets of Langerhans. The cells in these areas have special purposes: the alpha cells make glucagon, which raises the level of glucose in the blood; the beta cells make insulin; the delta cells make somatostatin; little is known about PP and D cells.

Pancreatin. An extract from pork pancreas.

Pantothenic acid. A B vitamin sometimes called B$_5$.

Para-amino-benzoic acid (PABA). A vitamin-like substance associated with the B-complex vitamins.

Parathyroid hormone. A hormone secreted by the parathyroid gland necessary for the regulation of blood calcium levels.

Pathogen. A microorganism that causes infection or disease.

Periodontal disease. Damage to the gums.

Peripheral neuropathy. Nerve damage, usually affecting the feet and legs. It causes pain, numbness, or a tingling feeling. Also called somatic neuropathy or distal sensory polyneuropathy.

Peripheral vascular disease (PVD). Disease in the large blood vessels of the arms, legs, and feet. People who have had diabetes for a long time may develop this because major blood vessels in the extremities are blocked and these limbs do not receive enough blood. The signs of PVD are aching pains in the arms, legs, and feet (especially when walking) and foot sores that heal slowly. This can best be avoided by taking good care of the feet, not smoking, and keeping blood pressure and diabetes under control.

Peroxide. The oxide that contains the most oxygen.

Pituitary gland. An endocrine gland in the small, bony cavity at the base of the brain. Often called "the master gland," it serves the body in many ways—in growth, in food use, and in reproduction.

Placebo. A dummy or look-alike pill used in double-blind studies. Neither the volunteers nor the scientists know the testing medication or the placebo until the code is broken at the end of the study.

Platelets. Cell fragments found in the blood.

Polycythemia. An excess of red blood cells.

Polydipsia. Great thirst, often a sign of diabetes.

Polyphagia. Great hunger, often a sign of diabetes. People with great hunger often lose weight.

Polysaccharide. A molecule containing many sugar molecules linked together.

Polyunsaturated fats. A type of fat that comes from vegetables, such as vegetable oils. These are omega-6 oils.

Polyuria. A need to urinate often, a common sign of diabetes.

Preeclampsia. A condition that some women with diabetes have during the late stages of pregnancy. Signs of this disorder include high blood pressure and swelling (edema) because the body cells are holding extra water.

Prostaglandins. Hormone-like substances from linoleic and linolenic acids that help in the contraction of smooth muscle and dilation of blood vessels.

Protein. One of the three main classes of food. Proteins are made of amino acids, which are called the building blocks of the cells. The cells need proteins to grow and to mend themselves. Main sources are meat, fish, poultry, and eggs.

Proteinuria. Too much protein in the urine. It may be a sign of kidney damage.

Prothrombin. A protein in the blood that is necessary for blood clotting.

Pruritus. Itching of skin, often as a symptom of diabetes.

Pyridoxine. Vitamin B_6.

Reagents. Strips or tablets that people use to test the level of glucose in blood and urine or the level of acetone in the urine.

Rebound. A swing to a high level of sugar in the blood after having a low level. *See also* Somogyi Effect.

Receptors. Areas on the outer part of a cell that allow the cell to join or bind with insulin that is in the blood. Also called insulin receptors.

Recommended dietary allowance (RDA). Suggested amounts of nutrients needed daily by individuals. This particular guide is being phased out, but it is still familiar to laypeople.

Regular insulin. Insulin that is fast acting.

Renal. Pertains to the kidneys.

Renal threshold. When the blood is holding so much of a substance, such as sugar, that the kidneys allow the excess glucose to spill into the urine. Also called kidney threshold, spilling point, and leak point.

Respiratory distress syndrome. Difficulty in breathing.

Retina. Center part of the back lining of the eye that senses light. It has many small blood vessels that are sometimes harmed when a person has had diabetes for a long time.

Retinol. Vitamin A.

Retinopathy. A disease of the small blood vessels in the retina of the eye. *See also* Diabetic Retinopathy.

Riboflavin. Vitamin B_2.

Risk factor. Anything that raises the chance that a person will get a disease. For example, with type 2 diabetes, people have a greater risk of getting the disease if they weigh more (20 percent or more) than they should.

Saccharide. Sugar molecule.

Satiety. A feeling of fullness.

Saturated fat. A type of fat that is solid at room temperature; usually derived from animal sources.

Secondary diabetes. When a person develops diabetes because of another disease or because of taking certain drugs or chemicals.

Serotonin. A neurotransmitter formed from the amino acid tryptophan. It regulates pain, mood, sleep, and appetite.

Serum. The fluid portion of blood that remains after clotting.

Shock. A person with diabetes can go into shock when the level of blood sugar drops suddenly. Also called insulin shock.

Somatostatin. A hormone made by the delta cells of the pancreas. It may control how the body secretes two other hormones, insulin and glucagon.

Somogyi effect. A swing to a high level of glucose in the blood from an extremely low level, usually occurring after an untreated insulin reaction during the night. The swing is caused by the release of stress hormones to counter low glucose levels. People who experience high levels of blood sugar in the morning may need to test their blood glucose levels in the middle of the night. If blood sugar levels are falling or low, adjustments in evening snacks or insulin doses may be recommended. Also called rebound.

Sorbitol. A sugar in alcohol.

Spilling point. When the blood is holding so much of a substance, such as glucose, that the kidneys allow the excess to spill into the urine. Also called renal threshold.

Statins. Drugs used to lower LDL cholesterol.

Steatorrhea. Excess fat in the stool.

Stiff hand syndrome. Thickening of the skin of the palm that results in loss of the ability to hold the hand straight. This condition occurs only in diabetics.

Strokes. Disease caused by damage to blood vessels in the brain. Depending on the part of the brain affected, a stroke can cause a person to lose the ability to speak or move a part of the body, such as an arm or leg. Usually only one side of the body is affected. *See also* Cerebrovascular Disease.

Subclinical deficiency. A deficiency of various nutrients that do not result in overt physical symptoms. You might have a vitamin C deficiency but not sufficient enough to cause scurvy.

Subcutaneous. Below the skin.

Sucrose. Table sugar. A form of sugar that the body must break down into a more simple form before the blood can absorb it and take it to the cells.

Sugar. A class of carbohydrates that tastes sweet. Sugar is a quick and easy fuel for the body to use. Types of sugar are lactose, glucose, fructose, and sucrose.

Sulfonylureas. Pills or capsules people take to lower the level of glucose (sugar) in the blood.

Symptom. A sign of disease. Frequent urination often is a symptom of diabetes.

Syndrome. A set of signs or a series of events occurring together to make up a disease or health problem.

Syndrome X. Now called metabolic syndrome.

Systemic. Conditions that affect the entire body. Diabetes is a systemic disease because it involves many parts of the body, such as the pancreas, eyes, kidneys, heart, and nerves.

Tachycardia. Unusually fast heart beat.

Thiamine. Vitamin B_1.

Thrombus. A blood clot that forms within an artery wall or cavity of the heart.

Tocopherol. Vitamin E.

Toxemia of pregnancy. A condition in pregnant women in which poisons, such as the body's waste products, build up and may cause harm to mother and fetus. The first signs of toxemia are swelling near the eyes and ankles (edema), headache, high blood pressure, and weight gain that the mother might confuse with the normal weight gain during pregnancy. The mother may have sugar and acetone in the urine.

Toxic. Harmful, having to do with poison.

Trans-fatty acid. A type of fat found in margarine.

Transient ischemic attack (TIA). Temporary problem, such as slurred speech or numbness of the arm, due to partial blockage of arteries to the brain.

Trauma. A wound, hurt, or injury to the body. Trauma can also be mental, such as when a person is under stress.

Triglyceride. A type of blood fat. The body needs insulin to remove this type of fat from the blood. When diabetes is under control and a person's weight is what it should be, the level of triglycerides in the blood is usually what it should be. Triglyceride levels around 100 mg/dl are considered normal.

Type 1 diabetes mellitus. Formerly called insulin-dependent diabetes.

Type 2 diabetes mellitus. Formerly called non-insulin-dependent diabetes.

Ubiquinone. A fat-soluble compound also called coenzyme Q, it is involved in the production of energy from carbohydrates. Coenzyme Q_{10} is being used to treat heart disease.

Ulcer. A break in the skin or a deep sore.

Ultralente insulin. A type of insulin that is long acting.

Unit of insulin. U-100 insulin means 100 units of insulin per milliliter (ml) or cubic centimeter (cc) of solution. Most insulin made in the U.S. is U-100.

Unsaturated fats. A type of fat, such as those from fish oils and vegetable oils.

Unstable diabetes. A type of diabetes when a person's blood sugar level often swings quickly from high to low and low to high. Also called brittle diabetes and labile diabetes.

Uptake. The absorption by a tissue of some substance, food, mineral, etc., and its permanent or temporary retention.

Urea. One of the chief waste products of the body. When the body breaks down food, it uses what it needs and throws the rest away as waste. The kidneys flush the waste from the body in the form of urea, which is in the urine.

Uremia. Urine in the blood.

Uric acid. The endproduct in the metabolism of purines, which is excreted in the urine. Excess blood levels are found in gout.

UTI. Urinary tract infection.

Vascular. Pertaining to the body's blood vessels (arteries, veins, and capillaries).

Vasoconstriction. A constriction of blood vessels.

Vasodilation. A dilation or expansion of blood vessels.

Vein. A blood vessel that carries blood to the heart.

Ventricle. One of the two lower chambers of the heart.

Visceral fat. Fat in the abdomen, which may be a risk factor for diabetes and heart disease.

Vitrectomy. Removing the gel from the center of the eyeball because it has blood and scar tissue in it that blocks sight. An eye surgeon replaces the clouded gel with a clear fluid. See also Diabetic Retinopathy.

Vitreous humor. The clear jelly (gel) that fills the center of the eye.

Void. To empty the bladder in order to obtain a urine sample for testing.

References

Chapter 1: What Is Diabetes?

1. U.S. Department of Health and Human Services, National Institutes of Health. "Diabetes Overview." Washington, DC: U.S. Department of Health and Human Services, National Institutes of Health, 2000.

2. Ibid.

3. Ibid.

4. Ensminger, A., et al. *Foods and Nutrition Encyclopedia.* Clovis, CA: Pegus Press, 1983, pp. 555ff.

5. Ibid.

6. American Diabetes Association. "National Diabetes Fact Sheet." Alexandria, VA: American Diabetes Association, 2005.

7. Ibid.

8. Klein, Samuel, et al. "Weight Management Through Lifestyle Modification for the Prevention and Management of Type 2 Diabetes: Rationale and Strategies. A Statement of the American Diabetes Association, the North American Association for the Study of Obesity, and the American Society for Clinical Nutrition." *American Journal of Clinical Nutrition* 80 (2004): 257–263.

9. Glumer, Charlotte, M.D., Ph.D., et al. "Risk Scores for Type 2 Diabetes Can Be Applied in Some Populations but not All." *Diabetes Care* 29 (2006): 410–414.

10. Lindquist, Christine H., et al. "Role of Dietary Factors in Ethnic Differences in Early Risk of Cardiovascular Disease and Type 2 Diabetes." *American Journal of Clinical Nutrition* 71 (2000): 725–732.

11. Center for Nutrition Policy and Promotion, U.S. Department of Agriculture. "Report Card on the Diet Quality of African-Americans." *Nutrition Week* 28:28 (July 1998): 4–5.

12 Cefalu, William T., M.D. "Glycemic Control and Cardiovascular Disease—Should We Reassess Clinical Goals?" *New England Journal of Medicine* 353:25 (December 2005): 2707–2708.

13 Alterman, Seymour L., M.D., and Donald A. Kullman, M.D. *How to Prevent, Control, and Cure Diabetes.* Hollywood, FL: Frederick Fell Publishers, 2000, p. 207.

14. American Diabetes Association. "Foot Care." Alexandria, VA: American Diabetes Association, undated.

15. Tapley, Donald F., M.D., et al. "Diabetes and Other Endocrine Disorders." In *Columbia University College of Physicians and Surgeons Complete Home Medical Guide.* New York: Crown, 1985, pp. 474ff.

16. Levin, Marvin E., M.D., and Michael A. Pfeiffer, M.D. *Uncomplicated Guide to Diabetes Complications.* Alexandria, VA: American Diabetes Association, 1998, pp. 304ff.

17. Katon, Wayne J., M.D., et al. "The Association of Comorbid Depression with Mortality in Patients with Type 2 Diabetes." *Diabetes Care* 28 (2005): 2668–2672.

18. Colchamiro, Russ. "Type 2 Diabetes Increases Risk of Dementia." *Medical Tribune* 41:1 (January 2000): 5.

19. Lopez, Livia A., M.D., et al. "Restless Leg Syndrome and Quality of Sleep in Type 2 Diabetes." *Diabetes Care* 28 (2005): 2633–2636.

Chapter 2: What Causes Diabetes?

1. Greenberg, Andrew S., and Martin S. Obin. "Obesity and the Role of Adipose Tissue in Inflammation and Metabolism." *American Journal of Clinical Nutrition* 83:Suppl (2006): 461S-465S.

2. Mokdad, Ali H., Ph.D., et al. "The Continuing Epidemics of Obesity and Diabetes in the United States." *Journal of the American Medical Association* 286:10 (September 2001): 1195–1200.

3. Farin, Helke M.F., et al. "Body Mass Index and Waist Circumference both Contribute to Differences in Insulin-Mediated Glucose Disposal in Non-Diabetic Adults." *American Journal of Clinical Nutrition* 83 (2006): 47–51.

4. Sullivan, Patrick W., Ph.D., et al. "Obesity, Inactivity, and the Prevalence of Diabetes and Diabetes-Related Cardiovascular Co-morbidities in the U.S.—2000–2002." *Diabetes Care* 28 (2005): 1599–1603.

5. Friedrich, M.J. "Epidemic of Obesity Expands Its Spread to Developing Countries." *Journal of the American Medical Association* 287:11 (March 2002): 1382ff.

6. Fernald, Lia C., Ph.D., et al. "High Prevalence of Obesity among the Poor in Mexico." *Journal of the American Medical Association* 291:21 (June 2004): 2544–2545.

7. Friedrich, M.J. "Epidemic of Obesity Expands Its Spread to Developing Countries." *Journal of the American Medical Association* 287:11 (March 2002): 1382ff.

8. Bes-Rastrollo, Maira, et al. "Predictors of Weight Gain in a Mediterranean

Cohort: The Seduimiento Universidad de Navarra Study." *American Journal of Clinical Nutrition* 83 (2006): 362-370.

9. Mooy, J.M., et al. "Prevalence and Determinants of Glucose Intolerance in a Dutch Caucasian Population. The Hoorn Study." *Diabetes Care* 18:9 (1995): 1270–1273.

10. Snijder, Marieke B., et al. "Associations on Hip and Thigh Circumference Independent of Waist Circumference with the Incidence of Type 2 Diabetes: The Hoorn Study." *American Journal of Clinical Nutrition* 77 (2003): 1192–1197.

11. Shimer, Porter. New Hope for People with Diabetes. Roseville, CA: Prima Publishing/Random House, 2001, pp. 4ff.

12. Stephenson, Joan, Ph.D. "Obesity-Diabetes Link." *Journal of the American Medical Association* 286:10 (September 2001): 1167.

13. Cox, Kay L., et al. "Independent and Additive Effects of Energy Restriction and Exercise on Glucose and Insulin Concentrations in Sedentary Overweight Men." *American Journal of Clinical Nutrition* 80 (2004): 308–316.

14. Redmon, J. Bruce, M.D., et al. "Two-Year Outcome of Combination of Weight Loss Therapies for Type 2 Diabetes." *Diabetes Care* 28 (2005): 1311– 1315.

15. Thorn, Lena M., M.D., et al. "Metabolic Syndrome in Type 1 Diabetes." *Diabetes Care* 28 (2005): 2019–2024.

16. Ford, E.S., et al. "Prevalence of the Metabolic Syndrome among U.S. Adults: Findings from the Third National Health and Nutrition Examination Survey." *Journal of the American Medical Association* 287 (2002): 356–359. Also, Sierra-Johnson, Justo, M.D., M.S., et al. "Correspondence between the Adult Treatment Panel III Criteria for Metabolic Syndrome and Insulin Resistance." *Diabetes Care* 29 (2006): 668–672. Also: "Expert Panel on Detection, Evaluation, and Treatment of High Blood Cholesterol in Adults: Executive Summary of the Third Report of the National Cholesterol Education Program (NCEP) Expert Panel in Adults (Adult Treatment Panel III)." *Journal of the American Medical Association* 285 (2001): 2486–2497.

17. Alterman, Seymour L., M.D., and Donald A. Kullman, M.D. *How to Prevent, Control, and Cure Diabetes.* Hollywood, FL: Frederick Fell Publishers, 2000, pp. 183–184.

18. Lorenzo, Carlos, M.D., et al. "Geographic Variations of the International Diabetic Federation and National Cholesterol Education Program-Adult Treatment Panel III Definitions of the Metabolic Syndrome in Non-Diabetic Subjects." *Diabetes Care* 29 (2006): 685–691.

19. Challem, Jack, Burton Berkson, M.D., and Melissa Diane Smith. *Syndrome X.* New York: John Wiley & Sons, 2000, pp. 32ff.

20. Hamilton, Kirk. "Syndrome X, Diet and Exercise." *Clinical Pearls.* Sacramen-

to, CA: I.T. Services, 2001; pp. 131-132. Also: Roberts, Karen, M.S., and Kathleen Dunn, MPH, R.D. "Syndrome X: Medical Nutrition Therapy." *Nutrition Reviews* 58:5 (2000): 154–160.

21. Roberts, Karen, M.S., and Kathleen Dunn, MPH, R.D. "Syndrome X: Medical Nutrition Therapy." *Nutrition Reviews* 58:5 (2000): 154–160.

22. Ibid.

23. Phillips, Robert H., Ph.D. *Coping with Diabetes.* New York: Avery/Penguin-Putnam, 2000; pp. 110-111.

24. Ibid.

25. Luna, Beatriz, Pharm.D., and Mark N. Feinglos, M.D. "Drug-Induced Hyperglycemia." *Journal of the American Medical Association* 286:16 (October 2001): 1945–1948.

26. Ibid.

27. Alterman, Seymour L., M.D., and Donald A. Kullman, M.D. *How to Prevent, Control, and Cure Diabetes.* Hollywood, FL: Frederick Fell Publishers, 2000, p. 96.

28. Riddle, Matthew C., M.D. "Impaired Insulin Secretion and Risk of Progressive Hyperglycemia." Paper read at the American Diabetes Association 60th Annual Scientific Session, June 9-13, 2000, San Antonio, Texas.

29. Ronzio, Robert A., Ph.D. *Encyclopedia of Nutrition and Good Health.* New York: Facts on File, 1997, p. 235.

30. Monnier, Louis, M.D., et al. "Activation of Oxidative Stress by Acute Fluctuations Compared with Sustained Chronic Hyperglycemia in Patients with Type 2 Diabetes." *Journal of the American Medical Association* 295:14 (2006): 1681–1687.

31. Atkins, Robert C., M.D. *Dr. Atkins' Health Revolution.* Boston: Houghton Mifflin, 1988, pp. 85–86.

32. Kronhausen, Eberhard, Ed.D., et al. *Formula for Life.* New York: William Morrow, 1989, pp. 259–260.

33. Gross, Lee S., et al. "Increased Consumption of Refined Carbohydrates and Epidemic of Type 2 Diabetes in the United States: An Ecologic Assessment." *American Journal of Clinical Nutrition* 79 (2004): 774–779.

34. Schulze, Matthias B., et al. "Glycemic Index, Glycemic Load, and Dietary Fiber Intake and Incidence of Type 2 Diabetes in Younger and Middle-Aged Women." *American Journal of Clinical Nutrition* 80 (2004): 348–356.

35. Gross, Lee S., et al. "Increased Consumption of Refined Carbohydrates and Epidemic of Type 2 Diabetes in the United States: An Ecologic Assessment." *American Journal of Clinical Nutrition* 79 (2004): 774–779.

36. Ibid.

37. Murray, Frank. *Program Your Heart for Health.* New York: Larchmont Books, 1977, pp. 185-186.

38. Wildey, M.B., et al. "Fat and Sugar Levels are High in Snacks Purchased from Student Stores in Middle Schools." *Journal of the American Diabetes Association* 100:3 (March 2000): 319–322.

39. Brennan, R.O., D.O. *Nutrigenetics.* New York: M. Evans, 1975, p. 35.

40. Crook, William G., M.D. *Tired—So Tired—and the "Yeast Connection."* Jackson, TN: Professional Books, 2001, pp. 138–139.

41. Hoffman, Ronald, L., M.D. *Intelligent Medicine.* New York: Simon & Schuster, 1997, pp. 102–103.

42. Gross, L.S., et al. "Increased Consumption of Refined Carbohydrates and the Epidemic of Type 2 Diabetes in the United States: An Ecological Assessment." *American Journal of Clinical Nutrition* 79 (2004): 774–779. See also: Jenkins, David J.A., et al. "Too Much Sugar, Too Much Carbohydrate, or Just Too Much." *American Journal of Clinical Nutrition* 79 (2004): 711–712.

43. Kristof, Nicholas D. "Hazardous to Your Health." *The New York Times* (April 11, 2006): A21.

44. MacLaren, Noel, M.D., and Mark Atkinson, Ph.D. "Is Insulin-Dependent Diabetes Mellitus Environmentally Induced?" *New England Journal of Medicine* 327:5 (July 1992): 348–349.

45. Scott, Fraser W., and Hubert Kolb. "Cow's Milk and Insulin-Dependent Diabetes Mellitus." *Lancet* 348 (August 1996): 613.

46. Akerblom, Hans K., et al. "Cow's Milk Protein and Insulin-Dependent Diabetes Mellitus." *Scandinavian Journal of Nutrition* 40 (1996): 98–103.

47. Virtanen, S.M., et al. "Diet, Cow's Milk, and the Risk of IDDM in Finnish Children." *Diabetologia* 37 (1994): 381–387.

48. Virtanen, S.M., et al. "Cow's Milk Consumption, Disease-Associated Auto-antibodies and Type 1 Diabetes Mellitus: A Follow-Up Study in Siblings of Diabetic Children." *Diabetic Medicine* 15 (1998): 730–738.

49. Hurley, Dan. "Studies Confirm Diabetes Risk from Cow's Milk in Infants." *Medical Tribune* (February 2, 1995): 11.

50. "Smoking and Diabetes." *Diabetes Care* 23 (2000): S63–S64.

51. Fox, Capri Gabrielle, Ph.D., et al. "Smoking and Incidence of Diabetes among U.S. Adults." *Diabetes Care* 28 (2005): 1501–1507.

52. "Doctors Link Diabetes and Secondhand Smoke." *The New York Times* (April 18, 2006): F8.

53. Facchini, Francesco, et al. "Insulin Resistance and Cigarette Smoking." *Lancet* 339 (May 1992): 1128–1138.

54. Hampton, Tracy, Ph.D. "Gene Variant Confers Risk of Diabetes." *Journal of the American Medical Association* 295:9 (March 2006): 997–998.

55. Vaarala, O., et al. "Environmental Factors in the Aetiology of Childhood Diabetes." *Diabetes and Nutrition Metabolism* 12:2 (1999): 75–85.

56. Seppa, Nathan. "Does Lack of Sleep Lead to Diabetes?" *Science News* 160:2 (July 2001): 31.

Chapter 3: The Way Forward

1. Cheraskin, Emanuel, M.D., D.M.D., W. Marshall Ringsdorf, Jr., M.S., D.M.D., and Emily L. Sisley, Ph.D. *Vitamin C Connection.* New York: Harper & Row, 1983, pp. 104–105.

2. Wylie Rosett, Judith, E.D.D., R.D. "Efficacy of Diet and Exercise in Reducing Body Weight and Conversion to Overt Diabetes." *Diabetes Care* 21 (1998): 334–335.

3. U.S. Department of Health and Human Services, National Institutes of Health. "Diabetes Overview." Washington, DC: U.S. Department of Health and Human Services, National Institutes of Health, November 2000.

Chapter 4: Why a Healthful Diet is Important

1. Nagourney, Eric. "New Findings on Diabetes and Diet." *The New York Times* (February 12, 2002): F7.

2. Ford, E.S., et al. "Fruit and Vegetable Consumption and Diabetes Mellitus Incidence among U.S. Adults." *Preventive Medicine* 32 (2001): 33–39.

3. "Diabetes Mellitus and Vegan Diet." *Nutrition Week* 29:35 (September 1999): 7.

4. Crane, Milton G., M.D., and Clyde Sample, R.D. "Regression of Diabetic Neuropathy with Total Vegetarian (Vegan) Diet." *Journal of Nutritional Medicine* 4 (1994): 431–436.

5. Kavita, M.S., et al. "Glycemic Response to Selected Cereal-Based South Indian Meals in Non-Insulin Dependent Diabetics." *Journal of Nutritional and Environmental Medicine* 7 (1997): 287–294.

6. Colditz, Graham A., et al. "Diet and the Risk of Clinical Diabetes in Women." *American Journal of Clinical Nutrition* 55 (1992): 1018–1023.

7. Sheard, Nancy F., Sc.D., R.D. "The Diabetic Diet: Evidence for a New Approach." *Nutrition Reviews* 53:1 (1995): 16–18.

8. Garg, Abhimanyu. "High Monounsaturated Fat Diets for Patients with Diabetes Mellitus." *American Journal of Clinical Nutrition* 67:Suppl (1998): 577S–582S.

9. Rodriguez-Villar, C., et al. "High-Monounsaturated Fat, Olive Oil-Rich Diet Has Effects Similar to a High-Carbohydrate Diet on Fasting and Postprandial State and Metabolic Profiles of Patients with Type 2 Diabetes." *Metabolism* 49:12 (December 2000): 1511–1517.

10. Tsihilas, E.B., et al. "Comparison of High- and Low-Glycemic-Index Breakfast Cereals with Monounsaturated Fat in the Long-Term Dietary Management of Type 2 Diabetes." *American Journal of Clinical Nutrition* 72 (2000): 439–449.

11. Parillo, M., et al. "A High-Monounsaturated Fat/Low Carbohydrate Diet Improves Peripheral Insulin Sensitivity in Non-Insulin Dependent Diabetes Patients." *Metabolism* 41:12 (December 1992): 1373–1378.

12. Rasmussen, Ole, et al. "Differential Effects of Saturated and Monounsaturated Fat on Blood Glucose and Insulin Response in Subjects with Non-Insulin Dependent Diabetes Mellitus." *American Journal of Clinical Nutrition* 63 (1996): 249–253.

13. Tuomilehto, J., et al. "Coffee Consumption as a Trigger for Insulin-Dependent Diabetes Mellitus in Childhood." *British Medical Journal* 300 (March 1990): 642–643.

14. "Anthocyanins and Blueberries." *Nutrition Week* 27:38 (October 1997): 7.

15. "Anti-Diabetic Activity Present in the Fruit Body of *Grifola Frondosa* (Maitake)." *Biological Pharmacology Bulletin* 17:8 (1994): 1106–1110.

16. McCullum, Christine, M.S., R.D. "How to 'Unmarket' Trans Fatty Acids Out of the Food Supply." *Nutrition Week* 26:7 (February 1996): 4–5.

17. Kronhausen, Eberhard, Ed.D., et al. *Formula for Life.* New York: William Morrow, 1989, pp. 306ff.

18. Brand-Miller, Janette, Ph.D., and Kaye Foster-Powell, B.Sc. "Diets with Low Glycemic Index: From Theory to Practice." *Nutrition Today* 34:2 (March/ April 1999): 66.

19. Murray, Michael, N.D., and Joseph Pizzorno, N.D. *Encyclopedia of Natural Medicine.* Rocklin, CA: Prima Publishing, 1998, p. 415.

20. Miller, J.C. "Importance of Glycemic Index in Diabetes." *American Journal of Clinical Nutrition* 59:Suppl (1994): 747S–752S.

21. Brand-Miller, Janette, M.D., and Kaye Foster-Powell, B.Sc. "Diets with a Low Glycemic Index: From Theory to Practice." *Nutrition Today* 34:2 (March/April 1999): 64–72.

22. Ostman, Elin M., et al. "Inconsistency between Glycemic and Insulinemic Response to Regular and Fermented Milk Products." *American Journal of Clinical Nutrition* 74 (2001): 96–100.

23. Foltz-Gray, Dorothy. "Against the Grain?" *Hippocrates* (November 1997): 54–61.

24. McLaren, D.S. "Not Fade Away—The Glycemic Index." *Nutrition* 16 (2000): 151–152.

25. Jenkins, David J.A., et al. "Low Glycemic Index: Lente Carbohydrates and Physiological Effects of Altered Blood Frequency." *American Journal of Clinical Nutrition* 59:Suppl (1994): 706S–709S.

26. Ronzio, Robert A., Ph.D. *Encyclopedia of Nutrition and Good Health.* New York: Facts on File, 1997, p. 273.

27. Soh, N.L., and J.C. Brand-Miller. "The Glycemic Index of Potatoes: The Effect of Variety, Cooking Method and Maturity." *European Journal of Clinical Nutrition* 53 (1999): 249–254.

28. Benzal, Sudodh, et al. "Glycemic Index of, and Insulin Response to, Some Food Items Consumed by Indians." *Medical Science Research* 25 (1997): 529–531.

29. Panlasigui, Leonara N., Ph.D., et al. "Extruded Rice Noodles: Starch Digestibility and Glycemic Response of Healthy and Diabetic Subjects with Different Habitual Diets." *Nutrition Research* 12 (1992): 1195–1204.

30. Perry, T., et al. "Glycemic Index of New Zealand Foods." *New Zealand Medical Journal* 113 (April 2000): 140–142.

31. Miller, Janette, et al. "Rice: A High or Low Glycemic Index Food?" *American Journal of Clinical Nutrition* 56 (1992): 1034–1036.

32. Janson, Michael, M.D. *Dr. Janson's New Vitamin Revolution.* New York: Avery/Penguin-Putnam, 2000, pp. 134–135.

33. Barclay, Alan W., BSC, et al. "Glycemic Index, Glycemic Load, and Glycemic Response are Not the Same." *Diabetes Care* 28 (2005): 1839.

34. Brand-Miller, Jennie C. "Postprandial Glycemia, Glycemic Index, and the Prevention of Type 2 Diabetes." *American Journal of Clinical Nutrition* 80 (2004): 243–244.

35. Adams, Ruth, and Frank Murray. *Good Seeds, The Rich Grains, The Hardy Nuts for a Healthier, Happier Life.* New York: Larchmont Books, 1973, pp. 7ff, 24ff, 33ff.

36. Liese, Angela D., et al. "Whole-Grain Intake and Insulin Sensitivity: The Insulin Resistance Atherosclerosis Study." *American Journal of Clinical Nutrition* 78 (2003): 965–971.

37. Sartorelli, Daniela Saes, et al. "Dietary Fiber and Glucose Tolerance in Japanese Brazilians." *Diabetes Care* 28 (2005): 2240–2242.

38. Fung, Teresa T., et al. "Whole-Grain Intake and the Risk of Type 2 Diabetes: A Prospective Study in Men." *American Journal of Clinical Nutrition* 76 (2002): 535–540.

39. Anderson, James W., and Tammy J. Hanna. "Whole Grains and Protection against Coronary Heart Disease: What Are the Active Components and Mechanisms?" *American Journal of Clinical Nutrition* 70 (1999): 307–308.

40. Ronzio, Robert A., Ph.D. *Encyclopedia of Nutrition and Good Health.* New York: Facts on File, 1997, pp. 175ff.

41. Behall, K., et al. "Mineral Balance in Adult Men: Effect of Four Refined Fibers." *American Journal of Clinical Nutrition* 46 (1987): 304–314.

42. Sahyouan, Nadine R., et al. "Whole-Grain Intake Is Inversely Associated with the Metabolic Syndrome and Mortality in Older Adults." *American Journal of Clinical Nutrition* 83 (2006): 124–131.

43. Jensen, Majken K., et al. "Whole Grains, Bran, and Germ in Relation to Homocysteine and Markers of Glycemic Control, Lipids and Inflammation." *American Journal of Clinical Nutrition* 83 (2006): 275–283.

44. Qi, Lu, M.D., Ph.D., et al. "Whole-Grain, Bran, and Cereal Fiber Intake and Markers of Systemic Inflammation in Diabetic Women." *Diabetes Care* 29 (2006): 207–211.

45. Murray, Michael, N.D., and Joseph Pizzorno, N.D. *Encyclopedia of Natural Medicine.* Rocklin, CA: Prima Publishing, 1998, p. 91.

46. Qi, Lu, M.D., Ph.D., et al. "Whole-Grain, Bran, and Cereal Fiber Intake and Markers of Systemic Inflammation in Diabetic Women." *Diabetes Care* 29 (2006): 207–211.

47. Chandalia, M., et al. "Beneficial Effects of High Dietary Fiber Intake in Patients with Type 2 Diabetes Mellitus." *New England Journal of Medicine* 342:19 (May 2000): 1392–1398.

48. Hallfrisch, Judith, et al. "Diets Containing Soluble Oat Extracts Improve Glucose and Insulin Responses of Moderately Hypercholesterolemic Men and Women." *American Journal of Clinical Nutrition* 61 (1995): 379–384.

49. Pick, Mary E., M.Sc., R.D., et al. "Oat Bran Concentrate Bread Products Improve Long-Term Control of Diabetes: A Pilot Study." *Journal of the American Dietetic Association* 96:12 (December 1996): 1254–1261.

50. Braten, J., et al. "Oat Gum Lowers Glucose and Insulin after an Oral Glucose Load." *American Journal of Clinical Nutrition* 53 (1991): 1425–1430.

51. Ebeling, P. et al. "Glucose and Lipid Metabolism and Insulin Sensitivity in Type 1 Diabetics: The Effect of Guar Gum." *American Journal of Clinical Nutrition* 43 (1988): 98–103.

52. Behall, K., et al. "Effect of Guar Gum on Mineral Balances in NIDDM Adults." *Diabetes Care* 12 (1989): 357–364.

53. Choe, M., and C. Kies. "Selenium Bioavailability: The Effect of Guar Gum Supplementation on Selenium Utilization in Human Subjects." *Nutrition Reports International* 39 (1989): 557–563.

54. Vuorinen-Markkola, Helena, et al. "Guar Gum and Insulin-Dependent Diabetes: Effects on Glycemic Control and Serum Lipoproteins." *American Journal of Clinical Nutrition* 56 (1992): 1056–1060.

55. Anderson, James W., et al. "Effects of Psyllium and Glucose and Serum Lipid Responses in Men and Type 2 Diabetes and Hypercholesterolemia." *American Journal of Clinical Nutrition* 70 (1999): 466–473.

56. Pastors, J., et al. "Psyllium Fiber Reduces Rise in Postprandial Glucose and Insulin Concentrations in Patients with Non-Insulin Dependent Diabetes." *American Journal of Clinical Nutrition* 53 (1991): 1431–1435.

57. Mahdi, G. et al. "Role of Chromium in Barley in Modulating the Symptoms of Diabetes." *Annals of Nutrition and Metabolism* 35 (1991): 65–70.

58. Anderson, James W. "High Fiber Diet for Diabetes: Safe and Effective Treatment." *Postgraduate Medicine* 88:2 (August 1990): 157–168.

59. Hurley, Jayne, and Stephen Schmidt. "Movie Theater Snacks." *Nutrition Action* (May 1994): 1, 9.

60. Hunninghake, Donald B., et al. "Hypercholesterolemic Effects of a Dietary Fiber Supplement." *American Journal of Clinical Nutrition* 59 (1994): 1050–1054.

Chapter 5: Vitamin A and the Carotenoids

1. Murray, Frank. *Program Your Heart for Health.* New York: Larchmont Books, 1997, pp. 291ff.

2. Berson, Eliot L., M.D. "A Randomized Trial of Vitamin A and Vitamin E Supplementation for Retinitis Pigmentosa." *Archives of Ophthalmology* 111 (June 1993): 761–772.

3. Goldberg, J., et al. "Factors Associated with Age-Related Macular Degeneration: An Analysis of Data from the First National Health and Nutrition Examination Survey." *American Journal of Epidemiology* 128:4 (1988): 700–710.

4. Cumming, R.G., et al. "Diet and Cataract: The Blue Mountain Eye Study." *Ophthalmology* 107:3 (March 2000): 450–456.

5. Denke, Margo A., M.D. "Diet and Nutrition." *Medical and Health Annual.* Chicago: Encyclopaedia Britannica, 1995, p. 268.

6. Kronhausen, Eberhard, Ed.D., et al. *Formula for Life.* New York: William Morrow, 1989, p. 257.

7. Ronzio, Robert A., Ph.D. *Encyclopedia of Nutrition and Good Health.* New York: Facts on File, 1997, p. 444.

8. Sibulesky, L., et al. "Safety of 7500 RE (25,000 IU) Vitamin A Daily in Adults with Retinitis Pigmentosa." *American Journal of Clinical Nutrition* 69 (1999): 656–663.

9. Landvik, Sharon, M.S., R.D. *Carotenoids Fact Book.* LaGrange, IL: VERIS Research Information Service, 1996.

10. Ibid.

11. Ford, E.S., et al. "Diabetes Mellitus and Serum Carotenoids: Findings from the Third National Health and Nutrition Examination Survey." *American Journal of Epidemiology* 149 (1999): 168–176.

12. Reunanen, A., et al. "Serum Antioxidants and Risk of Non-Insulin Dependent Diabetes Mellitus." *European Journal of Clinical Nutrition* 52 (1998): 89-93.

13. Kritchevsky, S.B., et al. "Provitamin A Carotenoid Intake and Carotid Artery Plaques: The Atherosclerosis Risk in Communities Study." *American Journal of Clinical Nutrition* 68 (1998): 726–733.

14. Jang, Y., et al. "Differences in Body Fat Distribution and Antioxidant Status in Korean Men with Cardiovascular Disease with or without Diabetes." *American Journal of Clinical Nutrition* 73 (2001): 68–74.

15. Dizon, Z.R., et al. "The Effect of a Low Carotenoid Diet on Malondialdehyde-Thiobarbituric Acid (MDA-TBA) Concentrations in Women: A Placebo-Controlled, Double-Blind Study." *Journal of the American College of Nutrition* 17 (1998): 54–58.

16. Klipstein-Grobush, Kerstin, et al. "Dietary Antioxidants and the Risk of Myocardial Infarction in the Elderly: The Rotterdam Study." *American Journal of Clinical Nutrition* 69 (1999): 261–266.

17. Landvik, Sharon, M.S., R.D. "Veris Research Summary." LaGrange, IL: VERIS Research Information Service, 1997.

18. Atkins, Robert C., M.D. *Dr. Atkins' Vita-Nutrient Solution.* New York: Simon & Schuster, 1998, p. 52.

19. Landvik, Sharon, M.S., R.D. *Carotenoids Fact Book.* LaGrange, IL: VERIS Research Information Service, 1996.

Chapter 6: The B-Complex Vitamins

1. Baker, Daniel, Pharm.D., and R. Keith Campbell. "Vitamin and Mineral Supplementation in Patients with Diabetes Mellitus." *Diabetes Educator* 18:5 (September/October 1992): 420–427.

2. Ibid.

3. Ibid.

4. Ibid.

5. Adams, Ruth, and Frank Murray. *Body, Mind and the B Vitamins.* New York: Larchmont Books, 1975, pp. 173–174.

6. Brady, Jennifer A., M.S., R.D., et al. "Thiamine Status, Diuretic Medications and the Management of Congestive Heart Failure." *Journal of the American Dietetic Association* 95 (1995): 541–544.

7. Hathcock, John N., Ph.D. *Vitamin and Mineral Safety.* Washington, DC: Council for Responsible Nutrition, 1997, p. 7.

8. *Food, The Yearbook of Agriculture.* Washington, DC: U.S. Department of Agriculture, 1959, pp. 142–143.

9. Ibid., p. 21.

10. Hathcock, John N., Ph.D. *Vitamin and Mineral Safety.* Washington, DC: Council for Responsible Nutrition, 1997, p. 7.

11. Hendler, Sheldon Saul, M.D., Ph.D. *Doctors' Vitamin and Mineral Encyclopedia.* New York: Simon & Schuster, 1990, p. 435.

12. Thompson, T. "Thiamine, Riboflavin and Niacin Content of the Gluten-Free Diet: Is There Cause for Concern?" *Journal of the American Dietetic Association* 99:7 (July 1999): 858–892.

13. Ensminger, A., et al. *Foods and Nutrition Encyclopedia.* Clovis, CA: Pegus Press, 1983, pp. 1588ff.

14. Knip, M., et al. "Safety of High-Dose Nicotinamide: A Review." *Diabetologia* 43 (2001): 1337–1345.

15. Probstfield, Jeffrey L., M.D. "Nicotinic Acid as a Lipoprotein-Altering Agent: Therapy Directed by the Primary Physician." *Archives of Internal Medicine* 154 (July 1994): 1557–1569.

16. Hoffer, Abram, M.D., Ph.D. *Orthomolecular Medicine for Physicians.* New Canaan, CT: Keats Publishing, 1989, pp. 42–43.

17. Cunningham, J.J. "Macronutrients as Nutraceutical Interventions in Diabetes Mellitus." *Journal of the American College of Nutrition* 17:1 (1998): 7–10.

18. Garg, Abhimayu, M.D., and Scott M. Grundy, M.D., Ph.D. "Nicotinic Acid as Therapy for Dyslipidemia in Non-Insulin-Dependent Diabetes Mellitus." *Journal of the American Medical Association* 264:6 (August 1990): 723–726.

19. Cleary, John P., M.D. "Vitamin B_3 in the Treatment of Diabetes Mellitus: Case Reports and Reviews of the Literature." *Journal of Nutritional Medicine* 1 (1990): 217–225.

20. Ibid.

21. Pozzilli, P., et al. "Nicotinamide Therapy in Patients with Newly-Diagnosed Type 1 Insulin-Dependent Diabetes." *Diabetologia* 31 (1988): A533.

22. Pozzilli, P., et al. "Double-Blind Trial of Nicotinamide in Recent-Onset Insulin-Dependent Diabetes Mellitus." *Diabetologia* 38:7 (1988): 848–852.

23. Pozzilli, P., et al. "Vitamin E and Nicotinamide Have Similar Effects in Maintaining Residual Beta Cell Function in Recent Onset Insulin-Dependent Diabetes (The IMDTAB IV Study)." *European Journal of Endocrinology* 137 (1997): 234–239.

24. Elam, Marshall B., Ph.D., M.D., et al. "Effect of Niacin on Lipid and Lipoprotein Levels and Glycemic Control in Patients with Diabetes and Peripheral Arterial Disease: The ADMIT Study: A Randomized Trial." *Journal of the American Medical Association* 284:10 (September 2000): 1263– 1270.

25. Hoffer, Abram, M.D., Ph.D. *Orthomolecular Medicine for Physicians*. New Canaan, CT: Keats Publishing, 1989, pp. 151–152.

26. Murray, Michael T., N.D. *Natural Alternatives to Over-the-Counter Prescription Drugs*. New York: William Morrow, 1994, p. 136.

27. Ensminger, A., et al. *Foods and Nutrition Encyclopedia*. Clovis, CA: Pegus Press, 1983, pp. 234ff.

28. Ellis, John M., M.D., and Jean Pamplin. *Vitamin B₆ Therapy*. New York: Avery Publishing Group, 1999, pp. 69ff.

29. Hamilton, Kirk. "Diabetes Mellitus and Vitamin B₆." *The Experts Speak*. Sacramento, CA: I.T. Services, 1996, pp. 102–103. Also: Mohan, Chandra, Ph.D. "Vitamin B₆ Metabolism and Diabetes." *Biochemical and Metabolic Biology* 52 (1994): 10–17.

30. Gaby, Alan, M.D. *B₆: The Natural Healer*. New Canaan, CT: Keats Publishing, 1987, pp. 107ff.

31. Ibid.

32. Bernstein, A., et al. "Treatment of Painful Diabetic Neuropathies with Vitamin B₆: A Clinical and Electrophysiologic Study." *FASEB Journal* 2 (1988): A438.

33. Hathcock, John N., Ph.D. *Vitamin and Mineral Safety*. Washington, DC: Council for Responsible Nutrition, 1997, p. 8.

34. *Food, The Yearbook of Agriculture*. Washington, DC: U.S. Department of Agriculture, 1959, pp. 147–148.

35. Araki, Atsushi, et al. "Plasma Homocysteine Concentrations in Japanese Patients with Non-Insulin-Dependent Diabetes Mellitus; Effect of Parenteral Cobalamin Treatment." *Atherosclerosis* 103 (1993): 149–157.

36. Murray, Michael T., N.D. *Diabetes and Hypoglycemia*. Rocklin, CA: Prima Publishing, 1994, pp. 99–100.

37. Hamilton, Kirk. "Diabetic Neuropathy, Vegetarian Diets and Vitamin B₁₂." *The Experts Speak*. Sacramento, CA: I.T. Services, 1996, pp. 104–105. Also: Crane, Milton, M.D. "Vitamin B₁₂ Studies in Total Nutrition." *Journal of Nutrition* 4 (1994): 419–430.

38. Chicola, Vincent F., M.D. "Vitamin B₁₂ Bats an Eye." *Cortlandt Forum* (July 1996): 122.

39. Hamilton, Kirk. "Diabetic Neuropathy, Vegetarian Diets and Vitamin B₁₂." *The Experts Speak*. Sacramento, CA: I.T. Services, 1996, pp. 104-105. Also: Crane, Milton, M.D. "Vitamin B₁₂ Studies in Total Nutrition." *Journal of Nutrition* 4 (1994): 419–430.

40. Ibid.

41. Hathcock, John N., Ph.D. *Vitamin and Mineral Safety*. Washington, DC: Council for Responsible Nutrition, 1957, p. 8.

42. *Food, The Yearbook of Agriculture*. Washington, DC: U.S. Department of Agriculture, 1959, pp. 146ff.

43. Woodside, Jayne V., et al. "Effect of B-Group Vitamins and Antioxidant Vitamins on Hyperhomo-cysteinemia: A Double-Blind, Randomized, Factorial-Design, Controlled Trial." *American Journal of Clinical Nutrition* 67:5 (May 1998): 858–866.

44. Brouwer, Ingeborg A., et al. "Low-Dose Folic Acid Supplementation Decreases Plasma Homocysteine Concentrations: A Randomized Trial." *American Journal of Clinical Nutrition* 69 (1999): 99–104.

45. Morrison, Howard I., Ph.D., et al. "Serum Folate and Risk of Fatal Coronary Heart Disease." *Journal of the American Medical Association* 275:24 (June 1996): 1893–1896.

46. Ubbink, Johan B., et al. "Vitamin B_{12} and Folate Nutritional Status in Men with Hyper-Homocysteinemia." *American Journal of Clinical Nutrition* 57 (1993): 47–53.

47. Ebly, E.M., et al. "Folate Status, Vascular Disease and Cognition in Elderly Canadians." *Age and Aging* 27 (1998): 485–491.

48. Hathcock, John N., Ph.D. *Vitamin and Mineral Safety*. Washington, DC: Council for Responsible Nutrition, 1997, p. 41.

49. Ensminger, A., et al. *Foods and Nutrition Encyclopedia*. Clovis, CA: Pegus Press, 1983, pp. 210ff.

50. *Prevention's Healing with Vitamins*. Emmaus, PA: Rodale Press, 1996, p. 220.

51. Golan, Ralph, M.D. *Optimal Wellness*. New York: Ballantine Books, 1995, pp. 188, 191–193, 360, 396.

52. Atkins, Robert C., M.D. *Dr. Atkins' Health Revolution*. Boston: Houghton Mifflin, 1988, pp. 102–103.

53. Hathcock, John N., Ph.D. *Vitamin and Mineral Safety*. Washington, DC: Council for Responsible Nutrition, 1997, p. 47.

54. Giller, Robert M., M.D., and Kathy Matthews. *Natural Prescriptions*. New York: Carol Southern Books, 1994, p. 72.

55. Golan, Ralph, M.D. *Optimal Wellness*. New York: Ballantine Books, 1995, pp. 188, 191–193, 360, 396.

56. Ronzio, Robert A., Ph.D. *Encyclopedia of Nutrition and Good Health*. New York: Facts on File, 1997, pp. 335-336.

57. Golan, Ralph, M.D. *Optimal Wellness*. New York: Ballantine Books, 1995, p. 192.

58. Caronel, F., et al. "Lipid-Lowering Treatment with Pantethine in Renal Transplant Patients." *Nephrologia* 15:1 (1995): 68–73.

59. Atkins, Robert C., M.D. *Dr. Atkins' Vita-Nutrient Solution*. New York: Simon & Schuster, 1998, pp. 84–85.

60. Ibid.

61. Murray, Michael T., N.D. *Natural Alternatives to Over-the-Counter and Prescription Drugs*. New York: William Morrow, 1994, p. 139.

62. Leung, Li-Hung, M.D. "A Stone that Kills Two Birds: Pantothenic Acid and the Treatment of Acne Vulgaris and Obesity." *Journal of Orthomolecular Medicine* 12:2 (1997): 99–114.

63. Hathcock, John N., Ph.D. *Vitamin and Mineral Safety*. Washington, DC: Council for Responsible Nutrition, 1997, p. 47.

64. Ensminger, A., et al. *Foods and Nutrition Encyclopedia*. Clovis, CA: Pegus Press, 1983, pp. 413ff.

65. Zeisel, Steven H., M.D., Ph.D. "Choline: An Important Nutrient in Brain Development, Liver Function and Carcinogenesis." *Journal of the American College of Nutrition* 11:5 (1992): 473–481.

66. Davis, Adelle. *Let's Get Well*. New York: New American Library, 1965, pp. 173–174, 194.

67. Atkins, Robert C., M.D. *Dr. Atkins' Vita-Nutrient Solution*. New York: Simon & Schuster, 1998, pp. 78-79.

68. Kang, Soo-Sang, et al. "Hyperhomocysteinemias: A Risk Factor for Occlusive Vascular Disease." *Annual Review of Nutrition* 12 (1992): 279–298.

69. Malinow, M.R., M.D. "Risk for Arterial Occlusive Disease: Is Hyperhomocysteinemia an Innocent Bystander?" *Canadian Journal of Cardiology* 7:9 (November 1991): VII–IX.

70. Ensminger, A., et al. *Foods and Nutrition Encyclopedia*. Clovis, CA: Pegus Press, 1983, pp. 1234ff.

71. Atkins, Robert C., M.D. *Dr. Atkins' Vita-Nutrient Solution*. New York: Simon & Schuster, 1998, pp. 80–82.

72. Davis, Adelle. *Let's Get Well*. New York: New American Library, 1965, p. 53.

73. Shamsuddin, AbulKalam M., M.D., Ph.D. *IP-6: Nature's Revolutionary Cancer-Fighter*. New York: Kensington Books, 1998, pp. 85–86.

74. Grafton, Gilliam, et al. "Effect of MG2 and NA+ Dependent Inositol Transport/Role for MG2 in Etiology of Diabetic Complications." *Diabetes* 41 (1992): 35–39.

75. Holub, Bruce J., Ph.D. "The Nutritional Importance of Inositol in the Phosphoinositides." *New England Journal of Medicine* 326:19 (May 1992): 1285–1287.

Chapter 7: Vitamin C

1. Rath, Matthias, M.D. *Cellular Health Series: The Heart.* Santa Clara, CA: MR Publishing, 2001, pp. 97ff.

2. Cunningham, John J., Ph.D. "The Glucose/Insulin System and Vitamin C Implementation in Insulin-Dependent Diabetes Mellitus." *Journal of the American College of Nutrition* 17:2 (1998): 105–108.

3. Cunningham, John J., Ph.D., et al. "Vitamin C: An Aldose Reductase Inhibitor that Normalizes Erythrocyte Sorbitol in Insulin-Dependent Diabetes Mellitus." *Journal of the American College of Nutrition* 13:4 (1994): 344–350.

4. Brazg, R., et al. "Effects of Dietary Antioxidants on LDL Cholesterol in Non-insulin Dependent Diabetics" *Clinical Research* 40 (1992): 103A.

5. Anderson, J.W., et al. "Antioxidant Supplementation Effects on Low-Density Lipoprotein Oxidation in Individuals with Type 2 Diabetes Mellitus." *Journal of the American College of Nutrition* 18:5 (1999): 451–461.

6. Roongpisuthipong, C., et al. "Vitamin Status in Elderly Diabetic Subjects." *FASEB Journal* 5 (1991): 1299A.

7. McAuliffe, A.V., et al. "Administration of Ascorbic Acid and an Aldose Inhibitor (Tolrestat) in Diabetes: Effect on Urinary Albumin Excretion." *Nephron* 80 (1998): 277–284.

8. Manson, J., et al. "A Prospective Study of Vitamin C and Incidence of Coronary Heart Disease in Women." *Circulation* 85 (1992): 865.

9. Osilesi, O., et al. "Blood Pressure and Plasma Lipids during Ascorbic Acid Supplementation in Borderline Hypertensive and Normotensive Adults." *Nutrition Research* 11 (1991): 405–412.

10. Farvid, Maryam Sadat, Ph.D., et al. "Comparison of the Effects of Vitamins and/or Mineral Supplementation on Glomerular and Tubular Dysfunction in Type 2 Diabetes." *Diabetes Care* 28 (2005): 2458–2464.

11. Millen, Amy E., et al. "Relation between Intake of Vitamins C and E and Risk of Diabetic Retinopathy in the Atherosclerosis Risk in Communities Study." *American Journal of Clinical Nutrition* 79 (2004): 865–873.

12. Iino, Kenzo, M.D., et al. "Serum Vitamin C Levels in Type 2 Diabetic Nephropathy." *Diabetes Care* 28 (2005): 2808.

13. Hathcock, John N., Ph.D. *Vitamin and Mineral Safety.* Washington, DC: Council for Responsible Nutrition, 1997, p. 34.

Chapter 8: Vitamin D

1. Ensminger, A., et al. *Foods and Nutrition Encyclopedia.* Clovis, CA: Pegus Press, 1983, pp. 2256ff.

2. Garrison, Robert J., M.A., R.Ph., and Elizabeth Somer, M.A., R.D. *Nutrition Desk Reference*. New Canaan, CT: Keats Publishing, 1995, pp. 78ff.

3. Ensminger, A., et al. *Foods and Nutrition Encyclopedia*. Clovis, CA: Pegus Press, 1983, pp. 2256ff.

4. Utiger, Robert D., M.D. "The Need for more Vitamin D." *New England Journal of Medicine* 338:12 (March 1998): 828–829.

5. Garrison, Robert J., M.A., R.Ph., and Elizabeth Somer, M.A., R.D. *Nutrition Desk Reference*. New Canaan, CT: Keats Publishing, 1995, pp. 78ff.

6. Marks, Robin, MPH, et al. "The Effect of Regular Sunscreen Use on Vitamin D Levels in an Australian Population." *Archives of Dermatology* 131 (April 1995): 415–421.

7. McKenna, M. "Differences in Vitamin D Status between Countries in Young Adults and the Elderly." *American Journal of Medicine* 93 (1992): 69–77.

8. Vaarala, O., et al. "Environmental Factors in the Aetiology of Childhood Diabetes." *Diabetes and Nutrition Metabolism* 12:2 (1999): 75–85.

9. Dahlquist, G., et al. "Vitamin D Supplement in Early Childhood and Risk of Type 1 (Insulin-Dependent) Diabetes Mellitus." *Diabetologia* 42 (1999): 51–54.

10. Holick, Michael F. "Too Little Vitamin D in Premenopausal Women: Why Should We Care?" *American Journal of Clinical Nutrition* 76 (2002): 3–4.

11. Baynes, K.C.R., et al. "Vitamin D, Glucose Tolerance and Insulinemia in Elderly Men." *Diabetologia* 40 (1997): 344–347.

12. Hamilton, Kirk. "Glucose Tolerance, Insulinemia and Vitamin D." *Clinical Pearls*. Sacramento, CA: I.T. Services, 1997, p. 305. Also: Boucher, B.J., M.D. "Vitamin D, Glucose Tolerance and Insulinemia in Elderly Men." *Diabetologia* 40 (1997): 344–347.

13. Grimes, David S., M.D. "Sunlight, Cholesterol and Coronary Heart Diseases." *Quarterly Journal of Medicine* 89 (1996): 579–589.

14. Watson, Karol E., M.D., et al. "Active Serum Vitamin D Levels Are Inversely Correlated with Coronary Calcification." *Circulation* 96 (1997): 1755–1760.

15. Adams, Ruth. *Complete Home Guide to All the Vitamins*. New York: Larchmont Books, 1975, pp. 196ff.

16. Ford, Earl S., M.D., MPH, et al. "Concentrations of Serum Vitamin D and the Metabolic Syndrome among U.S. Adults." *Diabetes Care* 28 (2005): 1228–1229.

17. Cigolini, Massimo, M.D., et al. "Serum 25-Hydroxyvitamin D_3 Concentrations and Prevalence of Cardiovascular Disease among Type 2 Diabetic Patients." *Diabetes Care* 29 (2006): 722–724.

18. Di Cesar, David J., et al. "Vitamin D Deficiency Is More Common in Type 2 than in Type 1 Diabetes." *Diabetes Care* 29 (2006): 174.

19. Utiger, Robert D., M.D. "The Need for More Vitamin D." *New England Journal of Medicine* 338:12 (March 1998): 828–829.

20. Hathcock, John N., Ph.D. *Vitamin and Mineral Safety.* Washington, DC: Council for Responsible Nutrition, 1997, p. 7.

Chapter 9: Vitamin E

1. Atkins, Robert C., M.D. *Dr. Atkins' Vita-Nutrient Solution.* New York: Simon & Schuster, 1999, pp. 108–109.

2. Ibid.

3. "Diabetes and Vitamin E." *Diabetes* (February 1995).

4. Phillips, Robert H., Ph.D. *Coping with Diabetes.* New York: Avery/Penguin-Putnam, 2000, p. 24.

5. Ibid.

6. Tapley, Donald F., M.D., et al. *Columbia University College of Physicians and Surgeons Complete Home Medical Guide.* New York: Crown, 1985, pp. 1493– 1494.

7. Baker, Daniel, Pharm.D., and R. Keith Campbell. "Vitamin and Mineral Supplementation in Patients with Diabetes Mellitus." *Diabetes Educator* 18:5 (September/October 1992): 420–427.

8. Jain, Sushil K., Ph.D., et al. "Effect of Modest Vitamin E Supplementation on Blood Glycolated Hemoglobin and Triglyceride Levels and Red Cell Indices in Type 1 Diabetic Patients." *Journal of the American College of Nutrition* 15:5 (1996): 1458–1461.

9. Paolisso, G., et al. "Pharmacologic Doses of Vitamin E Improve Insulin Action in Healthy Subjects and in Non-Insulin-Dependent Diabetic Patients." *American Journal of Clinical Nutrition* 57 (1993): 650–656.

10. Hamilton, Kirk. "Insulin Dependent Diabetes Mellitus, Vitamin E and Nicotinamide." *Clinical Pearls.* Sacramento, CA: I.T. Services, 1997, p. 315. Also: Pozzilli, Paolo, M.D. "Vitamin E and Nicotinamide Have Similar Effects in Maintaining Residual Beta Cell Function in Recent Onset Insulin-Dependent Diabetes." *European Journal of Endocrinology* 137 (1997): 234–239.

11. Davi, G., et al. "In Vivo Formation of 8-iso-prostaglandin E2 Alpha and Platelet Activation in Diabetes Mellitus." *Circulation* 99 (1990): 224–229.

12. Jain, S.K., et al. "Vitamin E Supplementation Restores Glutathione and Malondialdehyde to Normal Concentrations in Erythrocytes of Type 1 Diabetic Children." *Diabetes Care* 23 (2000): 1389–1394.

13. Devaraj, S., et al. "Low-Density Lipoprotein Post-secretory Modification, Monocyte Function and Circulating Adhesion Molecules in Type 2 Diabetic Patients with and without Macrovascular Complications: The Effect of Alpha-Tocopherol Supplementation." *Circulation* 102 (2000): 191–196.

14. Leppala, J.M., et al. "Vitamin E and Beta-Carotene Supplementation in High Risk of Stroke." *Archives of Neurology* 57 (2000): 1503–1509.

15. Wu, D., et al. "Vitamin E and Macrophage Cyclooxygenase Regulation in the Aged." *Journal of Nutrition* 131 (2001): 3825–3885.

16. Manzella, D., et al. "Chronic Administration of Pharmacologic Doses of Vitamin E Improves the Cardiac Autonomic Nerve System in Patients with Type 2 Diabetes." *American Journal of Clinical Nutrition* 73 (2001): 1052–1057.

17. Devaraj, S., et al. "Alpha Tocopherol Supplementation Decreases Serum C-Reactive Protein and Monocyte Interleukin-6 in Normal Volunteers and Type 2 Diabetic Patients." *Free Radical Biology and Medicine* 29 (2000): 790–792.

18. Engelen, W., et al. "Effects of Long-Term Supplementation with Moderate Pharmacologic Doses of Vitamin E Are Saturable and Reversible in Patients with Type 1 Diabetes." *American Journal of Clinical Nutrition* 72 (2000): 1142–1149.

19. Jialal, I., et al. "Is There a Vitamin E Paradox?" *Current Opinion in Lipidology* 12 (2001): 49–53.

20. Blumberg, Jeffrey, Ph.D. "The Requirement for Vitamins and Aging and Age-Associated Degenerative Conditions." *Vitamin Intake in Human Nutrition* 52 (1995): 108–115.

21. Bursell, S.E., et al. "High Dose Vitamin Supplementation Normalizes Retinal Blood Flow and Creatine Clearance in Patients with Type 1 Diabetes." *Diabetes Care* 22 (1999): 1215–1251.

22. Adams, Ruth, and Frank Murray. *Improving Your Health with Vitamin E.* New York: Larchmont Books, 1978, p. 122.

23. Ibid., p. 19.

24. Ibid., pp. 19–20.

25. Ibid., p. 120.

26. Park, Sunmin, and Soo Bong Choi. "Effects of Alpha-Tocopherol Supplementation and Continuous Subcutaneous Insulin Infusion on Oxidative Stress in Korean Patients with Type 2 Diabetes." *American Journal of Clinical Nutrition* 75 (2002): 728–733.

27. Hathcock, John N., Ph.D. Washington, DC: Council for Responsible Nutrition, 1997, p. 31.

Chapter 10: Minerals of Importance to Diabetics

1. Garrison, Robert, Jr., M.A., R.Ph., and Elizabeth Somer, M.A., R.D. *Nutrition Desk Reference.* New Canaan, CT: Keats Publishing, 1995, pp. 183–184.

2. Mertz, Walter, Ph.D. "Chromium in Human Nutrition: A Review." *Journal of Nutrition* 123 (1993): 626–633.

3. Bhanot, S., M.D. "Essential Trace Elements of Potential Importance in Nutritional Management of Diabetes Mellitus." *Nutrition Research* 14:4 (1994): 593–604.

4. Anderson, Richard A., Ph.D. "Chromium in the Prevention and Control of Diabetes." *Diabetes and Metabolism (Paris)* 26:1 (2000): 22–27.

5. Ibid.

6. Press, Raymond T., M.D. "The Effect of Chromium Picolinate on Serum Glucose, Glycosylated Hemoglobin and Cholesterol of Adult Onset Diabetics." Paper presented at a meeting of the Federation of American Societies for Experimental Biology, New Orleans, Louisiana, March 21, 1989.

7. Hellerstein, M.K. "Is Chromium Supplementation Effective in Managing Type 2 Diabetes?" *Nutrition Reviews* 56:10 (1998): 302–306.

8. Anderson, Richard A., Ph.D. "Nutritional Factors Influencing the Glucose/Insulin System: Chromium." *Journal of the American College of Nutrition* 16:5 (1997): 404–410.

9. Kuritzky, L., et al. "Improving Management of Type 2 Diabetes Mellitus: Chromium." *Hospital Practice* (February 15, 2000): 113–116.

10. Cefalu, W.T., et al. "Effect of Chromium Picolinate on Insulin Sensitivity In Vivo." *Journal of Trace Elements and Experimental Medicine* 12 (1999): 71–83.

11. Mahdi, G., et al. "Role of Chromium in Barley in Modulating the Symptoms of Diabetes." *Annals of Nutrition and Metabolism* 35 (1991): 65–70.

12. Gordon, J. "An Easy and Inexpensive Way to Lower Cholesterol." *Western Journal of Medicine* 154 (1991): 3.

13. Pineau, A., et al. "A Study of Chromium and Human Cataractous Lenses and Whole Blood of Diabetics, Senile and Normal Populations." *Biological Trace Element Research* 32 (1992): 133–138.

14. Kuritzky, L., et al. "Improving Management of Type 2 Diabetes Mellitus: Chromium." *Hospital Practice* (February 15, 2000): 113–116.

15. Garrison, Robert, Jr., M.A., R.Ph., and Elizabeth Somer, M.A., R.D. *Nutrition Desk Reference.* New Canaan, CT: Keats Publishing, 1995, p. 183.

16. Anderson, Richard A., Ph.D. "Chromium as an Essential Nutrient for Humans." *Regulatory Toxicology and Pharmacology* 26 (1997): 535–541.

17. Anderson, Richard A., Ph.D. "Nutritional Factors Influencing the Glucose/Insulin System: Chromium." *Journal of the American College of Nutrition* 16:5 (1997): 404–410.

18. Ding, W., et al. "Serum and Urine Chromium Concentrations in Elderly Diabetics." *Biological Trace Element Research* 63 (1998): 231–237.

19. Altura, Burton M., Ph.D., et al. "Magnesium Growing in Clinical Importance." *Patient Care* (January 15, 1994): 130–136.

20. Trehan, Shruti, M.D., et al. "Magnesium Disorders: What to Do When Homeostasis Goes Awry." *The Consultant* (November 1996): 2485–2497.

21. Altura, Burton M., Ph.D., et al. "Magnesium Growing in Clinical Importance." *Patient Care* (January 15, 1994): 130–136.

22. Kobayashi, T., et al. "Plasma and Erythrocyte Magnesium Levels Are Correlated with Oxygen Uptake in Patients with Non-Insulin Diabetes Mellitus." *Endocrine Journal* 45:2 (1998): 277–283.

23. Elamin, A., and T. Tuveno. "Magnesium and Insulin-Dependent Diabetes Mellitus." *Diabetes Research and Clinical Practice* 10 (1990): 203–209.

24. Rude, Robert K., M.D. "Magnesium Deficiency and Diabetes Mellitus: Causes and Effects." *Postgraduate Medicine* 92:5 (1992): 217–223.

25. Tosiello, Lorraine, M.D. "Hypomagnesaemia and Diabetes Mellitus." *Archives of Internal Medicine* 156 (June 1996): 1143–1148.

26. Song, Yiqing, M.D., et al. "Magnesium Intake, C-Reactive Protein, and the Prevalence of Metabolic Syndrome in Middle-Aged and Older U.S. Women." *Diabetes Care* 28 (2005): 1438–1444.

27. Yang, Chun-Y., Ph.D., et al. "Magnesium in Drinking Water and the Risk of Death from Diabetes Mellitus." *Magnesium Research* 12:2 (1999): 131– 137.

28. Kahn, Jason. "Magnesium Levels May Protect Risk of Type 2 Diabetes in Whites." *Medical Tribune* (July 1997): 16.

29. Bardicef, Mordechai, M.D., et al. "Extracellular and Intracellular Magnesium Depletion in Pregnancy and Gestational Diabetes." *American Journal of Obstetrics and Gynecology* 172:3 (1995): 1009–1014.

30. Tuvemo, T., et al. "Serum Magnesium and Protein Concentrations during the First Five Years of Insulin-Dependent Diabetes in Children." *Acta Pediatrica Supplement* 418 (1997): 7–10.

31. Paolisso, G., et al. "Magnesium and Glucose Homeostasis." *Diabetologia* 33 (1990): 501–514.

32. Nadler, Jerry, M.D. "Magnesium Lowers Blood Pressure in Type 2 Diabetes." *Practical Cardiology* 16:10 (October 1990): 4.

33. Eriksson, Johan, M.D., Ph.D. "Magnesium and Ascorbic Acid Supplementation in Diabetes Mellitus." *Annals of Nutrition and Metabolism* 39 (1995): 217–223.

34. Seelig, Mildred S., M.D., et al. "Low Magnesium: A Common Denominator in Pathologic Process in Diabetes Mellitus, Cardiovascular Disease and Eclampsis." *Journal of the American College of Nutrition* 11:5 (October 1992): 608/Abstract 39.

35. Lucas, Michael J., M.D., et al. "A Comparison of Magnesium Sulfate with Phenytoin for the Prevention of Eclampsia." *New England Journal of Medicine* 333:4 (July 1995): 201–205. Also: Duley, Lelia, and Richard Johanson. "Magne-

sium Sulfate for Preeclampsia and Eclampsia: The Evidence So Far." *British Journal of Obstetrics and Gynecology* 101 (July 1994): 565–567.

36. Browne, S.E., M.B. "The Case for Intravenous Magnesium Treatment of Arterial Disease in General Practice: Review of 34 Years of Experience." *Journal of Nutritional Medicine* 4 (1994): 169–177.

37. Ensminger, A., et al. *Foods and Nutrition Encyclopedia.* Clovis, CA: Pegus Press, 1983, pp. 1976ff.

38. Stapleton, S.R. "Selenium: An Insulin-Minetic." *Cellular and Molecular Life Sciences* 57 (2000): 1874–1879.

39. Ruiz, C., et al. "Selenium, Zinc and Copper in Plasma of Patients with Type 1 Diabetes Mellitus in Different Metabolic Control States." *Journal of Trace Elements in Medicine and Biology* 12 (1998): 91–95.

40. Simonoff, M., et al. "Serum and Erythrocyte Selenium in Normal and Pathological States in France." *Trace Elements in Medicine* 5:2 (1998): 64–69.

41. Osterode, W., et al. "Nutritional Antioxidants, Red Cell Membrane Fluidity an Blood Viscosity in Type 1 (Insulin Dependent) Diabetes Mellitus." *Diabetes Medicine* 13 (1996): 1044–1050.

42. Bluhm, G. "Selenium and Cardiovascular Disease." *Trace Elements in Medicine* 7:3 (1990): 139–145.

43. Kok, F., et al. "Decreased Selenium Levels in Acute Myocardial Infarction." *Journal of the American Medical Association* 261 (1989): 1161–1164.

44. Hamilton, Kirk. "Pancreatic (Acute) and Sodium Selenite." *The Experts Speak.* Sacramento, CA: I.T. Services, 1996, p. 174. Also: Kuklinski, Bodo, M.D. "Reducing the Lethality in Acute Pancreatitis with Sodium Selenite. Clinical Results of 4 Years Antioxidant Therapy." *Medizinische Klinik* 90:Suppl 1 (1995): 36–41.

45. Wright, Jonathan V., M.D., et al. "Improvement of Vision in Macular Degeneration Associated with Intravenous Zinc and Selenium Therapy." *Journal of Nutritional Medicine* 1 (1990): 133–138.

46. Ahlrot-Westerlund, Britt, M.D., et al. "Cataracts, Vitamin E, and Selenomethionine." *Acta Ophthalmology* 66:2 (April 1988): 237–238.

47. Rayman, Margaret P. "Dietary Selenium: Time to Act." *British Medical Journal* 314 (February 1997): 387–388.

48. Harland, Barbara F., Ph.D., R.D., et al. "Is Vanadium of Human Nutritional Importance Yet?" *Journal of the American Dietetic Association* 94:8 (August 1994): 891–895.

49. French, Rodney J., B.Sc., and Peter J.H. Jones, Ph.D. "Role of Vanadium in

Nutrition: Metabolism, Essentiality and Dietary Considerations." *Life Sciences* 52:4 (1993): 339–346.

50. Giller, Robert M., M.D., and Kathy Matthews. *Natural Prescriptions.* New York: Carol Southern Books, 1994, p. 116.

51. Clouatre, Dallas, Ph.D. *Anti-Fat Nutrients.* San Francisco: Pax Publishing, 1993, pp. 20ff.

52. Boden, Guenther, et al. "Effect of Vanadyl Sulfate on Carbohydrates and Lipid Metabolism in Patients with Non-Insulin Dependent Diabetes." *Metabolism* 45:9 (1996): 1130–1135.

53. Cusi, K., et al. "Vanadyl Sulfate Improves Hepatic and Muscle Insulin Sensitivity in Type 2 Diabetes." *Clinical Endocrinology and Metabolism* 86:3 (2001): 1410–1417.

54. Verma, Subodh, Ph.D., et al. "Nutritional Factors that Can Favorably Influence the Glucose/Insulin System: Vanadium." *Journal of the American College of Nutrition* 17:1 (1998): 11–18.

55. Cunningham, J.J. "Micronutrients as Nutraceutical Interventions in Diabetes Mellitus." *Journal of the American College of Nutrition* 17:1 (1998): 7–10.

56. Halberstam, Meyer. "Oral Vanadyl Sulfate Improves Insulin Sensitivity in NIDDM But Not in Obese Non-Diabetic Subjects." *Diabetes* 45 (1996): 659–666.

57. Roberts, Karen, et al. "Syndrome X: Medical Nutrition Therapy." *Nutrition Reviews* 58:5 (2000): 154–160.

58. French, Rodney, J., B.Sc., and Peter J.H. Jones, Ph.D. "Nutritional Aspects of Vanadium." *Nutrition Report* 11:7 (July 1993): 49, 56.

59. Badmaev, V., et al. "Vanadium: A Review of the Potential Role in the Fight against Disease." *Journal of Alternative and Complimentary Medicine* 5:3 (1999): 273–291.

60. Challem, Jack, Burton Berkson, M.D., and Melissa Diane Smith. *Syndrome X.* New York: John Wiley & Sons, 2000, p. 204.

61. Atkins, Robert C., M.D. *Dr. Atkins' Vita-Nutrient Solution.* New York: Simon & Schuster, 1998, pp. 148–151.

62. Hartland, Barbara F., Ph.D., R.D., et al. "Is Vanadium of Human Nutritional Importance Yet?" *Journal of the American Dietetic Association* 94:8 (August 1994): 891–895.

63. Hu, Min, et al. "Assisting Effects of Lithium on Hypoglycemic Treatment in Patients with Diabetes." *Biological Trace Element Research* 60 (1997): 131– 137.

64. Heiman, E.M. "Lithium-Aggravated Nocturnal Myoclonus and Restless Leg Syndrome." *American Journal of Psychiatry* 143:9 (September 1986): 1191– 1192.

65. Chausmer, Arthur B., M.D., Ph.D. "Zinc, Insulin and Diabetes." *Journal of the American College of Nutrition* 17:2 (1998): 109–115.

66. Brun, Jean-Frederic, et al. "Effects of Oral Zinc Gluconate on Glucose Effectiveness and Insulin Sensitivity in Humans." *Biological Trace Element Research* 47 (1995): 385–391.

67. Bhattacharyas, R.D., et al. "Significantly Altered Copper and Zinc Levels in Serum, Liver, Urine and Skeletal Muscle of Morbidly Obese Patients." *Journal of the American College of Nutrition* 7 (1988): 401.

68. Blostein-Fujii, Ashley, et al. "Short-Term Zinc Supplementation in Women with Non-Insulin Dependent Diabetes Mellitus: Effects on Plasma 5-Nucleotidase Activities, Insulin-Like Growth Factor 1 Concentrations and Lipoprotein Oxidation Rates in Vitro." *American Journal of Clinical Nutrition* 66 (1997): 639–642.

69. Haglund, Bengt, Ph.D., et al. "Evidence of a Relationship between Childhood-Onset Type 1 Diabetes and Low Groundwater Concentrations of Zinc." *Diabetes Care* 19:8 (August 1996): 873–875.

70. Marchesini, G., et al. "Zinc Supplementation Improves Glucose Disposal in Patients with Cirrhosis." *Metabolism* 47:7 (July 1998): 792–798.

71. Anderson, R.A., et al. "Potential Antioxidant Effects of Zinc and Chromium Supplementation in People with Type 2 Diabetes Mellitus." *Journal of the American College of Nutrition* 20:3 (2001): 212–218.

72. Singh, R.B., et al. "Current Zinc Intake and Risk of Diabetes and Coronary Artery Disease and Factors Associated with Insulin Resistance in Rural and Urban Populations of North India." *Journal of the American College of Nutrition* 17:6 (1998): 564–570.

73. Sandstead, Harold H., and Norman G. Egger. "Is Zinc Nutriture a Problem in Persons with Diabetes Mellitus?" *American Journal of Clinical Nutrition* 66 (1997): 681–682.

Chapter 11: Other Nutrients to Help Diabetics

1. Challem, Jack. "Beat Diabetes with Alpha-Lipoic Acid." *GreatLife* (November 2001): 34ff.

2. Packer, Lester, Ph.D., et al. "Alpha-Lipoic Acid as a Biological Antioxidant." *Free Radical Biology and Medicine* 19:2 (1995): 227–250.

3. Challem, Jack. "Beat Diabetes with Alpha-Lipoic Acid." *GreatLife* (November 2001): 34ff.

4. Khamaisi, M., et al. "Lipoic Acid Reduces Glycemia and Increases Muscle GLUT4 in Streptozotocin-Diabetic Rats." *Metabolism* 46 (1997): 763–768.

5. Konrad, Thomas, M.D., et al. "Alpha-Lipoic Acid Treatment Decreases Serum

Lactate and Pyruvate Concentrations and Improves Glucose Effectiveness in Lean and Obese Patients with Type 2 Diabetes." *Diabetes Care* 22:2 (1999): 280–287.

6. Hamdorf, G., M.D. "Thioctic Acid: A Rational Remedy for the Treatment of Diabetic Polyneuropathy." *Experimental Clinical Endocrinology and Diabetes* 104 (1995): 126–127.

7. Challem, Jack. "Beat Diabetes with Alpha-Lipoic Acid." *GreatLife* (November 2001): 34ff.

8. Hamdorf, G., M.D. "Thioctic Acid: A Rational Remedy for the Treatment of Diabetic Polyneuropathy." *Experimental Clinical Endocrinology and Diabetes* 104 (1995): 126–127.

9. Ibid.

10. Haak, E.S., et al. "The Effect of Alpha-Lipoic Acid on the Neurovascular Reflex Arc in Patients with Diabetic Neuropathy Assessed by Capillary Microscopy." *Microvascular Research* 58 (1999): 28–34.

11. Ziegler, Dan, M.D., and F. Arnold Gries. "Alpha-Lipoic Acid in the Treatment of Diabetic Peripheral and Cardiac Autonomic Neuropathy." *Diabetes* 46:Suppl 2 (September 1997): 562–566.

12. Melham, M.F., et al. "Effects of Dietary Supplementation of Alpha-Lipoic Acid on Early Glomerular Injury in Diabetes Mellitus." *Journal of the American Society of Nephrology* 12 (2001): 124–133.

13. Marangon, K., et al. "Comparison of the Effect of Alpha-Lipoic Acid and Alpha-Tocopherol Supplementation on Measures of Oxidative Stress." *Free Radical Biology and Medicine* 27 (1999): 1114–1121.

14. Werbach, Melvyn, M.D. *Healing with Food*. New York: HarperCollins, 1993, pp. 111, 121.

15. Low, P.A., et al. "The Roles of Oxidative Stress and Antioxidant Treatment in Experimental Diabetic Neuropathy." *Diabetes* 40:Suppl 2 (1997): S38– S42.

16. Lieberman, Shari, Ph.D., and Nancy Bruning. *The Real Vitamin and Mineral Book*. New York: Avery/Penguin, 2003, pp. 251–252.

17. Ensminger, A., et al. *Foods and Nutrition Encyclopedia*. Clovis, CA: Pegus Press, 1983, pp. 60ff.

18. Wernerman, J. "Documentation of Clinical Benefit of Specific Amino Nutrients." *Lancet* (September 5, 1998): 756–757.

19. Ronzio, Robert A., Ph.D. *Encyclopedia of Nutrition and Good Health*. New York: Facts on File, 1997, p. 19.

20. Atkins, Robert C., M.D. *Dr. Atkins' Vita-Nutrient Solution*. New York: Simon & Schuster, 1998, p. 186.

21. Wascher, T.C., et al. "Effects of Low-Dose L-arginine on Insulin-Mediated Vasodilation and Insulin Sensitivity." *European Journal of Clinical Investigation* 27 (1997): 690–695.

22. Franconi, Flavia. "Plasma and Platelet Taurine are Reduced in Subjects with Insulin Dependent Diabetes Mellitus: Effects of Taurine Supplementation." *American Journal of Clinical Nutrition* 61 (1995): 1115–1119.

23. Cangianno, C., et al. "Effects of Oral 5-Hydroxy-Tryptophan on Energy Intake and Macronutrient Selection in Non-Insulin-Dependent Diabetic Patients." *International Journal of Obesity* 22 (1998): 648–654.

24. Cannon, M.D., and F.Q. Nuttal. "The Metabolic Response to Dietary Protein in Subjects with Type 2 Diabetes." *Journal of the American College of Nutrition* 16:5 (1997): 478/Abstract 33.

25. Leverton, Ruth M. "Amino Acids." *Yearbook of Agriculture*. Washington, DC: U.S. Department of Agriculture, 1959, pp. 64ff.

26. Arsenio, L., et al. "An Investigation into the Therapeutic Effects of Phosphatidylcholine in Diabetes with Dyslipidemia." *La Clinica Therapeutica* 114:2 (July 1985): 117–127.

27. Sinatra, Stephen T., M.D. "Coenzyme Q_{10}-A Cardiologist's Commentary." *Natural Medicine Journal* 2:2 (February 1999): 9–15.

28. Ibid.

29. Atkins, Robert C., M.D. *Dr. Atkins' Vita-Nutrient Solution.* New York: Simon & Schuster, 1998, p. 248.

30. Liou, C.W., et al. "Correction of Pancreatic B-Cell Dysfunction with Coenzyme Q_{10} in a Patient with Miochondrial Encephalomyopathy, Lactic Acidosis and Stroke-Like Episodes Syndrome and Diabetes Mellitus." *European Neurology* 43 (2000): 54–55.

31. Sinatra, Stephen T., M.D. "Coenzyme Q_{10}-A Cardiologist's Commentary." *Natural Medicine Journal* 2:2 (February 1999): 9–15.

32. Langsjoen, Per H., et al. "Long-Term Efficacy and Safety of Coenzyme Q_{10} Therapy for Idiopathic Dilated Cardiomyopathy." *American Journal of Cardiology* 65 (February 1990): 521–523.

33. Ibid.

34. Mortensen, S.A., M.D. "Prospectives on Therapy of Cardiovascular Disease with Coenzyme Q_{10} (Ubiquinone)." *Clinical Investigator* 71 (1993): S116–S123.

35. Overvad, K., et al. "Coenzyme Q_{10} in Health and Disease." *European Journal of Clinical Nutrition* 53 (1999): 764–770.

36. Digiesi, V., et al. "Effect of Coenzyme Q_{10} on Essential Arterial Hypertension." *Current Therapeutic Research* 47:5 (May 1990): 841–845.

37. Digiesi, V., et al. "Mechanism of Action of Coenzyme Q_{10} in Essential Hypertension." *Current Therapeutic Research* 51:5 (May 1992): 668–672.

38. Kamikawa, T., et al. "Effects of Coenzyme Q_{10} on Exercise Tolerance in Chronic Stable Angina Pectoris." *American Journal of Cardiology* 56 (August 1985): 247–251.

39. Hamilton, Kirk. "Acute Myocardial Infarction and Antioxidants." *Clinical Pearls*. Sacramento, CA: I.T. Services, 1988, pp. 17–18. Also: Singh, Ram B. "Interventional Therapy with Mega Dose of Antioxidant Vitamins in Patients with Acute Myocardial Infarction: Could We Throw Caution to the Wind?" *American Journal of Cardiology* 80 (September 1997): 823–824.

40. Nash, Gerard K., D.O. "Whatever Happened to Coenzyme Q_{10}." *Cortlandt Forum* (February 1992): 48.

41. Judy, W.V., et al. "Myocardial Preservation in Therapy with Coenzyme Q_{10} during Heart Surgery." *Clinical Investigator* 71 (1993): S155–S161.

42. Atkins, Robert C. *Dr. Atkins' Vita-Nutrient Solution*. New York: Simon & Schuster, 1998, p. 250.

Chapter 12: Herbs

1. Mozersky, R.P. "Herbal Products and Supplemental Nutrients Used in the Management of Diabetes." *Journal of the American Osteopathic Association Suppl* 12 (December 1999): 54–59.

2. Ziyyat, A., et al. "Phytotherapy of Hypertension and Diabetes in Oriental Morocco." *Journal of Ethno-pharmacology* 58 (1997): 45–54.

3. Duke, James A., Ph.D. *Anti-Aging Prescriptions*. Emmaus, PA: Rodale, 2001, p. 349.

4. Murray, Frank. *Ampalaya: Nature's Remedy for Type 1 and Type 2 Diabetes*. Laguna Beach, CA: Basic Health Publications, 2006, pp. 21ff, 103ff.

5. Ibid.

6. Deal, Chad. L., M.D. "The Use of Tropical Capsaicin in Managing Arthritis Pain: A Clinician's Prospective." *Seminars in Arthritis and Rheumatism* 23:6 (June 1994): 48–52.

7. Sharma, R.D., et al. "Effect of Fenugreek Seed on Blood Glucose and Serum Lipids in Type 1 Diabetes." *European Journal of Clinical Nutrition* 44 (1990): 301–306.

8. Serraclara, Alicia, et al. "Hypoglycemic Action of an Oral Fig Leaf Decoction in Type 1 Diabetic Patients." *Diabetes Research and Clinical Practice* 39 (1998): 19–22.

9. Barrie, Stephen A., N.D., et al. "Effects of Garlic Oil on Platelet Aggregation, Serum Lipids and Blood Pressure in Humans." *Journal of Orthomolecular Medicine* 2:1 (1987): 187–192.

10. Pettit, J.L. "Ginseng." *Clinical Reviews* 10:8 (2000): 86–92.

11. Sotaniemi, Eero, M.D., Ph.D., et al. "Ginseng Therapy in Non-Insulin Dependent Diabetic Patients." *Diabetes Care* 18:10 (October 1995): 1373–1375.

12. Vuksan, V., et al. "American Ginseng (*Panax Quninquefolius L.*) Reduces Postprandial Glycemia in Non-Diabetic Subjects and Subjects with Type 2 Diabetes Mellitus." *Archives of Internal Medicine* 160 (April 2000): 1009-1013.

13. Walsh, N. "Asian Herb for Diabetes to Be Tested in Clinical Trial." *Family Practice News* 22 (April 2001): 37A–38A.

14. Duke, James A., Ph.D. *Anti-Aging Prescriptions*. Emmaus, PA: Rodale, 2001, pp. 350–351.

15. Duke, James A., Ph.D. *Green Pharmacy*. Emmaus, PA: Rodale, 1997, p. 165.

16. Velussi, Mari, M.D. "Silymarin Reduces Hyperinsulinemia, Malondialdehyde Levels and Daily Insulin Need in Cirrhotic Diabetic Patients." *Current Therapeutic Research* 53:5 (May 1993): 533–545.

17. Coriello, A., et al. "Red Wine Protects Diabetic Patients from Meal-Induced Oxidative Stress and Thrombosis Activation: A Pleasant Approach in the Prevention of Cardiovascular Disease in Diabetes." *European Journal of Clinical Investigation* 31:4 (2001): 322–328.

18. Rai, V., et al. "Effects of Ocimum Sanctum Leaf Powder on Blood Lipoproteins, Glycated Proteins and Total Amino Acids in Patients with Non-Insulin-Dependent Diabetes Mellitus." *Journal of Nutritional and Environmental Medicine* 7 (1997): 113–118.

Chapter 13: Why You Need to Exercise

1. Hill, James O. "Walking and Type 2 Diabetes." *Diabetes Care* 28 (2005): 1524–1525.

2. Di Loreto, Chiara, M.D., et al. "Make Your Diabetic Patients Walk." *Diabetes Care* 28 (2005): 1295–1302.

3. Irwin, Melinda L., Ph.D., MPH, et al. "Effects of Exercise on Total and Intra-Abdominal Body Fat in Postmenopausal Women: A Randomized Controlled Trial." *Journal of the American Medical Association* 289:3 (January 2003): 323–330.

4. Ibid.

5. Hamilton, Kirk. "Exercise is Medicine." *The Experts Speak*. Sacramento, CA: I.T. Services, 1997, p. 70. Also: Elrick, Harold, M.D. "Exercise is Medicine." *The Physician and Sports Medicine* 24:2 (February 1996): 72–78.

6. Wei, M., et al. "Cardio-respiratory Fitness and Physical Inactivity as Predictors of Mortality in Men with Type 2 Diabetes." *Annals of Internal Medicine* 132:8 (2000): 605–611.

7. Christensen, Damaris. "Walking and Eating for Better Health." *Science News* 160:10 (September 2001): 159.

8. Boule, Normand G., M.A., et al. "Effects of Exercise on Glycemic Control and Body Mass in Type 2 Diabetes Mellitus: A Meta-Analysis of Controlled Clinical Trials." *Journal of the American Medical Association* 286:10 (September 2001): 1218–1227.

9. Fahey, Patrick J., M.D., et al. "The Athlete with Type 1 Diabetes: Managing Insulin, Diet, and Exercise." *American Family Physician* (April 1996): 161ff.

10. Yamanouchi, Kunio, M.D., Ph.D. "Daily Walking Combined with Diet Therapy as a Useful Means for Obese, Non-Insulin Dependent Diabetes Mellitus Patients not only to Reduce Body Weight but also to Improve Insulin Sensitivity." *Diabetes Care* 18:6 (June 1995): 775–778.

11. Eriksson, J.G. "Exercise and the Treatment of Type 2 Diabetes Mellitus." *Sports Medicine* 27:6 (June 1999): 381–391.

12. Ibanez, Javier, M.D., Ph.D., et al. "Twice-Weekly Progressive Resistance Training Decreases Abdominal Fat and Improves Insulin Sensitivity in Older Men with Type 2 Diabetes." *Diabetes Care* 28 (2005): 662–667.

13. Ivy, John L. "Role of Exercise Training in the Prevention and Treatment of Insulin Resistance and Non-Insulin-Dependent Diabetes Mellitus." *Sports Medicine* 24:5 (1997): 321–336.

14. Mosher, Patricia E., Ed.D., et al. "Aerobic Circuit Exercise Training Effect on Adolescents with Well-Controlled Insulin-Dependent Diabetes Mellitus." *Archives of Physical Medicine and Rehabilitation* 79 (1998): 652–657.

15. Pramik, Mary Jean. "Exercise May Improve Insulin Sensitivity." *Medical Tribune* (June 18, 1996): 7.

16. Ibid.

17. Shahady, E.J. "Exercise as Medication: How to Motivate Your Patients." *Consultant* (November 2000): 2174–2178.

18. Villa-Caballero, L., et al. "Oxidative Stress, Acute and Regular Exercise: Are They Really Harmful in the Diabetic Patient?" *Medical Hypotheses* 55:1 (2000): 43-46.

Chapter 14: Treating Diabetes in Women and Children

1. Halton, Thomas L., et al. "Potato and French Fry Consumption and Risk of Type 2 Diabetes in Women." *American Journal of Clinical Nutrition* 83 (2006): 284–290.

2. Hu, Frank B., M.D., et al. "Diet, Lifestyle and the Risk of Type 2 Diabetes in Women." *New England Journal of Medicine* 345:11 (September 2001): 790–797.

3. Peterson, Charles M., M.D., and Lois Jovanovic-Peterson, M.D. "Randomized Crossover Study of 40 percent Versus 55 percent Carbohydrate Weight Loss Strategies in Women with Previous Gestational Diabetes Mellitus and Non-Diabetic Women of 130-200 percent Ideal Body Weight." *Journal of the American College of Nutrition* 14:4 (1995): 369–375.

4. Dabelea, Dana, M.D., Ph.D., et al. "Increasing Prevalence of Gestational Diabetes Mellitus over Time and by Birth Cohort." *Diabetes Care* 28 (2005): 579–584.

5. Schaefer-Graf, Ute M., M.D., et al. "Birth Weight and Parental BMI Predict Overweight in Children from Mothers with Gestational Diabetes." *Diabetes Care* 28 (2005): 1745–1750.

6. Downs, Danielle Symons, Ph.D., and Jan S. Ulbrecht, M.D. "Understanding Exercise Beliefs and Behaviors in Women with Gestational Diabetes Mellitus." *Diabetes Care* 29 (2006): 236–240.

7. Rodekamp, Elke, et al. "Long-Term Impact of Breast-Feeding on Body Weight and Glucose Tolerance in Children with Diabetic Mothers." *Diabetes Care* 28 (2005): 1457–1462.

8. Kleinfield, N.R. "Diabetes Is Seen as a Rising Risk in Mothers-to-Be." *The New York Times* (February 18, 2006): 1, B3.

9. Stortmeyher, Elsa S., Ph.D., et al. "Middle-Aged Premenopausal Women with Type 1 Diabetes Have Lower Bone Mineral Density and Calcaneal Quantitative Ultrasound than Non-diabetic Women." *Diabetes Care* 29 (2006): 306–311.

10. Coulsten, Ann. "Cardiovascular Disease Risk in Women with Diabetes Needs Attention." *American Journal of Clinical Nutrition* 79 (2004): 931–932.

11. Tanasescu, Mihaela, et al. "Dietary Fat and Cholesterol and the Risk of Cardiovascular Disease among Women with Type 2 Diabetes." *American Journal of Clinical Nutrition* 79 (2004): 999–1005.

12. Baker, H., et al. "Thiamin Status of Gravidas Treated for Gestational Diabetes Mellitus Compared to Their Neonates at Parturition." *International Journal of Vitamin and Nutrition Research* 70:6 (2000): 317–320.

13. Aharoni, A., et al. "Hair Chromium Content of Women with Gestational Diabetes Compared with Non-diabetic Pregnant Women." *American Journal of Clinical Nutrition* 55 (1992): 104–107.

14. Pittas, Anastassios, G., M.D., et al. "Vitamin D and Calcium Intake in Relation to Type 2 Diabetes in Women." *Diabetes Care* 29 (2006): 650–656.

15. Liu, Simin, M.D., Sc.D., et al. "Dietary Calcium, Vitamin E, and the Prevalence of Metabolic Syndrome in Middle-Aged and Older U.S. Women." *Diabetes Care* 28 (2005): 2926–2932.

16. Knight, K., et al. "Calcium Supplementation on Normotensive and Hypertensive Pregnant Women." *American Journal of Clinical Nutrition* 55 (1992): 891–895.

17. Jovanovic-Peterson, Lois, M.D. "Vitamin and Mineral Deficiencies which May Predispose to Glucose Tolerance of Pregnancy." *Journal of the American College of Nutrition* 15:1 (1996): 14–20.

18. Salmerton, Jorge, et al. "Dietary Fat Intake and Risk of Type 2 Diabetes in Women." *American Journal of Clinical Nutrition* 73 (2001): 1019–1026.

19. Stene, L.C., et al. "Use of Cod Liver Oil During Pregnancy Associated with Lower Risk of Type 1 Diabetes in the Offspring." *Diabetologia* 43 (2000): 1093–1098.

20. Hu, F.B., et al. "Physical Activity and Risk for Cardiovascular Events in Diabetic Women." *Annals of Internal Medicine* 134:2 (2001): 96–105.

21. Ludwig, David S., M.D., and Cara B. Ebbeling, Ph.D. "Type 2 Diabetes Mellitus in Children." *Journal of the American Medical Association* 286:12 (September 2001): 1427–1430.

22. Ibid.

23. Lee, Joyce M., M.D., et al. "An Epidemiologic Profile of Children with Diabetes in the U.S." *Diabetes Care* 29 (2006): 420–421.

24. Ludwig, David S., M.D., Ph.D., and Cara B. Ebbeling, Ph.D. "Overweight Children and Adolescents." *New England Journal of Medicine* 353:10 (September 2005): 1070.

25. Huerta, Milagros G., M.D., et al. "Magnesium Deficiency Is Associated with Insulin Resistance in Obese Children." *Diabetes Care* 28 (2005): 1175– 1181.

26. Baker, Barbara. "Infant Vitamins May Protect against Diabetes." *Family Practice News* (July 15, 1996): 4.

27. Thernlund, Gunilla, M.D., et al. "Psychological Stress and the Onset of Insulin-Dependent Diabetes Mellitus in Children." *Diabetes Care* 18 (1995): 1323–1329.

28. Rensch, Michael J., M.D., et al. "Gluten-Sensitive Enteropathy in Patients with Insulin-Dependent Diabetes Mellitus." *Annals of Internal Medicine* 124:6 (March 1996): 564–567.

29. Calero, P., et al. "IgA Antigliadin Antibodies as a Screening Method for Non-Overt Celiac Disease in Children with Insulin-Dependent Diabetes Mellitus." *Journal of Pediatric Gastroenterology and Nutrition* 23 (1996): 29–33.

30. Murray, Joseph A., et al. "Effect of a Gluten-Free Diet on Gastrointestinal Symptoms of Celiac Disease." *American Journal of Clinical Nutrition* 79 (2004): 669–673.

31. Sanchez-Albisua, I., et al. "Celiac Disease in Children with Type 1 Diabetes Mellitus: The Effect of the Gluten-Free Diet." *Diabetes Medicine* 22 (2005): 1079–1082.

32. Lalla, Evanthia, DDS, et al. "Periodontal Changes in Children and Adolescents with Diabetes." *Diabetes Care* 29 (2006): 295–299.

33. Pettit, David J. "Breastfeeding and Incidence of Non-Insulin-Dependent Diabetes Mellitus in Pima Indians." *Lancet* 350 (July 1997): 166–168.

34. Virtanen, S.M., et al. "In Children or Parents' Coffee or Tea Consumption Associated with the Risk of Type 1 Diabetes Mellitus in Children." *European Journal of Clinical Nutrition* 48 (1994): 279–285.

35. Stene, Lars C., et al. "Use of Cod Liver Oil during the First Year of Life is Associated with Lower Risk of Childhood-Onset Type 1 Diabetes: A Large, Population-Based, Case-Control Study." *American Journal of Clinical Nutrition* 78 (2003): 1128–1134.

Chapter 15: High Blood Pressure

1. Roccella, Edward J., Ph.D., M.P.H., et al. "Hypertension." *Medical and Health Annual.* Chicago: Encyclopaedia Britannica 1994, pp. 333ff.

2. Osborne, Carl G., D.V.M., et al. "Evidence for the Relationship of Calcium to Blood Pressure." *Nutrition Reviews* 54:12 (December 1996): 365–381.

3. Roccella, Edward J., Ph.D., M.P.H., et al. "Hypertension." *Medical and Health Annual.* Chicago: Encyclopaedia Britannica 1994, pp. 333ff.

4. Alterman, Seymour L., M.D., and Donald A. Kullman, M.D. *How to Prevent, Control, and Cure Diabetes.* Hollywood, FL: Frederick Fell Publishers, 2000, p. 207.

5. Landsberg, Lewis. "Insulin and Hypertension: Introduction." *Proceedings of the Society for Experimental Biology and Medicine* 208:4 (1995): 315–316.

6. Maruno, Yoshiko, M.D., et al. "Hyperinsulinemia in Relation to Hypertension and Other Coronary Risk Factors in Japanese Men." *Japanese Heart Journal* 38:5 (September 1997): 685–696.

7. Appel, Lawrence J., M.D., et al. "A Clinical Trial of the Effects of Dietary Patterns on Blood Pressure." *New England Journal of Medicine* 336 (April 1997): 1117–1124.

8. Moline, J., et al. "Dietary Flavonoids and Hypertension: Is There a Link?" *Medical Hypotheses* 55:4 (2000): 306–309.

9. Ronzio, Robert A., Ph.D. *Encyclopedia of Nutrition and Good Health.* New York: Facts On File, 1997, pp. 180–181.

10. Simons, Morton, et al. "Diet and Blood Pressure in Children and Adolescents." *Pediatric Nephrology* 11 (1997): 244–249.

11. Sacks, F.M., et al. "Effects on Blood Pressure of Reduced Dietary Sodium and the Dietary Approaches to Stop Hypertension (DASH) Diet." *New England Journal of Medicine* 344:1 (January 2001): 3–10.

12. "Blood Pressure and Potassium." *International Journal of Clinical Practice* 51 (1997): 219–222.

13. "Blood Pressure and Potassium." *Nutrition Week* 30:42 (November 2000): 7.

14. Silagy, Christopher A., and Andrew W. Neil. "Meta-Analysis of the Effects of Garlic on Blood Pressure." *Journal of Hypertension* 12 (1994): 463–468.

15. Jee, S., et al. "The Effects of Chronic Coffee Drinking and Blood Pressure: A Meta-Analysis of Controlled Clinical Trials." *Hypertension* 33 (February 1999): 647–652.

16. Rakie, V., et al. "Effects of Coffee on Ambulatory Blood Pressure in Older Men and Women." *Hypertension* 33 (February 1999): 869–873.

17. Duffy, S.J., et al. "Treatment of Hypertension with Ascorbic Acid." *Lancet* 354 (December 1999): 2048–2049.

18. Stampler, J., et al. "Antioxidants Protective Against Rising Blood Pressure." *Circulation* 89:2 (1994): 932.

19. Wirell, M.P., et al. "Nutritional Dose of Magnesium in Hypertensive Patients on Beta Blockers Lowers Systolic Blood Pressure: A Double-Blind Cross-Over Study." *Journal of Internal Medicine* 236 (1994): 189–195.

20. Nadler, Jerry, M.D. "Magnesium Lowers Blood Pressure in Type 2 Diabetes." *Practical Cardiology* 16:10 (October 1990): 4.

21. Knight, Kathy B., and Robert E. Keith "Calcium Supplementation on Normotensive and Hypertensive Pregnant Women." *American Journal of Clinical Nutrition* 55 (1992): 891–895.

22. Ibid.

23. Knight, Kathy B., and Robert E. Keith. "Effects of Oral Calcium Supplementation via Calcium Carbonate Versus Diet on Blood Pressure and Serum Calcium in Young, Normotensive Adults." *Journal of Optimal Nutrition* 3:4 (1994): 152–158.

24. Digiesi, V., et al. "Mechanism of Action of Coenzyme Q_{10} in Essential Hypertension." *Current Therapeutic Research* 51:5 (May 1992): 668-672.

25. Digiesi, V., et al. "Effect of Coenzyme Q_{10} on Essential Arterial Hypertension." *Current Therapeutic Research* 47:5 (May 1990): 841–845.

26. Knapp, Howard R., M.D. "Fatty Acids and Hypertension." *World Review of Nutrition and Diet* 76 (1994): 9–14.

27. Levinson, Paul D., et al. "Effects of N-3 Fatty Acids in Essential Hypertension." *American Journal of Public Health* 13 (1990): 754–760.

28. Faivelson, Saralie. "Fiber and Fruit Protects Against Hypertension." *Medical Tribune* 33:22 (November 26, 1992): 1.

29. "Pregnancy, Hypertension and Vitamin E." *Nutrition Week* 28:36 (September 18, 1998): 7.

30. Lenfant, Claude, M.D. "The Sixth Report of the Joint National Committee on Prevention, Detection, Evaluation and Treatment of High Blood Pressure." *Archives of Internal Medicine* 157 (November 1997): 2413–2446.

31. Arroll, Bruce, M.B., et al. "Salt Restriction and Physical Activity in Treated Hypertensives." *New Zealand Medical Journal* (July 14, 1995): 266–268.

32. Lenfant, Claude, M.D. "The Sixth Report of the Joint National Committee on Prevention, Detection, Evaluation and Treatment of High Blood Pressure." *Archives of Internal Medicine* 157 (November 1997): 2413–2446.

33. Nurminen, M.L., et al. "Dietary Factors in the Pathogenesis and Treatment of Hypertension." *Annals of Medicine* 30 (1998): 143–150.

Chapter 16: The Complications of Cardiovascular Disease

1. Tapley, Donald F., M.D., et al. *Columbia University College of Physicians and Surgeons Complete Home Medical Guide.* New York: Crown, 1985, p. 481.

2. Ibid.

3. Ibid.

4. Ibid.

5. Seppa, Nathan. "Poor Glucose Metabolism Risks Clots." *Science News* 157:5 (January 29, 2000): 77.

6. Seppa, Nathan. "Glucose Control Spares Arteries in Diabetes." *Science News* 159:26 (June 30, 2001): 406.

7. Christensen, Damaris. "Inflammation Linked to Diabetes." *Science News* 160:6 (August 11, 2001): 89.

8. Kretchmer, Norman. "Nutrition is the Keystone of Prevention." *American Journal of Clinical Nutrition* 60:1 (1994): 1.

9. Folz-Gray, Dorothy. "Against the Grain?" *Hippocrates* (November 1997): 54–61.

10. Adams, Ruth, and Frank Murray. *Improving Your Health with Zinc.* New York: Larchmont Books, 1978; pp. 108–109, 114–115.

11. Folz-Gray, Dorothy. "Against the Grain?" *Hippocrates* (November 1997): 54–61.

12. Gazis, Anastasios, et al. "Vitamin E and Cardiovascular Protection in Diabetes: Antioxidants May Offer Particular Advantage in this High-Risk Group." *British Medical Journal* 314 (June 1997): 1845–1846.

13. Rude, Robert K., M.D. "Magnesium Deficiency and Diabetes Mellitus: Causes and Effects." *Postgraduate Medicine* 92:5 (October 1992): 217–223.

14. Mertz, Walter. "Chromium in Human Nutrition: A Review." *Journal of Nutrition* 123 (1993): 626–633.

15. Ceriello, A., et al. "Red Wine Protects Diabetic Patients from Meal-Induced Oxidative Stress and Thrombosis Activation: A Pleasant Approach to the Prevention of Cardiovascular Disease in Diabetes." *European Journal of Investigation* 31:4 (2001): 322–328.

16. Adams, Ruth, and Frank Murray. *Improving Your Health with Zinc.* New York: Larchmont Books, 1978; pp. 108–109, 114–115.

17. Adams, Ruth, and Frank Murray. *Is Low Blood Sugar Making You a Nutritional Cripple?* New York: Larchmont Books, 1975, pp. 18ff.

18. Hu, F.B., et al. "Physical Activity and Risk for Cardiovascular Events in Diabetic Women." *Annals of Internal Medicine* 134:2 (January 2001): 96–105.

Chapter 17: High Cholesterol

1. Clayman, Charles B., M.D. (medical editor). *American Medical Association Home Medical Encyclopedia.* New York: Random House, 1989, p. 275.

2. Murray, Frank. *Program Your Heart for Health.* New York: Larchmont Books, 1977, pp. 210ff, 262ff.

3. Coons, Callie Mae. *Food, Yearbook of Agriculture.* Washington, DC: U.S. Department of Agriculture, 1959, various pages.

4. Murray, Frank. *Program Your Heart for Health.* New York: Larchmont Books, 1977, pp. 210ff, 262ff.

5. Coons, Callie Mae. *Food, Yearbook of Agriculture.* Washington, DC: U.S. Department of Agriculture, 1959, various pages.

6. Murray, Frank. *Program Your Heart for Health.* New York: Larchmont Books, 1977, pp. 210ff, 262ff.

7. Ostlund, R.E., et al. "Sitostanol Administered in Lecithin Micelles Potentially Reduces Cholesterol Absorption in Humans." *American Journal of Clinical Nutrition* 70 (1999): 826–831.

8. Ibid.

9. King, James M., M.D., et al. "Evaluation of Effects of Unmodified Niacin on Fasting and Postprandial Plasma Lipids and Normolipidemic Men with Hypaoalpha Alipoproteinemia." *American Journal of Medicine* 97 (October 1994): 323–331.

10. Guyton, J.R., et al. "Extended-Release Niacin vs. Gemfibrozil for the Treatment of Low Levels of High-Density Lipoprotein Cholesterol." *Archives of Internal Medicine* 160 (April 2000): 1177–1184.

11. Zema, M.J. "Gemfibrozil, Nicotinic Acid and Combination Therapy in

Patients with Isolated Hypoalphalipoproteinemia: A Randomized, Open-Label, Crossover Study." *Journal of the American College of Cardiology* 35:3 (March 2000): 640–646.

12. Lupton, Joanne R., Ph.D. "Cholesterol-Lowering Effects of Barley Bran Flour and Oil." *Journal of the American Dietetic Association* 95 (1994): 65–70.

13. Gerhardt, Ann L., and Noreen B. Gallo. "Full-Fat Rice Bran and Oat Bran Similarly Reduce Hypercholesterolemia in Humans." *Journal of Nutrition* 128 (1998): 865–869.

14. Anderson, J.W., et al. "Long-Term Cholesterol-Lowering Effects of Psyllium as an Adjunct to Diet Therapy in the Treatment of Hypercholesterolemia." *American Journal of Clinical Nutrition* 71 (2000): 1433–1438.

15. Goel, Vinti, Ph.D., et al. "Cholesterol Lowering Effects of Rhubarb Stalk Fiber in Hypercholesterolemic Men." *Journal of the American College of Nutrition* 16:6 (1997): 600–604.

16. Zoler, M.L. "Cholestin Cuts Serum Cholesterol by 20%–30%." *Family Practice News* (May 15, 1999): 30–31.

17. Edwards, K., et al. "Effect of Pistachio Nuts on Serum Lipid Levels in Patients with Moderate Hypercholesterolemia." *Journal of the American College of Nutrition* 18:3 (1999): 229–232.

18. Abbey, Mavis, et al. "Partial Replacement of Saturated Fatty Acids with Almonds or Walnuts Lowers Total Plasma Cholesterol and Low-Density Lipoprotein Cholesterol." *American Journal of Clinical Nutrition* 59 (1994): 995–999.

19. Warshafsky, S., et al. "Effect of Garlic on Total Serum Cholesterol: A Meta-Analysis." *Annals of Internal Medicine* 119:7 Part I (October 1993): 599–605.

20. Saba, Paolo, et al. "A Pilot Study of the Effects of Omega-3 Polyunsaturated Fatty Acids on Blood Lipids in Hyperlipidemic Patients." *Current Therapeutic Research* 55:4 (April 1994): 408–415.

21. Hermann, J., et al. "Effects of Chromium Supplementation on Plasma Lipids, Apolipoproteins and Glucose in Elderly Subjects." *Nutrition Research* 14:5 (May 1994): 671–674.

22. Anderson, J.W., and S.E. Gilliland. "Effects of Fermented Milk (Yogurt) Containing Lactobacillus Acidophilus L1 on Serum Cholesterol in Hypercholesterol Humans." *Journal of the American College of Nutrition* 18:1 (1999): 43–50.

23. Mani, U.V., et al. "Long-Term Effect of Cereal-Pulse Mix (Diabetic Mix) Supplementation on Serum Lipid Profile in Non-Insulin Dependent Diabetes Mellitus Patients." *Journal of Nutritional and Environmental Medicine* 7 (1997): 163–168.

24. Shane, Jan M., et al. "Corn Bran Supplementation of a Low-Fat Controlled

Diet Lowers Serum Lipids in Men with Hypercholesterolemia." *Journal of the American Dietetic Association* 95:1 (January 1995): 40–45.

25. National Cholesterol Education Program (NCEP). "NCEP Issues Major New Cholesterol Guidelines." National Institutes of Health (NIH) News Release (May 15, 2001). Also: Cleeman, James I., M.D., et al. "Executive Summary of the Third Report of the National Cholesterol Education Program (NCEP) Expert Panel on Detection, Evaluation and Treatment of High Blood Cholesterol in Adults (Adult Treatment Panel III)." *Journal of the American Medical Association* 285:19 (May 2001): 2486ff. Pace, Brian, M.A., et al. "Cholesterol and Atherosclerosis." *Journal of the American Medical Association* 285:19 (May 2001): 2536.

26. Ashen, M., et al. "Low HDL Cholesterol Levels." *New England Journal of Medicine* 353:12 (September 2005): 1252–1258.

27. Ibid.

Chapter 18: High Triglycerides

1. Tapley, Donald F., M.D., et al. *Columbia University College of Physicians and Surgeons Complete Home Medical Guide.* New York: Crown, 1985, p. 481.

2. Leverton, Ruth M. "Amino Acids." *Food: The Yearbook of Agriculture.* Washington, DC: U.S. Department of Agriculture, 1959, p. 76.

3. Miller, Michael, M.D., et al. "Normal Triglyceride Levels and Coronary Artery Disease Events: The Baltimore Coronary Observational Long-Term Study." *Journal of the American College of Cardiology* 31:6 (May 1988): 1252– 1257.

4. Sharma, R.D., et al. "Effect of Fenugreek Seed on Blood Glucose and Serum Lipids in Type 1 Diabetes." *European Journal of Clinical Nutrition* 44 (1990): 301–306.

5. Singh, R.B., et al. "Can Dietary Magnesium Modulate Blood Lipids?" *Journal of the American College of Nutrition* 9:5 (1990): 527/Abstract 23.

6. Tornvall, Per, et al. "Normalization of Composition of Very Low Density Lipoproteins in Hypertriglyceridemia by Nicotinic Acid." *Atherosclerosis* 84 (1990): 219–227.

7. "Heart Attack." *New Scientist* 162:2187 (May 1999): 25.

8. Roche, H.M., and Gibney, M.J. "Effect of Long-Chain-3 Polyunsaturated Fatty Acids on Fasting and Postprandial Triglyceride Metabolism." *American Journal of Clinical Nutrition* 71:Suppl (2000): 232S–237S.

9. Grimsgaard, Sameline, et al. "Highly Purified Eicosapentaenoic Acid and Docosahexaenoic Acid in Humans Have Similar Triglyceride Lowering Effects but Divergent Effects on Serum Fatty Acids." *American Journal of Clinical Nutrition* 66 (1997): 649–659.

10. Stark, K.D., et al. "Effect of a Fish-Oil Concentrate on Serum Lipids in Post-menopausal Women Receiving and not Receiving Hormone Replacement Therapy in a Placebo-Controlled, Double-Blind Trial." *American Journal of Clinical Nutrition* 72 (2000): 389–394.

11. Flaten, Hugo, et al. "Fish Oil Concentrate: Effects on Variables Related to Cardiovascular Disease." *American Journal of Clinical Nutrition* 52 (1990): 300–306.

12. Hau, Man-Fai, et al. "Effects of Fish Oil on Oxidation on Resistance of VLDL in Hypertriglyceridemic Patients." *Arteriosclerosis, Thrombosis and Vascular Biology* 16 (1996): 1197–1202.

13. Patti, L., et al. "Long-Term Effects of Fish Oil on Lipoprotein Subfractions and Low Density Lipoprotein Size in Non-Insulin Dependent Diabetic Patients with Hypertriglyceridemia." *Atherosclerosis* 146 (1999): 361–367.

Chapter 19: Eye Problems

1. American Diabetes Association. "Eye Care and Retinopathy." Alexandria, VA: American Diabetes Association, 1997.

2. Tapley, Donald F., M.D., et al. *Columbia University College of Physicians and Surgeons Complete Home Medical Guide*. New York: Crown, 1985, p. 669.

3. Cellini, M., et al. "The Use of Polyunsaturated Fatty Acids in Ocular Hypertension: A Study with Blue-on-Yellow Perimetry." *Acta Ophthalmology Scandinavia* (1999): 54–55.

4. Virno, M., et al. "Oral Treatment of Glaucoma with Vitamin C." *The Eye, Ear Nose and Throat Monthly* 46 (December 1967): 1502–1508.

5. Linner, E. "The Pressure Lowering Effect of Ascorbic Acid in Occular Hypertension." *Acta Ophthalmology* 47:III (1969): 685–689.

6. Filina, A.A., and N.A. Sporova. "Effect of Lipoic Acid on Tyrosine Metabolism in Patients with Open-Angle Glaucoma." *Vestn Ofalmol* 107:3 (May-June 1991): 19–21.

7. Samples, J.R., et al. "Effects of Melatonin on Intracellular Pressure." *Current Eye Research* 7:7 (1988): 649–653.

8. Taylor, Allen, M.D. "Nutritional and Environmental Influences on Risk for Cataract." *Nutritional and Environmental Influences on the Eye* 4 (1999): 53–93.

9. Tavani, Alessandra, Sc.D., et al. "Food and Nutrient Intake and Risk of Cataract." *Annals of Epidemiology* 6 (1996): 41–46.

10. Taylor, Allen, M.D., and Thomas Nowell. "Oxidative Stress and Antioxidant Function in Relation to Risk for Cataract." *Advances in Pharmacology* 38 (1997): 515–536.

11. Hankinson, S., et al. "Nutrient Intake and Cataract Extraction in Women: A Prospective Study." *British Medical Journal* 305 (1992): 335–339.

12. Brown, L., et al. "A Prospective Study of Carotenoid Intake and Risk of Cataract Extraction in U.S. Men." *American Journal of Clinical Nutrition* 70 (1999): 517–524.

13. Hammond, B.R., Jr., et al. "Carotenoids in the Retina and Lens: Possible Acute and Chronic Effects on Human Visual Performance." *Archives of Biochemistry and Biophysics* 385 (2001): 41–46.

14. Bernstein, P.S., et al. "Identification and Quantification of Carotenoids and Their Metabolites in the Tissues of the Human Eye." *Experimental Eye Research* 72 (2001): 215–223.

15. "Cataracts, Lutein and Zeazanthin." *Tufts University Health and Nutrition Letter* 17:10 (December 1999): 1.

16. Olmedilla, B., et al. "Lutein in Patients with Cataracts and Age-Related Macular Degeneration: A Long-Term Supplementation Study." *Journal of the Science of Food and Agriculture* 81 (2001): 904–909.

17. Obrosova, I., et al. "Diabetes-Induced Changes in Lens Antioxidant Status, Glucose Utilization and Energy Metabolism: Effect of DL-Alpha-Lipoic Acid." *Diabetologia* 41 (1998): 1442–1450.

18. Jacques, P., et al. "Vitamin Intake and Senile Cataract." *Journal of the American College of Nutrition* 6 (1987): 435.

19. Seth, R.K., et al. "Protective Function of Alpha-Tocopherol against the Process of Cataractogenesis in Humans." *Annals of Nutrition and Metabolism* 43 (1999): 268–289.

20. Leske, M.C., et al. "Antioxidant Vitamins and Nuclear Opacities." *Ophthalmology* 105 (1998): 831–836.

21. Hamilton, Kirk. "Cataract and Vitamin C." *Clinical Pearls.* Sacramento, CA: I.T. Services, 2000, pp. 90–91. Also: Simon, Joel A., M.D. "Serum Ascorbic Acid and Other Correlates of Self-Reported Cataract among Older Americans." *Journal of Clinical Epidemiology* 52:12 (1999): 1207–1211.

22. Cumming, R.G., et al. "Diet and Cataract: The Blue Mountain Eye Study." *Ophthalmology* 107:3 (March 2000): 450–456.

23. Mares-Perlman, J.A., et al. "Vitamin Supplement Use and Incident Cataracts in Population-Based Study." *Archives of Ophthalmology* 118 (November 2000): 1556-1563.

24. Ahlrot-Esterlund, Britt, M.D., and Ake Norrby. "Remarkable Success of Antioxidant Treatment (Selenomethionine and Vitamin E) to a 34-year-old

Patient with Posterior Subcapsular Cataract, Keratoconus, Severe Atopic Eczema and Asthma." *Acta Ophthalmology* 66:2 (April 1988): 237–238.

25. Spadea, L., and E. Balestrazzi. "Treatment of Vascular Retinopathies with Pycnogenol." *Phytotherapy Research* 15 (2001): 219–223.

26. De Valk, H.W. "Magnesium in Diabetes Mellitus." *Netherlands Journal of Medicine* 54 (1999): 139–146.

27. Vaccaro, O., et al. "Plasma Homocysteine and Its Determinants in Diabetic Retinopathy." *Diabetes Care* 23:7 (2000): 1026–1027.

28. Hoffman, Ronald L., M.D. *Intelligent Medicine.* New York: Simon & Schuster, 1997, p. 282.

29. Bunce, G.E. "Nutrition and Eye Disease of the Elderly." *Journal of Nutritional Biochemistry* 5 (1994): 66–77.

30. Newsome, David A., M.D. "Role of Antioxidants in Macular Degeneration: An Update." *Ophthalmic Practice* 12:4 (1994): 169–171.

31. Ibid.

32. Mares-Perlman, J.A., et al. "Lutein and Zeaxanthin in the Diet and Serum and Their Relation to Age-Related Maculopathy in the Third National Health and Nutrition Examination Survey." *American Journal of Epidemiology* 153 (2001): 424–432.

33. Bone, R.A., et al. "Macular Pigment in Donor Eyes with and without AMD: A Case-Control Study." *Investigative Ophthalmology and Visual Science* 42 (2001): 235–240.

34. Landrum, J.T., and R.A. Bone. "Lutein, Zeaxanthin and the Macular Pigment." *Archives of Biochemistry and Biophysics* 385 (2001): 28–40.

35. Berendschot, T.T., et al. "Influence of Lutein Supplementation on Macular Pigment, Assessed with Two Objective Techniques." *Investigative Ophthalmology and Visual Science* 41 (2000): 3322–3326.

36. Rozankowska, M.B., et al. "Interaction of Carotenoids with Other Antioxidants in Protection of the Retina against Oxidative Damage." *Investigative Ophthalmology and Visual Science* 41:Suppl (2000): S601.

37. Christen, William G., Sc.D., et al. "A Prospective Study of Cigarette Smoking and Risk of Age-Related Macular Degeneration in Men." *Journal of the American Medical Association* 276:14 (October 1996): 1147–1151. Also: Seddon, Johanna F., M.D. "A Prospective Study of Cigarette Smoking and Age-Related Macular Degeneration in Women." *Journal of the American Medical Association* 276:14 (October 1996): 1141–1146.

38. Dagnelie, G., et al. "Lutein Improves Visual Function in Some Patients with

Retinal Degeneration: A Pilot Study via the Internet." *Optometry* 71 (2000): 147–164.

39. The Age-Related Eye Disease Study Research Group. "A Randomized, Placebo-Controlled, Clinical Trial of High-Dose Supplementation with Vitamins C and E, Beta-Carotene and Zinc for Age-Related Macular Degeneration and Vision Loss." *Archives of Ophthalmology* 119 (2001): 1417–1436.

40. Belda, J.I., et al. "Serum Vitamin E Levels Negatively Correlate with Severity of Age-Related Macular Degeneration." *Mechanisms of Aging and Development* 107 (1999): 159–164.

41. Delcourt, C., et al. "Age-Related Macular Degeneration and Antioxidant Status in the POLA Study." *Archives of Ophthalmology* 117 (1999): 1384–1390.

Chapter 20: Foot Problems

1. American Diabetes Association. "Foot Care." Alexandria, VA: American Diabetes Association, undated.

2. Scheffler, Neil M., D.P.N. "Diabetic Neuropathy." *Diabetes Wellness Letter* 6:10 (2000): 4, 8.

3. Ibid.

4. Abuaisha, B.B., et al. "Acupuncture for the Treatment of Chronic Painful Peripheral Diabetic Neuropathy: A Long-Term Study." *Diabetes Research and Clinical Practice* 39 (1998): 115–121.

5. Adams, Ruth, and Frank Murray. *Improving Your Health with Vitamin E.* New York: Larchmont Books, 1978, pp. 43–44.

6. Ibid., pp. 120ff.

7. Petrassi, C., et al. "Pycnogenol in Chronic Venous Unsufficiency." *Phytomedicine* 7 (2000): 383–388.

8. Browne, S.E. "The Case for Intravenous Magnesium Treatment of Arterial Disease in General Practice: Review of 34 Years of Experience." *Journal of Nutritional Medicine* 4 (1994): 169–177.

9. Clayman, Charles B., M.D. (medical editor). *American Medical Association Home Medical Encyclopedia.* New York: Random House, 1989, pp. 474–475.

10. American Diabetes Association. "Foot Care." Alexandria, VA: American Diabetes Association, undated.

Chapter 21: Kidney Disease

1. Tapley, Donald F., M.D., et al. "Diabetes and Other Endocrine Disorders." *Columbia University College of Physicians and Surgeons Complete Home Medical Guide.* New York: Crown, 1985, pp. 474ff.

2. Kakkar, Rakesh, et al. "Antioxidant Defense System in Diabetic Kidney." *Life Sciences* 60:9 (1997): 667–679.

3. Tapley, Donald F., M.D., et al. "Diabetes and Other Endocrine Disorders." *Columbia University College of Physicians and Surgeons Complete Home Medical Guide*. New York: Crown, 1985, pp. 474ff.

4. Klahr, Saulo, M.D. "Progression of Kidney Disease May Be Preventable." *Kidney/90/Medical Report* 7:4 (July/August 1990): 6–7.

5. Altman, Lawrence K. "Blasting of Kidney Stones Has Risks, Study Reports." *The New York Times* (April 10, 2006): A18.

6. Hamilton, Kirk. "Renal Disease, Diabetes and Protein Restriction." *The Experts Speak*. Sacramento, CA: I.T. Services, 1997, p. 115. Also: Pedrini, Michael T., M.D., et al. "The Effect of Dietary Protein Restriction on the Progression of Diabetic and Non-Diabetic Renal Disease: A Meta-Analysis." *Annals of Internal Medicine* 124:7 (April 1996): 627–632.

7. Pedrini, Michael T., M.D., et al. "The Effect of Dietary Protein Restriction on the Progression of Diabetic and Non-Diabetic Renal Diseases: A Meta-Analysis." *Annals of Internal Medicine* 124:7 (April 1996): 627–632.

8. Khajehdeni, P., et al. "A Randomized, Double-Blind, Placebo-Controlled Trial of Supplementary Vitamins E, C and Their Combination for Treatment of Hemodialysis Cramps." *Nephrology, Dialysis Transplantation* 16 (2001): 1447–1451.

9. Hanck, A., M.D. "Vitamin Intake under CAPD." *Niren-Und Hochduckkrankheiten* 21:Suppl 1 (May 1992): S64–S69.

10. Schmicker, Richard. "Nutritional Treatment of Hemodialysis and Peritoneal Dialysis Patients." *Artificial Organs* 19:8 (1995): 837–841.

11. Triolo, Luigi, M.D., et al. "Serum Coenzyme Q_{10} and Uremic Patients and Chronic Hemodialysis." *Nephron* 66 (1994): 153–156.

12. Trachtman, H., and Sturman, J.A. "Taurine: A Therapeutic Agent in Experimental Kidney Disease." *Amino Acids* 11 (1996): 1–13.

Chapter 22: Thyroid Gland Complications

1. Clayman, Charles B., M.D. *American Medical Association Home Medical Encyclopedia*. New York: Random House, 1989, pp. 985ff.

2. Ibid.

3. Barnes, Broda O., M.D., and Lawrence Galton. *Hypothyroidism: The Unsuspected Illness*. New York: Thomas V. Crowell, 1976, pp. 214ff.

4. Ibid.

5. Bartalena, Luigi, et al. "Cigarette Smoking and the Thyroid." *European Journal of Endocrinology* 133 (1995): 507–512.

6. Barnes, Broda O., M.D., and Lawrence Galton. *Hypothyroidism: The Unsuspected Illness.* New York: Thomas V. Crowell, 1976, pp. 214ff.

7. Whitaker, Julian, M.D. *Dr. Whitaker's Guide to Natural Healing.* Rocklin, CA: Prima Publishing, 1995, pp. 282–283.

8. Katz, Ronald D.O., and Robert Goldman, M.D. *Stopping the Clock.* New Canaan, CT: Keats Publishing, 1996, p. 175.

9. Murray, Michael, N.D., and Joseph Pizzorno, N.D. *Encyclopedia of Natural Medicine.* Rocklin, CA: Prima Publishing, 1998, p. 562.

10. Pimenta, W.P., et al. "The Assessment of Zinc Status by the Zinc Tolerance Test and Thyroid Disease." *Trace Elements in Medicine* 9:1 (1992): 34-37.

11. Weeber, Kenneth A., M.D. "Subclinical Thyroid Dysfunction." *Archives of Internal Medicine* 157 (May 1997): 1065-1068.

12. Cooper, Catherine. "Overtreating Hypothyroidism is an Easy, Insidious Mistake." *Family Practice News* (June 1, 1993): 5.

Chapter 23: Impotence

1. Levin, Marvin E., M.D., and Michael A. Pfeiffer, M.D. *Uncomplicated Guide to Diabetes Complications.* Alexandria, VA: American Diabetes Association, 1998, pp. 304ff.

2. Thompson, Ian M., M.D., et al. "Erectile Dysfunction and Subsequent Cardiovascular Disease." *Journal of the American Medical Association* 294:23 (December 2005): 2996–3002.

3. Wei, Ming, et al. "Total Cholesterol and High Density Lipoprotein Cholesterol as Important Predictors of Erectile Dysfunction." *American Journal of Epidemiology* 140:10 (1994): 930–937.

4. Esposito, Katherine, M.D., et al. "High Proportions of Erectile Dysfunction in Men with the Metabolic Syndrome." *Diabetes Care* 28 (2005): 1201– 1203.

5. De Berardis, Giorgia, et al. "Longitudinal Assessment of Quality of Life in Patients with Type 2 Diabetes and Self-Reported Erectile Dysfunction." *Diabetes Care* 28 (2005): 2637–2643.

6. Giller, Robert M., M.D., and Kathy Matthews. *Natural Prescriptions.* New York: Carol Southern Books, 1994, pp. 206ff.

7. Khan, Jason. "Smoking May Increase Risk of Impotence." *Medical Tribune* (January 19, 1995): 5.

8. Feinstein, Alice (editor). *Prevention's Healing with Vitamins.* Emmaus, PA: Rodale, 1996, p. 334.

9. Hoffman, Ronald L., M.D. *Intelligent Medicine.* New York: Simon & Schuster, 1997, p. 253.

10. Giller, Robert M., M.D., and Kathy Matthews. *Natural Prescriptions*. New York: Carol Southern Books, 1994.

11. Kalter-Leibovici, Ofra, M.D., et al. "Clinical, Socioeconomic, and Lifestyle Parameters Associated with Erectile Dysfunction among Diabetic Men." *Diabetes Care* 28 (2005): 1739–1744.

12. Whitaker, Julian, M.D. *Dr. Whitaker's Guide to Natural Living*. Rocklin, CA: Prima Publishing, 1995, pp. 284ff.

13. Pfeiffer, Carl C., Ph.D., M.D. *Mental and Elemental Nutrients*. New Canaan, CT: Keats Publishing, 1975, pp. 469ff.

14. Mindell, Earl, R.Ph., Ph.D. *Earl Mindell's Vitamin Bible for the 21st Century*. New York: Warner Books, 1999, p. 281.

15. Ito, T., et al. "The Effects of ArginMax, a Natural Dietary Supplement for Enhancement of Male Sexual Function." *Hawaii Medical Journal* 57 (December 1998): 741–744.

16. Kronhausen, Eberhard, Ed.M., et al. *Formula for Life*. New York: William Morrow, 1989, pp. 552–553.

17. Rowland, David L., Ph.D., et al. "Yohimbine, Erectile Capacity, and Sexual Response in Men." *Archives of Sexual Behavior* 26:1 (1997): 49–62.

18. Teloken, Claudio, et al. "Therapeutic Effects of High Dose Yohimbine Hydrochloride on Organic Erectile Dysfunction." *Journal of Urology* 159 (January 1998): 122–124.

19. Murray, Frank. *100 Super Supplements for a Longer Life*. New York: McGraw-Hill, 2000, pp. 171ff.

20. James A. Duke, Ph.D. *Green Pharmacy*. Emmaus, PA: Rodale, 1997, p.232.

Index

About the Author

A former editor of *Better Nutrition, GreatLife,* and *Let's Live* (England) magazines, Frank Murray is the author or coauthor of 48 books on health and nutrition, including *100 Super Supplements for a Longer Life* (McGraw-Hill), available in English and Chinese; *Health Benefits Derived From Sweet Orange* and *Ampalaya: Nature's Remedy for Type 1 and Type 2 Diabetes,* both published by Basic Health Publications. He is a member of the American Botanical Council and the New York Academy of Sciences. Mr. Murray lives in New York.